HOSPITAL
PHARMACY

HOSPITAL PHARMACY

William E. Hassan, Jr., Ph.D., LL.B.

Director, Peter Bent Brigham Hospital
Formerly Adjunct Professor of Hospital Pharmacy
Massachusetts College of Pharmacy

Third Edition

With 97 Illustrations

Lea & Febiger

Philadelphia 1974

Library of Congress Cataloging in Publication Data

Hassan, William E.
  Hospital pharmacy.

  1. Hospital pharmacies.   [DNLM: 1. Hospital pharmacy service.
WX 179 H353h 1973]
RA975.5.P5H3   1973   658′.91′6154   73-4909
ISBN 0-8121-0415-3

First Edition, 1965
Second Edition, 1967
Reprinted September, 1968
Third Edition, 1973

Library of Congress Catalog Card Number 73-4909

Published in Great Britain by Henry Kimpton Publishers, London

Printed in the United States of America

PREFACE

Since the publication of the first edition of HOSPITAL PHAR-MACY in 1965, the institutional practice of pharmacy has made great progress. Professional pharmacists now practice in hospitals, extended care facilities, nursing homes, neighborhood health centers and satellite clinics. Within these environments, pharmacists contribute to the triad of *patient care, teaching* and *research* through clinical programs involving the taking of patient drug histories, maintaining patient drug profiles and providing surveillance for drug interactions. Also, of great importance are programs in unit dose dispensing, preparation of hyperalimentation fluids, drug abuse education, drug utilization review and the development of systems for the control of drugs covered by the Controlled Substances Act of 1970.

Notwithstanding the above cited developments within the profession, the original purposes and scope of the book as well as my philosophy relative to the methodology of presentation have not changed. Thus, new material has been added and no longer pertinent subjects have been deleted. Hopefully, the end result is a useful text which permits the teacher the opportunity to provide the student with academically cogent supplementary data via classroom lectures, yet provides the practitioner guidance in the development of a pharmaceutical service to meet the needs of the particular institution served.

Thanks and appreciation are hereby extended to all of my friends and colleagues who have offered their counsel and suggestions for the improvement of the book. All material quoted from the American Society of Hospital Pharmacists is copyrighted by the American Society of Hospital Pharmacists and used with their permission.

WILLIAM E. HASSAN, JR.

Boston, Massachusetts

CONTENTS

Chapter

1

Introduction

THE specialty of hospital pharmacy has been defined as follows[1]:

> . . . the department or service in a hospital which is under the
> direction of a professionally competent, legally qualified pharma-
> cist, and from which all medications are supplied to the nursing
> units and other services, where special prescriptions are filled for
> patients in the hospital, where prescriptions are filled for
> ambulatory patients and out-patients, where pharmaceuticals are
> manufactured in bulk, where narcotic and other prescribed drugs
> are dispensed, where biologicals are stored and dispensed, where
> injectable preparations should be prepared and sterilized, and
> where professional supplies are often stocked and dispensed.

With such a broad definition of purpose, one might wonder about
the origin of this branch of the profession of pharmacy. According to
Urdang,[2] the hospital pharmacist was the first recognized representative
of the pharmaceutical profession. He states that hospital pharmacists
were employed in the hospitals which were a part of many early mona-
steries. Many of the descriptions of these old hospitals include a
description of the "apothecary shop" and its garden for the cultivation
of the medicinal herbs.

From this ancient period, hospital pharmacy passes into the early
American era, 1752 to be exact, when Pennsylvania Hospital, the first
in North America was opened, with Jonathan Roberts as its hospital
pharmacist. Since this historic date, over two hundred years have
passed, and a number of outstanding persons associated with hospital
pharmacy have received professional recognition and the accolade of
pharmaceutical historians.

The greatest strides in the profession were made in the early 1940's.
It was during this period that the American Society of Hospital Pharmacists was formed, August 21, 1942. Besides the formation of a
distinct professional society the other major contributing factors were
the publishing of the Society's official organ, the *American Journal of
Hospital Pharmacy,* the formation of affiliated chapters at the state

level, the acceptance of the Society as a member of the United States Pharmacopoeial Convention, the affiliation of the Society with the American Pharmaceutical Association, the establishment of minimum standard for pharmacies in hospitals, the institution of internships and training programs in connection with accredited colleges of pharmacy, and the institutes or "refresher courses" which the Society has co-sponsored with the American Pharmaceutical Association and other hospital organizations. These are only a few of the many advances made by this hitherto unheard-of body of pharmacists. It is no wonder that those who have watched this remarkable progress during the past decade foresee an even brighter and more successful future.

During the past fifteen years, hospitalization has developed into one of the nation's major enterprises. In 1971[3] there were approximately 7,000 hospitals registered by the American Hospital Association. The total bed capacity of these hospitals was stated to be 1,319,339 beds and approximately 94,000 bassinets. These hospitals handled 30,602,094 admissions and cared for 3,465,000 births. The average daily census for the year was 1,237,000 which represents a percentage daily occupancy for the period of 79.5 per cent. In caring for these patients, the hospitals are stated to have purchased in excess of $500,000,000 worth of pharmaceuticals and related products.

Many modern hospital administrators, after surveying this tremendous purchase and use of drugs, have suddenly realized that only trained pharmaceutical personnel are capable of storing, handling, pricing, and dispensing these products. As a result, many hospitals have retained the services of a pharmacist either on a full-time or part-time basis.

The presence of adequate pharmaceutical personnel in many hospitals has benefited both patient and staff members, for hospital manufacture of various pharmaceutical products as well as parenteral solutions has reduced the cost of medication. In addition, it enables the members of the staff to prescribe mixtures which require compounding skill. Also, hospital pharmacists have become involved in the preparation of hyperalimentation products, dialysis fluids, intravenous additive programs, unit dose packaging and unit dose dispensing. Without the knowledge possessed by a trained pharmacist, these preparations could not be properly or safely prepared in the hospital.

Whereas in the past, pharmacists acted as pharmacologic advisor to the physician concerning the pharmacology, toxicology, and posology of the new classes of drugs, today this clinical role has expanded to the point where it is a specialty unto itself. These clinical pharmacists are involved in the preparation of patient drug profiles, recording patient drug history, advising physicians of possible drug-drug interactions and drug effects on clinical laboratory test results.

Because of their special training, hospital pharmacists are now serving on the faculties of many of the hospital schools of nursing, teaching courses in pharmaceutical mathematics and pharmacology. This particular duty helps immeasurably to strengthen the professional bond between these two allied health professions.

In addition, the hospital pharmacists of today's hospitals serve on such vital committees as the Pharmacy and Therapeutics Committee, the Safety Committee, Committee on Standardization, the Antibiotics Committee, the Committee on Environmental Sepsis and the Policy Committee of the Administrative Staff.

These paragraphs have briefly summed up the past and present of hospital pharmacy. Consideration must now be given to its future.

The American Hospital Association has registered 7,097 hospitals. Of these, about 1000 hospitals are more than 200-bed capacity, whereas the remainder of them have 100 or fewer beds. It is in the hospitals of no more than 100 beds that the greatest challenge for providing adequate pharmaceutical services exists. Statistics show that less than 70 per cent of all hospitals possess a pharmacy.

With these figures in mind, it would seem that the profession of hospital pharmacy must now satisfy a newly recognized need, that of placing a hospital pharmacist in every hospital throughout the country. This is necessary since the hospital pharmacist, in his new role, is a vital link in the chain of health professions dedicated to the care of hospitalized patients.

Another advantage to the hospital resulting from the specialized training of the hospital pharmacist manifests itself in the smaller hospital. In these institutions, the individual serving as a hospital pharmacist may also serve as an assistant to the administrator, purchasing agent, supervisor of the central sterile supply room and in some instances as a laboratory technician. By combining his duties, a hospital pharmacist is within the financial reach of every hospital, irrespective of size.

Archambault,[4] in a study on the manpower needs of hospital pharmacists, arrived at the conclusion that there is an annual need for more than 400 hospital pharmacists.

Competition for the services of qualified hospital pharmacists by hospitals is best evidenced by a perusal of some of the listings in hospital journals. It will be noted that many positions are available and range from staff pharmacist to Chief Pharmacist. Salaries range from $10,000 to $30,000 or more depending upon the size of the hospital. Some of the inducements offered include four weeks' vacation with pay, three weeks' sick leave, meals free while on duty, 100 per cent hospitalization, 25 per cent discount on hospitalization for immediate family, pension plan, and nine to eleven paid holidays. The work week ranged from a low of thirty-five hours to a high of forty-four hours with the majority of institutions adhering to the standard forty hours.

Dr. Charles Letourneau[5] a consultant in hospital administration and Editorial Director of the Journal, *Hospital Management,* wrote—

> ". . . the function of the hospital pharmacist is vital not only to the professional care of the patient but to the management of the hospital as well. The management function of the hospital pharmacist is a relatively recent concept which is rapidly achieving recognition in the hospital field. Hospital administration is the coordination of men, money and materials to provide facilities to assist a physician to treat his patient. The pharmacist participates in hospital administration in addition to his professional obligations."

Don Francke,[6] then Editor of the *American Journal of Hospital Pharmacy,* advanced in an editorial the concept of establishing a School of Hospital Pharmacy as an integral part of a major university with established schools of medicine, dentistry, nursing, public health and a large teaching hospital.

The idea of such a school marshals the interest of the academically minded members of our profession and this exciting possibility may some day materialize.

Should the profession meet the challenge of the future, the opportunities and resources of hospital pharmacy would be greatly increased. With this increase, it is inevitable that new young blood must be attracted to the profession in sufficient quantity to make this a profession with a notable past, a noble and invigorating present, and a brilliant future.

Goals for Hospital Pharmacy

The American Society of Hospital Pharmacists has developed a statement on the *Goals for Hospital Pharmacy* which are consistent with its constitutional objectives. The six goals promulgated should be the focus of attention for the hospital pharmacists of the future and are therefore cited.[7]

Coordinated plans must be drawn and implemented to:

1. Teach hospital pharmacists by word and precept the philosophy and ethics of hospital pharmacy as one of the healing arts and their personal, individual accountability to assume responsibility for professional practice.
2. Strengthen and expand the scientific and professional aspects of the practice of hospital pharmacy, including the consulting

role of the hospital pharmacist, his teaching role, and his activities in the field of investigation and research.

3. Strengthen and perfect the administrative or management skills and tools essential to the hospital pharmacist in his role as a department head.

4. Attract a greater number of well-trained pharmacists to hospital practice, including those with specialized education and training in hospital pharmacy.

5. Promote payment of realistic salaries to hospital pharmacists in both staff and managerial positions in order to attract and retain the services of career personnel.

6. Utilize the resources of hospital pharmacy to assist in the development and improvement of the profession as a whole.

Minimum Standards

The original *Minimum Standard for Pharmacies in Hospitals* was developed and adopted by the American College of Surgeons in 1935. A revised version was adopted by the American Society of Hospital Pharmacists in 1950 and such was approved by the American Pharmaceutical Association. Later, a *"Guide to Application"* for each of the six sections of the *Minimum Standard* was appended as supplementary material. This *"Guide to Application"* was developed by the American Society of Hospital Pharmacists without approval from other organizations. Thus, there is an important differentiation which must be recognized between the two documents—the former is an official document, whereas the latter is supplementary information.

Because the new practitioner and the student may not have available to them the journals carrying the *Minimum Standard for Pharmacies in Hospitals with Guide to Application,* they are hereinafter reproduced in detail.[8]

MINIMUM STANDARD FOR PHARMACIES IN HOSPITALS WITH GUIDE TO APPLICATION*

1. Organization

There shall be a properly organized pharmacy department under the direction of a professionally competent, legally qualified pharmacist whose training in hospital pharmacy conforms to the standards herein established by the AMERICAN SOCIETY OF HOSPITAL PHARMACISTS.

*The Guide to Application of the Minimum Standard for Pharmacies in Hospitals is an elaboration for the guidance of administrators and examiners, as well as hospital pharmacists. The Guide has not been submitted to the various organizations for approval. Note that the Standard appears in large type with the elaboration in small type following each section of the Standard.

ELABORATION ON ORGANIZATION: The director of pharmacy service shall be responsible to the proper administrative authority of the hospital for developing, supervising and coordinating all the activities of the pharmacy department.

Obviously the pharmacy department must be integrated with the general services supplied by the hospital of which it is a part. Where outpatient service is given, the hospital pharmacy should include outpatient prescription service. A general compounding and dispensing laboratory is a prime essential for any hospital pharmacy service. Where manufacturing is carried on on more than a small compounding and dispensing scale, a separate manufacturing laboratory must be available. Where the pharmacy is depended upon for the storage and supply of ordinary and extraordinary medical and surgical equipment, facilities for storage and handling such equipment must be adequate and should not encroach upon the space required for good pharmaceutical technic. Where the pharmacy is depended upon for scientific, administrative, mechanical and educational activities not usually associated with the practice of pharmacy, adequate facilities for such activities must be available.

Departmentalization of the hospital pharmacy should follow good administrative procedure integrated with the administration of the hospital in general.

The organizational structure of the pharmacy department will vary in different hospitals, depending upon the size and character of the institution and it is not the intent of the Minimum Standard to cast all pharmacy departments in the same mold, although it is its intent to assure the establishment of fundamental principles which will enable competent pharmacists to operate with sufficient freedom to supply the demand for adequate pharmaceutical service.

2. Policies

The director of pharmacy service, with approval and cooperation of the director of the hospital, shall initiate and develop rules and regulations pertaining to the administrative policies of the department. The director of pharmacy service, with the approval and cooperation of the Pharmacy and Therapeutics Committee, shall initiate and develop rules and regulations pertaining to the professional policies of the department.

ELABORATION ON POLICIES: Only those orders and prescriptions originating within the hospital should be dispensed by the hospital pharmacy. Prescriptions written by physicians who are not members of the hospital staff should not be dispensed by the hospital pharmacy. Regulations pertaining to the dispensing of medications to hospital personnel should be formulated and enforced.

Administrative and professional policies may of necessity overlap. This is unavoidable in the formulation of any set of standards. The spirit of this Standard is one of helpful cooperation and this should be kept in mind by the administrator, the pharmacist, and the examiner when the Standard is interpreted. Reference to policy may occur in other sections of the elaboration of this Standard because it may be more appropriate to refer to it there.

3. Personnel

The director of pharmacy service shall be well-trained in the specialized functions of hospital pharmacy and shall be a graduate of an accredited college of pharmacy or meet an equivalent standard of training and experience as set forth in the supplement to these standards. He shall have such assistants as the volume of work in the pharmacy may dictate. These assistants shall include an adequate number of additional licensed pharmacists and such other personnel as the activities of the pharmacy may require to supply pharmaceutical services of the highest quality. All members of the staff of the pharmacy shall be competent, of good moral character and mentally and physically fit to perform their duties acceptably.

ELABORATION ON PERSONNEL: The personnel listed below represent the ultimate in hospital pharmacy staffing and it is realized that varying numbers and components of pharmacy staffs will be required, based on size and scope of operations of each activity.

1. Director of pharmacy service
2. One or more assistant directors of pharmacy service
3. Staff pharmacists
4. Residents (where a hospital pharmacy residency program, preferably a program accredited by the AMERICAN SOCIETY OF HOSPITAL PHARMACISTS, exists)
5. Personnel trained in nonprofessional functions
6. Clerical help

The director of pharmacy service, the assistant director(s) of pharmacy service and the staff pharmacists shall be graduates of colleges of pharmacy accredited by the American Council on Pharmaceutical Education, and currently licensed in one of the 50 states, the District of Columbia, or territories of the United States. (If graduation was prior to accrediting activity by the Council, the college shall have been a member of the American Association of Colleges of Pharmacy.) The director of pharmacy service shall have a Bachelor of Science degree and at least one year's experience in hospital pharmacy. The additional pharmacists, whenever possible, shall have had experience in hospital pharmacy and preferably shall have completed an approved hospital pharmacy residency. This applies especially to the director and assistant director(s) of pharmacy service. Licensed pharmacists actively engaged in the practice of hospital pharmacy on or before January 1, 1950, who do not hold a Baccalaureate degree, may satisfy the personnel requirements in part by evidence of extensive experience in hospital pharmacy, professional ability, membership in professional and scientific societies and with evidence in writing of their efficiency and capacity in hospital pharmacy as presented to the administration, superintendent, chief of service or medical staff.

Directors of pharmacy service who have completed a three-year course and who do not have a B.S. degree shall have had five years' experience in hospital pharmacy. Those who have completed a two-year course in pharmacy, but have not received a B.S. degree shall have had ten years experience in hospital pharmacy. In small hospitals where it may not be economically feasible to have a pharmacist devote full time to purely pharmaceutical matters, it is recommended that the pharmacist be a full-time staff member and assigned additional related collateral duties. In smaller organizations in which a pharmacist cannot be utilized on a full-time basis even with related collateral duties, a qualified pharmacist should be employed for a portion of each day. Consideration shall be given not only to the professional competence of licensed pharmacists, but to personality traits which will materially influence compatibility and cooperation with other members of the professional hospital staff. All licensed pharmacists shall be urged to maintain membership in the American Pharmaceutical Association, the AMERICAN SOCIETY OF HOSPITAL PHARMACISTS and other professional pharmaceutical societies and participate actively in their functions.

The selection of residents shall be on the basis of minimum standards established for the overall residency program. In all instances, incumbents shall be graduates and, where possible, licensed pharmacists, and shall be assigned duties commensurate with their schooling and training.

Clerical and stenographic assistance shall be provided to assist with records, reports and correspondence.

In view of their numerous contacts with members of the professional staff in the hospital, personnel trained in nonprofessional functions, whose work shall be largely of a mechanical and janitorial nature and incident or preparatory to the work of a pharmacist, shall be carefully selected. In order to insure the best pharmaceutical service as a protection to the patient, these nonprofessionals shall not be assigned duties which should be performed only by professionally trained, licensed pharmacists.

The hospital shall provide rules for employee conduct and the director of pharmacy service shall be responsible for the enforcement of such rules within the pharmacy.

The employment and discharge of employees in the pharmacy department shall be only on the recommendation of the director of pharmacy service.

A licensed pharmacist shall be on duty at all hours when the pharmacy is open and provision should be made for emergency pharmaceutical service.

4. Facilities

Adequate pharmaceutical and administrative facilities shall be provided for the pharmacy department, including especially: (A) the necessary equipment for the compounding, dispensing and manufacturing of pharmaceuticals and parenteral preparations, (B) bookkeeping supplies and related materials and equipment necessary for the proper administration of the department, (C) an adequate library and filing equipment to make information concerning drugs readily available to both pharmacists and physicians, (D) special locked storage space to meet the legal requirements for storage of narcotics, alcohol and other prescribed drugs, (E) a refrigerator for the storage of thermolabile products, (F) adequate floor space for all pharmacy operations and the storage of pharmaceuticals at a satisfactory location provided with proper lighting and ventilation.

ELABORATION ON FACILITIES: In those states where minimum equipment lists have been provided by the boards of pharmacy and other agencies controlling the practice of pharmacy, such minimum equipment must be available in the pharmacy for proper compliance with state laws and/or regulations.

Adequate office furniture, stationery, bookkeeping and stenographic supplies shall be provided. The systems of communication, messenger and delivery service maintained by the hospital shall extend to the pharmacy.

A modern pharmaceutical library shall be maintained. As a minimum, latest editions of the following shall be available:

United States Pharmacopeia
National Formulary
New Drugs
United States Dispensatory
American Hospital Formulary Service

Also, the library should contain recent editions of text and reference books covering the following fields:

Pharmacy: theoretical and practical
Chemistry: general, organic, pharmaceutical and biological
Pharmacology, toxicology and therapeutics
Bacteriology
Biological stains and staining techniques
Sterilization and disinfection
Medical dictionary

The following journals shall be available:

International Pharmaceutical Abstracts
Journal of the American Pharmaceutical Association
Journal of Pharmaceutical Sciences
American Journal of Hospital Pharmacy
Journal of the American Medical Association

There should be maintained files containing literature on newer therapeutic agents, the house organs of pharmaceutical manufacturers, and their catalogs and price lists.

Floor space in the pharmacy should be guided by the suggested standards of the Hospital Facilities Division of the Public Health Service and approved by the AMERICAN SOCIETY OF HOSPITAL PHARMACISTS.*

5. Responsibilities

The director of pharmacy service shall be responsible for: (*A*) the preparation and sterilization of injectable medication when manufactured in the hospital, (*B*) the manufacture of pharmaceuticals, (*C*) the dispensing of drugs, chemicals, and pharmaceutical preparations, (*D*) the filling and labeling of all drug containers issued to services from which medication is to be administered, (*E*) necessary inspection of all pharmaceutical supplies on all services, (*F*) the maintenance of an approved stock of antidotes and other emergency drugs, (*G*) the dispensing of all narcotic drugs and alcohol and the maintenance of a perpetual inventory of them, (*H*) specifications both as to quality and source for purchase of all drugs, chemicals, antibiotics, biologicals and pharmaceutical preparations used in the treatment of patients, (*I*) furnishing information concerning medications to physicians, interns and nurses, (*J*) establishment and maintenance, in cooperation with the accounting department, of a satisfactory system of records and bookkeeping in accordance with the policies of the hospital for (1) charging patients for drugs and pharmaceutical supplies, (2) maintaining adequate control over the requisitioning and dispensing of all drugs and pharmaceutical supplies, (*K*) planning, organizing and directing pharmacy policies and procedures in accordance with the established policies of the hospital, (*L*) maintenance of the facilities of the department, (*M*) cooperation in teaching courses to students in the school of nursing and in the medical intern training program, (*N*) implementing the decisions of the Pharmacy and Therapeutics Committee (*O*) the preparation of periodic reports on the progress of the department for submission to the administrator of the hospital.

ELABORATION ON RESPONSIBILITIES: Following the principles of good management, the pharmacist should be assigned specific responsibilities together with the proper authority to carry them out.

*Currently the AMERICAN SOCIETY OF HOSPITAL PHARMACISTS recommends the suggested standards of the Hospital Facilities Division of the Public Health Service.

The pharmacist is best qualified by education, training and experience to assume responsibility for the preparation and sterilization of injectable medication. The manufacture of injectable medication is a major responsibility which should be assigned only to those legally and professionally qualified. It is unwise for the hospital to place itself in an untenable position, legally and morally, by assigning this responsibility to unqualified and unlicensed personnel. By the same standard the pharmacist is the individual who should prepare the specifications for purchase of these medicaments if they are not manufactured in the hospital.

It is self evident that the manufacture of pharmaceuticals and the dispensing of drugs, chemicals and pharmaceutical preparations should be the responsibility solely of the pharmacist and should not be entrusted to unqualified personnel.

The proper filling and labeling of all drug containers is an important task which should be centralized. Many errors leading to results detrimental and even fatal to the patient have resulted from the improper practice of assigning this responsibility to others. An inspection of pharmaceutical supplies on all services should be made with sufficient frequency to insure that medications are properly labeled and that the drugs being used have not deteriorated nor in any other manner become unfit for use. Normally a monthly inspection should be sufficient.

If 24-hour pharmaceutical service cannot be provided by licensed pharmacists, it is the responsibility of the pharmacy to make emergency drugs available for rapid procurement at all times when the pharmacy is closed.

Narcotic drugs should be dispensed in strict accordance with Federal and State narcotic regulations. The pharmacist should, at all times, keep narcotic drugs in a locked compartment. He should maintain a perpetual record of the stock on hand and should record all narcotic drugs dispensed in such a manner that the final disposition of any particular item may be readily traced. The same procedure should apply to other regulated drugs under Federal and State laws.

The pharmacist should furnish specifications for the purchase of all drugs, chemicals and pharmaceutical preparations even though a purchasing agent may do the actual procurement through a centralized department. Since the pharmacist has the responsibility for the compounding, dispensing and manufacture of the drugs used in the hospital he should also have the authority to specify the drugs to be purchased. In large institutions with centralized purchasing, the pharmacist and the purchasing agent should work hand-in-hand, each recognizing the importance of the function of the other. In such a system it is essential that the pharmacist state the specifications for drugs to be purchased and to have authority to reject any article below standard or not complying with specifications so that the purchasing agent may be guided and assisted in his function. The pharmacist will also, in certain instances, wish to consult with the Pharmacy and Therapeutics Committee concerning specifications for drugs.

Since the potency of many drugs is affected by temperature, light, moisture and other conditions, the pharmacist should establish storage specifications for labile products and should be provided with adequate refrigeration facilities so that the pharmaceuticals affected by heat may be properly preserved.

The pharmacy should be the hospital's center for information concerning drugs. The pharmacist should be thoroughly familiar with the library at his disposal (as detailed in the section on facilities) so that, upon request, information may be secured promptly. Also, the pharmacist should be responsible for the systematic arrangement of this library and for additions to it as necessary. The pharmacy should, if possible, publish a circular or bulletin containing information on new drugs. This should be circulated to members of the medical and nursing staffs. Representatives from pharmaceutical firms calling on members of the hospital staff should make the pharmacy their first point of call to acquaint the pharmacist with the products they would like to promote, to learn how the products fit into the overall pharmacy policy, and to become conversant with the regulations regarding the procedures to be followed when promoting pharmaceutical specialties in the hospital.

The establishment and maintenance of proper business records in the pharmacy is one of the major administrative duties of the pharmacist. The purpose of such records is to aid the pharmacist and the hospital administration in evaluating the efficiency and economy with which the pharmacy department is being operated, to insure that adequate direct or indirect charges for medication are apportioned, and to prevent needless waste through adequate control over the requisitioning and dispensing of medication and related supplies.

The accounting department should assist the pharmacist in establishing a proper system of business records. Charges for drugs and related supplies issued by the pharmacy to patients or to other units of the hospital should be credited to the pharmacy. All invoices for drugs and related supplies should be charged to the pharmacy. Administrative expense and other services rendered to the pharmacy should be charged to it. Services rendered by the pharmacy to other units of the hospital should be credited to the pharmacy.

A proper system of records supplies to the pharmacist basic information pertaining to the unit cost of drugs whether manufactured or purchased. It should include a consideration of inventory, turnover or stock, distribution of supplies, drug cost, departmental overhead, administrative costs, operating expense per patient day and the cost of drugs per patient day. A separate stock card should be provided for each item purchased or manufactured. The card should include definite information including a description or specification of the item, date manufactured or purchased, quantity, source of supply, unit cost, requisition number and/or order number.

In planning, organizing and directing pharmacy policies and procedures in accordance with the established policies of the hospital, the pharmacist should proceed in such a manner as to assure the best pharmacy service to the patient and at the same time to establish an efficient and economical department of the hospital. To accomplish this he must develop work schedules, routines and procedures within the department and also he must work cooperatively with other departments which constantly obtain service for the patient through the pharmacy. In establishing pharmacy policies he will be guided by the advice of the Pharmacy and Therapeutics Committee, by the administrative officer of the hospital, and in certain instances by other specialized departments of the institution.

Maintenance of facilities of the pharmacy include responsibility for assuring orderliness, cleanliness, and sanitary procedures as well as keeping all equipment in good working order.

It is especially advantageous that the pharmacist be assigned to instruct student nurses in pharmacology since, in addition to possessing a basic knowledge of the action and uses of drugs, he has a more particularized acquaintance of the preparations, dosage forms and storage requirements of drugs used in the hospital.

After the Pharmacy and Therapeutics Committee has made its decisions regarding the addition or deletion of drugs approved for use in the hospital, or has passed other recommendations regarding pharmacy policy and such recommendations have received approval, it shall be the responsibility of the pharmacist to carry out the recommendations.

The pharmacist should prepare reports on the progress of the pharmacy department and submit them to the director of the hospital. These reports may be rendered monthly, quarterly or yearly depending upon the requirements of the hospital. Reports should include a summary of the professional and administrative activities of the department for the fiscal period involved.

6. Pharmacy and Therapeutics Committee

There shall be a Pharmacy and Therapeutics Committee, which shall hold at least two regular meetings annually and such additional meeting as may be required. The members of the committee shall be chosen from the several divisions of the medical staff. The director of pharmacy service shall be a member of the committee and shall serve as its secretary. He shall keep a transcript of proceedings and shall forward a copy to the proper governing authority of the hospital. The purpose of the committee shall be (A) to develop a formulary of accepted drugs for use in the hospital, (B) to serve as an advisory group to the hospital pharmacist on matters pertaining to the choice of drugs to be stocked, (C) to evaluate clinical data concerning drugs requested for use in the hospital, (D) to add to and to delete from the list of drugs accepted for use in the hospital, (E) to prevent unnecessary duplication in the stock of the same basic drug and its preparations and (F) to make recommendations concerning drugs to be stocked on the nursing units and other services.

ELABORATION ON PHARMACY AND THERAPEUTICS COMMIT-
TEE: This committee is an advisory group of the medical staff
and serves as the organizational line of communication between
the medical staff and the pharmacy department. It is also a
policy-making body to the medical staff and to the administration
of the hospital on all matters related to the use of drugs, including investigational drugs.

The hospital formulary system is a method whereby the medical staff of a hospital, working through the Pharmacy and Therapeutics Committee, evaluates, appraises and selects from among
numerous available medicinal agents and dosage forms those that
are considered most useful in patient care. The hospital formulary is a continually revised compilation of pharmaceuticals
which reflects the current clinical judgment of the medical staff.

The terms of office of the several members of the committee
should be staggered. This will prevent the appointment at one
time of an entirely new and inexperienced committee.

The committee should meet preferably once a month, but
not less than twice annually. Medical staff members should
present, in writing, their requests to the committee for action.
The committee meetings should precede staff meetings by a sufficient interval of time to allow the secretary to make up reports.
Reports of committee meetings and actions taken should be
presented by the secretary to the medical staff meetings. These
reports should include additions to the formulary, deletions from
the formulary, reasons for not including requested items and all
other actions taken by the committee.

Further information on the Pharmacy and Therapeutics Committee, the hospital formulary system, and the use of investigational drugs in hospitals may be obtained from three documents available from the AMERICAN SOCIETY OF HOS-
PITAL PHARMACISTS: (1) Statement on the Pharmacy and
Therapeutics Committee, (2) Statement of Guiding Principles
on the Operation of the Hospital Formulary System, and (3)
Statement of Principles Involved in the Use of Investigational
Drugs in Hospitals.

Abilities Required of Hospital Pharmacists

The American Society of Hospital Pharmacists and the American
Association of Colleges of Pharmacy, recognizing the specialty of
hospital pharmacy and the fact that qualified practitioners must be
specially educated, have developed and approved a *Statement on the
Abilities Required of Hospital Pharmacists.*

For the convenience of the practitioner and student, the *Statement*
is hereinafter reproduced.[9]

THE PRIME OBJECTIVE OF EDUCATION for specialization in hospital
pharmacy is to prepare qualified pharmacists to render all elements
of institutional pharmaceutical service in the interest of better patient

care. A foundation based on a broad general and strong professional education is necessary to the realization of this objective.

Specifically the well-qualified hospital pharmacist must have:

1. A Thorough Knowledge of Drugs and Their Actions

A basic understanding of the biological and physical sciences is a necessary part of the hospital pharmacist's background.

The close association of the hospital pharmacist with the medical staff requires him to be knowledgeable in the chemistry, pharmacology, toxicology, routes of administration, stability and other information relating to drugs.

The hospital serves as an educational laboratory for physicians in training and the pharmacist carries an obligation to provide authoritative information on drugs to help in the training of this group. Moreover, new developments in drug therapy often take place in hospitals which again requires the pharmacist to serve as the focal point for information concerning proper drug usage.

His ability to give help relating to proper handling of drugs is a unique feature of his pharmacy practice and calls for skills and knowledge not ordinarily expected of pharmacists practicing outside the hospital environment. For example, radioisotopes are not encountered ordinarily by pharmacists outside of the hospital environment. Similarly, drugs under experimental investigation are not encountered elsewhere. The hospital pharmacist must be able to provide information and assistance in the proper handling of these and similar drugs if proper patient service is to be rendered.

Hospital staffs are made up essentially of specialists, and therefore it is not unusual that the medical team members look to the pharmacist as a colleague with a highly specialized background and knowledge of drugs. He applies his knowledge in individual contacts with physicians, as well as in his relationship with the Pharmacy and Therapeutics Committee, by making, for example, comparisons of the data on drug actions, dosage, toxicity, and relative costs. He is relied upon to determine and assure the pharmaceutical quality of drugs he dispenses, particularly when responsibility for brand selection is delegated to the pharmacist by the medical staff and when use of nonproprietary terminology is an accepted practice.

2. Ability to Develop and Conduct a Pharmaceutical Manufacturing Program

This ability is necessary because drugs in large quantities are needed to meet the drug requirements of the large numbers of hospitalized patients served from the hospital pharmacy. The pharmacist must be able to evaluate the relative savings that may be possible by manufacturing drugs in bulk quantities. He must be able to assess the economic factors involved since cost of providing labor and controls may dictate purchase from outside sources of supply. His ability to assess all factors relating to the manufacturing process is required for an intelligent decision. His knowledge of the availability and sources of drugs is intimately associated with the proper management of this program.

The medical staff often requests the pharmacist to prepare drugs in forms which are not commercially available. Therefore, the pharmacist must be prepared to supply this service and to offer a flexibility that is not ordinarily expected of pharmacists in other circumstances. To be able to render this service the hospital pharmacist must have readily available the equipment and trained personnel required. This point is emphasized since the hospital is a site for investigational procedures involving new drugs and new applications of known drugs.

3. An Intimate Knowledge of Control Procedures

Understanding of controls means to the hospital pharmacist not only ability to interpret data and carry out chemical, biological and physical tests establishing the purity of a drug product, but also the establishment of internal controls for distribution of drugs.

a. Quality Control. An essential part of a hospital pharmacist's responsibility is the development and writing of specifications for drugs to be purchased and dispensed by the hospital pharmacy. This requires a thorough knowledge of all pharmaceutical properties necessary to assure a quality product as well as the standards of strength and purity available in official compendia. He should also have knowledge and ability to determine conformance to specifications of the drugs he receives. Moreover, the pharmacist must be able to determine and carry out control procedures on his own products.

It should be emphasized that evaluation of quality controls of the manufacturer of drugs is as important to the hospital pharmacist as the actual performance of control procedures carried out on drugs manufactured in the pharmacy. Ability to evaluate controls properly is important in selecting manufactured drugs since quality must determine whether the drug should be stocked in the pharmacy.

b. Control of Distribution Throughout the Hospital. This phase of his responsibility is unique because of special distribution problems relating to drugs in the hospital situation. Indeed, it can vary from hospital to hospital depending upon the type and size of hospital involved. Sizable quantities of drugs often physically located outside of the pharmacy at nursing stations, supply rooms and clinical units. The necessity of having controls for internal distribution of drugs is therefore a special problem of the hospital pharmacist.

The hospitalized patient who may require intensive drug therapy requires control procedures which will allow rapid re-checks of drug source and quality. The potentialities of "automated" dispensing at nursing stations brings further emphasis to the establishment of correct controls for drug distribution in this situation.

4. Ability to Conduct and Participate in Research

The hospital pharmacist's research role may fall in one or both of two broad categories. They are: (a) participation, as the pharmaceutical team member, in medical research, and (b) performance of pharmaceutical research. In some instances these may be combined.

In his role as *participant in medical research,* the hospital pharmacist collaborates with the principal investigator or serves as a co-investigator, in designing and conducting research activities involving the use of drugs. In double blind research studies, the pharmacist may hold the only key to the identity of drugs being used. The pharmacist maintains information on the chemistry, pharmacology, posology, and toxicology of compounds under investigation. Familiarity with and ability to search medical and pharmacy journals for information is required in this role; equally important is the ability to comprehend, interpret, apply, and transmit the information to others.

The hospital pharmacist may perform *pharmaceutical research* related to improving the usefulness of pharmaceutical preparations; developing methods for preserving and stabilizing drugs and pharmaceuticals; improving vehicles and bases; improving taste; and increasing therapeutic effectiveness. When a drug is first developed, or is being initially evaluated, the hospital pharmacist may develop additional dosage forms or means of administration. He may also develop various bases, vehicles or combinations for comparison of degree of absorption of medicinal components in internal preparations, and speed, completeness of release, or effectiveness of active ingredients from internal or external preparations.

In both of these roles, the pharmacist must have a basic understanding of the scientific method so that he can properly evaluate research data and design experiments that will provide information from which valid conclusions may be drawn.

5. Ability to Conduct Teaching and In-Service Training Programs

The chief pharmacist, or other hospital pharmacists under his direction, plans and presents the pharmaceutical contribution to the teaching program in hospitals. He may prepare lectures and demonstrations for the nursing staff covering such topics as storage of drugs, drug usage, dosage forms, and pharmaceutical mathematics, involving conversions, percentage solutions, and calculation of doses. Topics such as prescription writing, drug usage, and incompatibilities may be presented to the medical staff or to medical interns and residents.

The chief pharmacist also is responsible for indoctrinating new personnel and for carrying on a continuous training program for staff pharmacists. In hospitals having pharmacy residencies or internships, the hospital pharmacist must develop well planned and coordinated training programs so that the period of internship or residency is a meaningful educational experience to future practitioners of hospital pharmacy rather than one confined to simpler duties and menial tasks in the pharmacy. In hospitals having pharmacy residencies or internships combined with academic programs, the hospital pharmacist must have a thorough understanding both of his own hospital program and the course material and objectives of the academic phase to assist in coordinating one with the other.

6. Ability to Administer and Manage a Hospital Pharmacy

Broad areas of a hospital pharmacist's administrative and management responsibilities include planning and integrating pharmacy policies, budgeting, stock control, maintenance of records and preparation of reports. The hospital pharmacist must be thoroughly familiar with the organization of a hospital, staff and line relationships, and appropriate lines of communication. He coordinates pharmacy activities with medical, nursing and other services, and with the administrative elements of the hospital. He must be able to prepare suitable written communications to the hospital staff in order to bring to their attention pertinent matters affecting their relationship to the pharmacy.

The chief pharmacist usually is responsible for interviewing, selecting and evaluating personnel for work in the pharmacy. He organizes and schedules the work of pharmacy personnel. He is responsible for their training and development, and in most cases prepares performance ratings and initiates promotions. He must be a capable and understanding supervisor.

The chief pharmacist is responsible for the justification, accountability, and expenditure of pharmacy funds. He must be able to analyze and interpret prescribing trends and the economic impact of new drug developments, which for budgeting purposes are translated to his forecast of future drug expenditures. He must maintain an adequate system of stock and inventory control.

Chief pharmacists keep records on all pharmacy operations which may be required legally or administratively. The data collected are translated, by the hospital pharmacist, into periodic or special reports to management. Reports may include, but usually are not limited to, reports on prescriptions filled, controlled drugs dispensed, drug purchases, inspections, improvements in operations.

In hospitals in which patients are charged for drugs, hospital pharmacists develop or participate in development of policies relating to charges made for pharmaceutical services.

In general, the pharmacy must be administered in an efficient, business-like way as a professional component in a complex organizational setting.

Summary

IN ORDER TO MEET the demands of change brought about by the rapid progress in medical care, the pharmacist must endeavor to keep pace. If he is to fit into this changing pattern, he may have to convince his associates who are not aware of the advantages accruing from superior pharmaceutical service.

The opportunity to utilize all of these skills may not be present in all hospitals due to a variety of reasons. In some instances the administrator and staff or the *pharmacist* may be lacking in necessary vision to see the importance and advantages of complete and proper pharmaceutical service.

It must be understood that no one person may possess all of the abilities cited or opportunities to exercise them. Certainly a teaching or research hospital of large size provides more opportunity to utilize these skills. All hospital pharmacists should, however, develop minimal skills in each area and be capable of becoming expert in any one or several of them. This certainly requires more than casual acquaintance with a broad area of knowledge and emphasizes the need for a sound professional education resting on a firm base of physical and biological sciences.

Finally, any education is a prelude to a lifetime experience of learning. With the rapid progress in the pharmaceutical and medical sciences, the ability to read and understand and interpret the professional and technical literature is imperative. In fact, it means that hospital pharmacists must maintain a regular program of reading. Similarily, added importance is associated with his participation in more formal programs of continuing education. Not only does this mean participation in seminars and courses directly associated with pharmacy, but also in the over-all hospital program directed to all staff members through departmental seminars and other educational media. It is this continuing growth and association as a colleague on the health team that will enable the pharmacist in today's hospital to provide superior pharmacy service in years to come.

Research in Hospital Pharmacy

It has been stated that for hospital pharmacy to continue its advancement as a contributing member of the health professions, it must encourage its practitioners towards greater participation in research.

To achieve this objective the American Society of Hospital Pharmacists issued a *Statement on Research in Hospital Pharmacy* which recommends the following:[10]

1. The Director of Pharmacy Services should establish research to improve patient care as one of the formal objectives of his department.
2. The Director of Pharmacy Services should establish a Research Unit of the Department of Pharmacy, either as a separate unit or combined with the Analytical Unit.
3. The Director of Pharmacy Services should select a competent, well-motivated pharmacist with the proper educational background to direct the research activities of the department.
4. The Director of Pharmacy Services associated with a research hospital should develop research programs related to the hospital's objective and employ a full-time research pharmacist to carry them out.
5. The Director of Pharmacy Services in all hospitals where research is an objective should become more active in collaborative research projects with the medical and allied professional staffs and with administrative personnel of the hospital.
6. The Director of Pharmacy Services should seek outside grants for support of patient related and non-patient related research projects to be conducted by the research unit.

Scope of Hospital Pharmacy Research

The hospital pharmacist who possesses adequate education and training can conduct a protracted investigation in the various scientific disciplines which comprise the profession of pharmacy. In addition, the hospital pharmacist may become involved in research pertaining to the packaging, distribution, manufacture and storage of pharmaceutical preparations. There exists also the opportunity to develop new dosage forms, improve existing ones and to develop new and more accurate methods for analyzing the final product.

Some writers even suggest that the hospital pharmacist and/or the clinical pharmacist become involved, along with other members of the hospital's clinical research team, in studies on the absorption, distribution and excretion of drugs and their metabolites. The feeling being that these pharmacists possess the analytical chemical knowledge to make a worthy contribution in this type of applied research.

By the same token, many hospital pharmacists are capable of conducting a studious inquiry into problems of pharmaceutical administration, quality control, professional practice, and the sociological aspects of patient care as they relate to the practice of hospital pharmacy.

Pharmaceutical Services in Accredited Hospitals

The Joint Commission on Accreditation of Hospitals was incorporated in 1952 through a joint effort of the primary associations of North American medicine and hospitals for the purpose of encouraging the voluntary attainment of uniformly high standards of institutional medical care. The founding sponsors of the Joint Commission on Accreditation of Hospitals were the American College of Surgeons, the American College of Physicians, the American Hospital Association, the American Medical Association and the Canadian Medical Association.

One of the fundamental purposes of the Commission was "To establish standards for the operation of hospitals and other health care facilities and services." Because pharmacy is an essential aspect of institutional health care services, it falls within the purview of the Joint Commission on Accreditation of Hospitals accreditaton program.

Accordingly, the following standards and their interpretations are published verbatim from the *Accreditation Manual for Hospitals 1970.*[11]

Standard I

The pharmaceutical service shall be directed by a professionally competent and legally qualified pharmacist. It shall be staffed by a sufficient number of competent personnel, in keeping with the size and scope of services of the hospital.

INTERPRETATION: There shall be a director of the pharmaceutical service who is legally and professionally qualified, and who is responsible to the chief executive officer. The director should be a graduate of a recognized college of pharmacy and may be employed either part time or full time as the activity of the service requires. He should be oriented to the specialized functions of hospital pharmacies or have completed a hospital pharmacy residency program approved by the American Society of Hospital Pharmacists. The director of pharmaceutical service should be assisted by additional qualified pharmacists and ancillary personnel as needed.

If trained pharmacy assistants are employed, they should be carefully selected and shall work under the supervision of a pharmacist. They shall not be assigned duties that should be performed only by registered pharmacists. Clerical and stenographic assistance should be provided as needed to assist with records, reports and correspondence.

The organizational structure of the pharmaceutical service will vary, depending upon the size and complexity of the hospital. If the hospital does not have an organized pharmacy, pharmaceutical service shall be obtained from another hospital having such service, or from a community pharmacy. Prepackaged drugs then should be stored in, and distributed from, the hospital drug storage area under the supervision of the director of pharmaceutical service.

Standard II

There shall be equipment and supplies provided for the professional and administrative functions of the pharmaceutical service, as required to ensure patient safety through the proper storage and dispensing of drugs.

INTERPRETATION: Hospitals with an organized pharmaceutical service should have the necessary equipment and physical facilities for compounding and dispensing drugs, including parenteral preparations.

Drugs stored within the pharmacy, and throughout the hospital, must be under the supervision of the pharmacist. They must be stored under proper conditions of sanitation, temperature, light, moisture, ventilation, segregation and security. There should be adequate and properly controlled drug preparation areas, as well as locked storage areas, on the nursing units. These areas, which should be well lighted, should be located in a place where the nursing personnel will not be interrupted when handling drugs. The pharmacist, or his designee, must make periodic inspections of all drug storage and medication centers on nursing care units. A record of these inspections should be maintained in order to verify that:

Disinfectants and drugs for external use are stored separately from internal and injectable medications.

Drugs requiring special conditions for storage to ensure stability are properly stored. For example, biologicals and other thermolabile medications should be stored in a separate compartment within a refrigerator that is capable of maintaining the necessary temperature.

No outdated drugs are stocked.

Distribution and administration of controlled drugs are adequately documented.

Emergency drugs are in adequate and proper supply.

Metric-apothecaries' weight and measure conversion charts posted wherever they are needed.

Materials and equipment necessary for the administration of the service should be provided. Effective messenger and delivery service should connect the pharmacy with appropriate parts of the hospital.

Up-to-date pharmaceutical reference material should be provided in order to furnish the medical and nursing staffs with adequate information concerning drugs. As a minimum the following should be available: *United States Pharmacopeia, National Formulary, American Hospital Formulary Service,* and *A.M.A. Drug Evaluations.**

In addition, there should be current editions of text and reference books covering theoretical and practical pharmacy; general, organic, pharmaceutical and biological chemistry; toxicology; pharmacology; bacteriology; sterilization and disinfection; as well as other related matters important to good patient care. Authoritative, current antidote information should be readily available in the pharmacy for emergency reference, along with the telephone number of the regional poison control center.

Standard III

The scope of the pharmaceutical service shall be consistent with the medication needs of the patients and shall include a program for the control and accountability of drug products throughout the hospital.

INTERPRETATION: Policies and procedures relative to the selection and distribution, as well as to the safe and effective use,

---

* *American Hospital Formulary Service* (Washington, D.C.: Society of Hospital Pharmacists, 1959).

A.M.A. Drug Evaluations (Chicago: American Medical Association, 1970).

National Formulary (Easton, Pa.: Mack Publishing Co., 1970).

U.S. Pharmacopeia (Easton, Pa.: Mack Publishing Co., 1965).

of drugs shall be developed by the medical staff in cooperation with the pharmacist and with representatives of other disciplines, as necessary. Such policies and procedures should be approved by the medical staff. All drugs and chemicals should be obtained and used in accordance with these established policies. Such products shall meet the standards of quality of the *United States Pharmacopeia* or *National Formulary*. Drugs for bona fide clinical investigations may be exceptions.

Within this framework, the director of the pharmaceutical service should be responsible for at least the following:

Preparing and sterilizing parenteral medications that are manufactured in the hospital.

Admixture of parenteral products, when feasible.

Manufacturing pharmaceuticals when this is done in the hospital.

Establishing specifications for the procurement of all approved drugs, chemicals and biologicals.

Participating in the development of a hospital formulary. The existence of a hospital formulary does not preclude the use of unlisted drugs.

Dispensing drugs and chemicals.

Filling and labeling all drug containers issued to departments/services from which medications are to be administered.

Implementing the decisions of the pharmacy and therapeutics committee.

Maintaining and keeping available the approved stock of antidotes and other emergency drugs, both in the pharmacy and in patient care areas. Authoritative, recent antidote information, as well as the phone number of the regional poison control center, should be readily available in the areas where these drugs are stored.

Maintaining records of the transactions of the pharmacy as required by law and as necessary to maintain adequate control and accountability of all drugs. This should include a system of controls and records for the requisitioning and dispensing of supplies to nursing care units and to other departments/services of the hospital as well as records of all prescription drugs dispensed.

Cooperating in the teaching and research programs of the hospital.

Standard IV

Written policies and procedures that pertain to the intrahospital drug distribution system shall be developed by the medical staff in cooperation with the pharmacist and representatives of other disciplines, as necessary.

INTERPRETATION: Drug compounding and dispensing shall be restricted to the pharmacist, or to his designee under the direct supervision of the pharmacist. It is desirable for the pharmacist to review the prescriber's original order, or a direct copy, before the initial dose of medication is dispensed.

Written policies and procedures that are essential for patient safety, and for the control and accountability of drugs, should include, but should not be limited to, provision that:

All drugs shall be labeled adequately, including the addition of appropriate accessory or cautionary statements, as indicated.

Discontinued and outdated drugs and containers with worn, illegible or missing labels shall be returned to the pharmacy for proper disposition.

Only the pharmacist, or authorized pharmacy personnel under the direction and supervision of the pharmacist, shall dispense medications, make labeling changes, or transfer medications to different containers.

Only prepackaged drugs shall be removed from the pharmacy when the pharmacist is not available. These drugs shall be removed only by a designated nurse or physician, and in amounts sufficient for immediate therapeutic needs. A record of such withdrawals shall be made.

There shall be a drug recall procedure that can be readily implemented.

Standard V

Written policies and procedures that govern the safe administration of drugs shall be developed by the medical staff in cooperation with the pharmacist and with representatives of other disciplines, as necessary.

INTERPRETATION: Written policies, which are essential for the safe administration of drugs to patients, shall include at least the following:

Drugs shall be administered only upon the order of an individual who has been assigned clinical privileges or who is an authorized member of the house staff.

All medications shall be administered by appropriately licensed personnel in accordance with any laws and regulations governing such acts.

Acceptable precautionary measures for the safe admixture of parenteral products shall be developed. Whenever drugs are added to intravenous solution, a distinctive supplementary label shall be affixed that indicates the name and amount of the drug added, the date and time of the addition and the name of the person who prepared the admixture.

Each dose of medication administered shall be properly recorded in the patient's medical record.

Medication errors and drug reactions shall be reported immediately to the practitioner who ordered the drug. An entry of the medication given and/or the drug reaction shall be properly recorded in the patient's medical record. Hospitals are encouraged to report any unexpected or significant adverse drug reactions to the Hospital Reporting Program of the Federal Food and Drug Administration and to the manufacturer.

If patients bring their own drugs into the hospital, these drugs shall not be administered unless they can be identified, and written orders to administer these specific drugs are given by the responsible practitioner. If the drugs that the patient brought to the hospital are not to be used while he is hospitalized, they should be packaged, sealed, stored and returned to the patient at the time of discharge if such action is approved by the responsible practitioner.

Self-administration of medications by patients shall be permitted only when specifically ordered by authorized house staff members and/or individuals who have been granted clinical privileges.

Investigational drugs properly labeled shall be used only under the direct supervision of the principal investigator and should be approved by an appropriate medical staff committee. Nurses may administer these drugs only after they have been given basic pharmacologic information about the drug. A central unit should be established where essential information on investigational drugs is maintained.*

Orders involving abbreviations and chemical symbols should be carried out only if the abbreviations and symbols appear on a standard list approved by the medical staff.

SELECTED REFERENCES

1. ZOPF, LOUIS C.: The Pharmacist's Role in Comprehensive Health Care, Pharmaceutical Marketing & Media, 4:1:9, Jan. 1969.
2. CAMPBELL, NORMAN A. and HASSAN, WILLIAM E.: Institutional Pharmacy: Specialty or Basic Discipline, Am. J. Pharm. Ed., 33:2:61, Feb. 1969.
3. NIGHTINGALE, CHARLES H.: The "Clinical" Concept of Pharmacy, Pharmaceutical Marketing & Media, 4:8:21, Aug. 1971.
4. Institutional Pharmacy Practice in the 1970's. Reprint Series 72/2 August 1972, Pub. No. 73-3001 Dept. HEW, Health Services and Mental Health Administration National Center for Health Services Research and Development, Rockville, Maryland 20852.

* For further guidance, refer to *Statement of Principles Involved in the Use of Investigational Drugs in Hospitals*, approved by the American Hospital Association and the American Society of Hospital Pharmacists. (Washington, D.C.: The Society, 1957).

BIBLIOGRAPHY

1. COOKE, E. F., and MARTIN, E. W.: *Remington's Practice of Pharmacy,* 10th Ed. Easton, The Mack Publishing Co., 1951.
2. URDANG, GEORGE: Foreword to Ten Years of the American Society of Hospital Pharmacists, The Bulletin, A.S.H.P., 9:1:281, 1952.
3. Hospital Statistics 1971, American Hospital Association, Chicago, Illinois.
4. ARCHAMBAULT, GEORGE F.: Needs for Hospital Pharmacists in the United States 1957–1970, Am. J. Hosp. Pharm., 15:2:131, 1958.
5. LETOURNEAU, CHARLES U.: The Hospital Pharmacist Needs Management Skills, Am. J. Hosp. Pharm., 16:2:73, 1959.
6. FRANCKE, DON E.: Editorial—An American School of Hospital Pharmacy, Am. J. Hosp. Pharm., 16:2:53, 1959.
7. Goals for Hospital Pharmacy, Am. J. Hosp. Pharm., 21:11:535, 1964.
8. Minimum Standard for Pharmacies in Hospitals with Guide to Application, American Society of Hospital Pharmacists Reprinted 1-1-66.
9. Statement on the Abilities Required of Hospital Pharmacists, Am. J. Hosp. Pharm., 19:9:493, 1962.
10. Statement on Research in Hospital Pharmacy, Am. J. Hosp. Pharm., 21: 11:537, 1964.
11. Accreditation Manual for Hospitals 1970, Joint Commission on Accreditation of Hospitals, 654 No. Michigan Ave., Chicago, Illinois 60611.

Chapter

2

The Hospital and Its Organization

"The hospital is a complex organization utilizing combinations of intricate, specialized scientific equipment, and functioning through a corps of trained people educated to the problems of modern medical science. These are all welded together in the common purpose of restoration and maintenance of good health.

The hospital, as an organization, provides special facilities and trained personnel to facilitate the work of the physician in his primary position involving care of the patient who is the focal point about which all activities of the hospital revolve. In the delivery of medical services to patients, therefore, the medical and associated technical staff of nurses, dietitians etc. become a most important factor. The character and extent of hospital services are adjusted continuously to keep abreast of changes and advances in medical science.

Although primary emphasis is placed on the care of bed patients, the frontier of the hospital in recent years has been extended from the sick person in the hospital bed, to the potentially sick person in his normal living situation. Hospitals have been assuming more and more responsibility for programs of preventive medicine. They serve as the medium in many communities through which the professional staffs and official health agencies pool their efforts for improvement of the public health."[1]

Because of the specific scope of this volume, only a general view of the complex organizational structure of a hospital will be presented. Those desiring a more comprehensive treatment of the subject are referred to McGibony's *Principles of Hospital Administration*[2] and MacEachern's treatise, *Hospital Organization and Management.*[3]

Classification of Hospitals

Hospitals may be classified in many different ways and any single institution may fall into more than one grouping. For example, the Peter Bent Brigham Hospital is a "private, non-profit, teaching hospital." The following is a brief general classification schedule which will serve to classify the great majority of hospitals:

HOSPITAL CLASSIFICATIONS

CLINICAL	OWNERSHIP & CONTROL
General Medical & Surgical	*Governmental*
Specialty	Army, Navy, Veterans
MEDICINE	Administration
Internal Medicine	Public Health Service
Psychiatric & Nervous Diseases	State
Tuberculosis	County
Communicable Diseases	City
Pediatrics	*Non-Government*
SURGERY	Private for profit
Orthopedic	Non-profit
Gynecologic	Church
Otolaryngologic	Fraternal order
MATERNITY	Community
Length of Stay	Non-profit private
Short term	*BY ACCREDITATION* *
Long term (Chronic)	Accredited (2 years)
Custodial (Long term)	Accredited (1 year)
	Non-accredited

*Joint Commission on Accreditation of Hospitals

What are teaching hospitals? A major teaching hospital is one which, like the Peter Bent Brigham Hospital, is used extensively for the clinical instruction of medical school students. A minor teaching hospital is used only for a limited amount of student instruction, such as occasional demonstrations or clinics.

Traditionally, teaching hospitals are places where the new medical graduate seeks postgraduate training. He almost always undergoes one year of hospital training as an intern. He may frequently spend two or more additional years in a hospital as a resident in some specialty, such as internal medicine, surgery, pediatrics or radiology. On the other hand, some community hospitals maintain intern and residency programs. When they exist, however, they tend to be far less complete than in the teaching institution.

Numerically, teaching hospitals represent approximately 350 of the nation's 7123 registered hospitals. However, they care for a little over one of every five hospitalized Americans.

Industry also recognizes the importance of the teaching hospital by virtue of the special coverage it receives from the company's medical service representatives as well as its desire to financially support both educational and research programs.

Because teaching hospitals provide a higher standard of medical care than is normally found in the community, third party payors have been, in recent years, reimbursing these hospitals at a higher rate than small suburban institutions with no teaching-research programs.

Most young physicians entering practice look for locations in a teaching hospital because such institutions assure them of the most contemporary educational opportunities coupled with broad experiences in the clinical care of patients, teaching and research.

Organizational Pattern

The organizational pattern of a hospital does not differ from that of any industrial plant. The apparent difference is superficial and deals only with the nomenclature of the positions. For example, the Director or Administrator of a hospital may be the Executive Vice-President or the General Manager of the commercial entity. Two organizational charts are presented in Figures 1 and 2. Obviously, the smaller the hospital the fewer the administrative positions of associate or assistant director and conversely, the very large institutions may further sub-divide the general areas of clinical and administrative services into smaller units under the aegis of assistant directors. The corporation and the board of trustee segment of the organization is standard for all private hospitals. Governmental hospitals usually have a board of trustees but no corporate body.

Governing Body and Management

One of the purposes of the Joint Commission on the Accreditation of Hospitals is "to establish standards for the operation of hospitals and other health care facilities and services."[4] To accomplish this, the Joint Commission on the Accreditation of Hospitals has adopted the following principle:[5]

> There shall be an organized governing body, or designated person(s) so functioning, that has overall responsibility for the conduct of the hospital in a manner consonant with the hospital's objective of making available high quality patient care.

The resulting application of this principle is that hospitals, in general, are legally organized as CORPORATIONS according to the corporate laws of the State in which they operate, although a few of the privately owned and operated units still function under a partnership agreement. The total number of members in each corporation will vary from hospital to hospital.

Because the corporation may consist of a large number of people from widely scattered areas, a representative group, from within the corporate membership, is elected to a board of trustees. This group is also known as the governing board, board of governors, board of managers or board of directors.

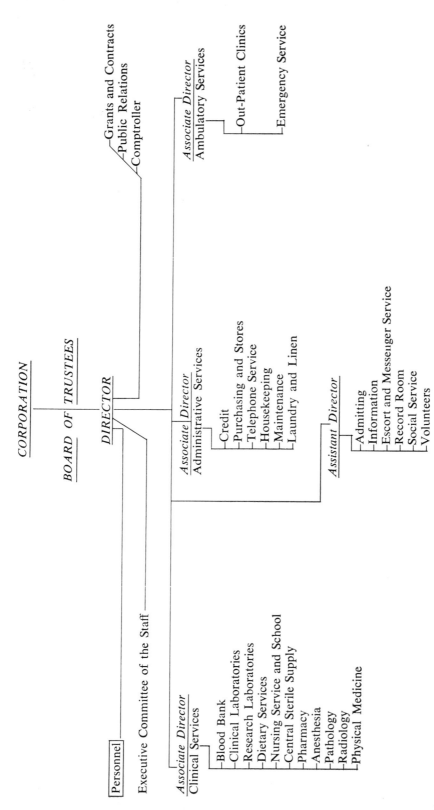

CORPORATION

BOARD OF TRUSTEES

DIRECTOR

Executive Committee of the Staff

Personnel

Grants and Contracts
Public Relations
Comptroller

Associate Director
Ambulatory Services
- Out-Patient Clinics
- Emergency Service

Associate Director
Administrative Services
- Credit
- Purchasing and Stores
- Telephone Service
- Housekeeping
- Maintenance
- Laundry and Linen

Assistant Director
- Admitting
- Information
- Escort and Messenger Service
- Record Room
- Social Service
- Volunteers

Associate Director
Clinical Services
- Blood Bank
- Clinical Laboratories
- Research Laboratories
- Dietary Services
- Nursing Service and School
- Central Sterile Supply
- Pharmacy
- Anesthesia
- Pathology
- Radiology
- Physical Medicine

Fig. 1. Administrative Organization Chart

31

Generally, the above board includes a broad representation of the community served by the hospital and its members are selected for their ability to contribute to its effective management.

It is required, both by State laws and the Joint Commission on the Accreditation of Hospitals, that the governing body adopt by-laws identifying the purposes of the hospital and the means of fulfilling them. Included in the by-laws are the following:[6]

(i)   definition of the powers and duties of the governing body officers, committees and chief executive officer.
(ii) qualifications for governing body membership.
(iii) method of selection of membership.
(iv) tenure.
(v)   committees—kinds, appointment and membership tenure.

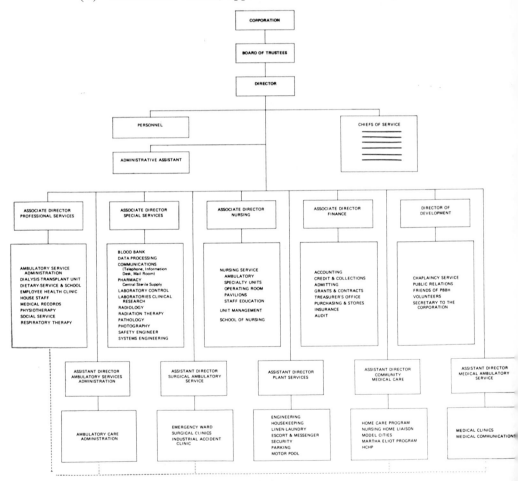

FIG. 2. Large Hospital Administrative Chart.

The by-laws also describe the authority delegated to the chief executive officer (Director or Administrator) and to the medical staff. It should be clear to the student that such a delegation of authority does not preclude the governing body from exercising the control and authority required to meet its responsibility for the conduct of the hospital. The governing body always has the right to rescind any such delegation.

As part of the organizational process, the governing body elects its officers and causes to be appointed a wide variety of committees necessary for the discharge of its duties. These may include an Executive Committee, Building Committee, Investment and Finance Committee and a Joint Conference Committee.

The governing body of the hospital has, through its chief executive officers, a number of obligations best exemplified by recording Standards V through X of the J.C.A.H.[7]

Standard V

The governing body, through its chief executive officer, shall provide appropriate physical resources and personnel required to meet the needs of the patients, and shall participate in planning to meet the health needs of the community.

Standard VI

The governing body, through its chief executive officer, shall take all reasonable steps to conform to all applicable federal, state and local laws and regulations, including those relating to licensure, fire inspection and other safety measures.

Standard VII

The governing body, through its chief executive officer, shall provide for the control and use of the physical and financial resources of the hospital.

Standard VIII

The governing body shall delegate to the medical staff the authority to evaluate the professional competence of staff members and applicants for staff privileges; it shall hold the medical staff responsible for making recommendations to the governing body concerning initial appointments, reappointments and the assignment or curtailment of privileges.

Standard IX

The medical staff by-laws, rules and regulations shall be subject to governing body approval, which shall not be unreasonably withheld. These shall include an effective formal means for the medical staff to participate in the development of hospital policy relative to both hospital management and patient care.

Standard X

The governing body shall require that the medical staff establish controls that are designed to ensure the achievement and maintenance of high standards of professional ethical practices.

The Administration

The active management of hospitals is delegated, by the board of trustees, to the administrator and his staff of associates, assistants, supervisors and department heads.

It should be noted that the Director of the Pharmacy Service (Pharmacist-in-Chief) reports to the assistant or associate director responsible for the clinical services of the hospital. Too often, the pharmacy is considered a business type of service and is assigned to the division of administrative services. Grouping the pharmacist with the housekeeper, laundry manager and maintenance group does irreparable harm to the professional stature of the pharmacist and damages his rapport with the other members of the clinical group.

The administrator of a hospital is especially trained for his position. Today, most of the new appointees to the top post in hospitals are graduates of special programs and hold the *Master of Hospital Administration* degree. The lack of such a degree does not preclude other qualified individuals from being appointed administrator. In addition, many boards of trustees require that the administrator be a *Fellow* of the American College of Hospital Administrators.

The main function of the administrator is to enforce trustee policy in the daily management routine. In addition, he must play an active role in community public relations as well as liaison between the medical staff and the board of trustees. In commenting upon the expanding role of the hospital administrator, Cordes[8] has stated . . .

> ". . . the hospital administrator of today must know and understand his community, its people, their historical traditions, the value structure that is at work, the resources available, and the weaknesses to be reckoned with in any course of action. Armed with this knowledge and understanding, he must educate the community to his enterprise, its goals, its problems, its needs, and its opportunities for contribution to the community . . ."

The modern hospital administrator can be described as a specialist in administration, as an educator, as a community adviser and as an organizer. Reporting to the governing body, he bears responsibility for the operation of the entire institution, assuring the medical and scientific staffs, the trustees and the patients of the highest possible standards of both service and economy. Within the hospital he plans, directs and coordinates activities which outside the institution would be complete entities in themselves: food service, laundry, pharmacy, out-patient clinic. The future of the institution depends, in significant measure, on the vision of the hospital administrator.[9]

Medical Staff

Clearly, every hospital must have a medical staff that is responsible for the quality of all medical care provided to patients and for the ethical conduct and professional practices of its membership.

Generally, medical staff membership is limited to individuals who are fully licensed to practice medicine or dentistry. As a body, this group usually organizes itself to provide for the election or appointment of officers and committees whose function it is to create and maintain an optimal level of professional performance of its membership.

The framework of the medical staff will vary from hospital to hospital due to the varying size and activities of the hospital and the staff. However, the staff may be divided into the following categories: active medical staff; associate medical staff; courtesy medical staff; consulting medical staff and honorary medical staff.

The active medical staff is responsible for the delivery of the preponderance of medical service within the hospital and is most involved in the organizational and administrative duties pertaining to the medical staff.

The associate medical staff consists of individuals who are being considered for advancement to the active medical staff. These practitioners are appointed and assigned to the various services in the same manner as are members of the active medical staff.

The courtesy medical staff consists of practitioners who are eligible for staff membership, who are given privileges to admit an occasional patient to the hospital. Courtesy staff members may neither vote nor hold office in the medical staff organization.

The consulting medical staff consists of medical practitioners of recognized professional ability who are not members of the preceding categories of staff membership.

The honorary medical staff consists of former staff members, retired or emeritus, and of other practitioners whom the medical staff chooses to honor.

The Clinical Departments

The degree of departmentalization of the clinical divisions of the hospital depends almost entirely upon the degree of specialization of the medical staff. In the very small communities, one would expect to find two major departments in a hospital—medicine and surgery. Supportive services such as radiology and pathology are also offered but are generally limited in their capability to provide service. In those areas where there are two or more small hospitals, it is common to have a single department of pathology or radiology servicing both institutions. However, in the large metropolitan areas the hospital staff is highly specialized and therefore greater sub-divisions within a particular department.

Generally, the department of medicine includes the following sub-divisions:

Internal Medicine	Geriatrics
Allergy	Pediatrics
Cardiology	Gastroenterology
Infectious Diseases	Neurology
Dermatology	Psychiatry
Endocrinology	Pulmonary Diseases

The department of surgery is generally divided into the following:

General Surgery	Otolaryngology
Orthopedic Surgery	Plastic Surgery
Neurological Surgery	Proctology
Obstetrics & Gynecology	Thoracic Surgery
Ophthalmology	Urology
Dental & Oral Surgery	

In addition there may be a division of general practice as well as a division of physical medicine and rehabilitation within the hospital.

Each of these sub-divisions usually has a chief-of-service who in turn is responsible to the departmental chief. In addition, the medical staff is organized in such a manner as to provide fair representation of each individual on the staff through to the administration and the governing body.

It should be clear to the student that the larger and more specialized medical staff is indicative of the fact that the institution is a teaching hospital. Because the description "teaching hospital" has been misused, the American Hospital Association describes such an institution in the following manner:[10,11]

> A hospital that allocates a substantial part of its resources to conduct, in its own name or in formal association with a college or courses of instruction in the health disciplines that lead to the granting of recognized certificates, diplomas, or degrees, or that are required for professional certification or licensure, is a teaching hospital.

The association also placed the following interpretation on the definition:

> The allocation of resources and facilities, personnel, and funds must be adequate to demonstrate the discharge of teaching programs.

Educational programs or courses of instruction are "formal" when based upon published or recorded curricula covering specified periods of study and have faculty qualification and student admission requirements established or agreed to by the hospital. They are not work and learn or on the job training arrangements that primarily augment the hospital's capability to provide services. Further, the hospital controls, or agrees to, the appointment of faculty and selection of students except during the term of agreements that gives a college or medical school exclusive authority therefore.

Certificates, degrees, or diplomas must be recognized and accepted by national educational agencies, professional qualifying bodies, or state approving authorities. This implies that the courses or educational programs need standards generally recognized in the health field.

The teaching hospital affords the hospital pharmacists with innumerable opportunities to participate in and to develop educational programs. The literature is replete with articles describing endeavors by hospital pharmacists in the teaching of various subjects to student nurses, conducting in-service programs for graduate nurses and practical nurses, developing seminars on the pharmacology of drugs for interns, residents and senior staff physicians, training undergraduate and graduate students in hospital pharmacy and participating in the training of students in hospital administration.

Because of the unique training of the professional hospital pharmacist, he can make noteworthy contributions towards the fulfillment of the criteria required for an institution to qualify as a teaching hospital.

The Supporting Services

To those unfamiliar with the hospital environment, it would seem as though the hospital consisted of the clinical departments only. Actually, the clinical departments would be unable to function without the supporting services. Amongst the supporting services are the nursing department, the dietary service, laboratory services, the medical records department, the blood bank, the central sterile supply, and the social service department.

There are other services clinically essential to the operation of the hospital such as the maintenance and engineering divisions. However, for the purpose of this text only the former will be discussed.

Nursing Service

Much has been written relative to the progress that has been made in the field of medicine during the past decade. This revolution in medical care has had its effect on the other health professions. For nursing, keeping pace with medicine has meant many changes in practice. The nursing team, made up of workers with varying degrees of nursing skill and directed by a professional nurse, now replaces the single nurse who once did everything for the patient. Today's nursing practitioner recognizes social, psychological, or religious problems with the patient that might influence his physical well

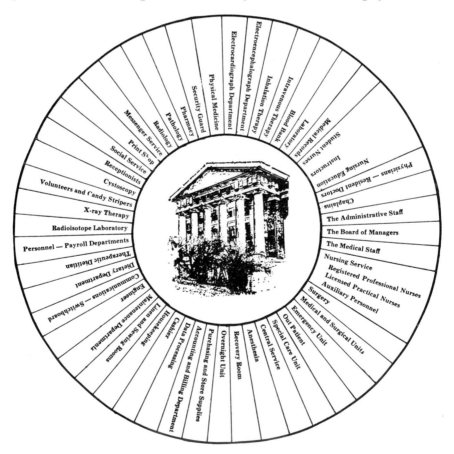

Fig. 3. The Hospital . . . A Multiple Service Unit.

being and refer those that lie outside the province of nursing to the person most competent to deal with them. Helping the patients to help themselves is another new element of nursing practice, added because of increased emphasis on self care by the patient as an aid to early recovery. The new patterns of nursing service thus brought about are often misunderstood by the public when the changes and the reasons behind them are not explained. Thus in 1964, The National League for Nursing directed a statement concerning the basic assumptions which one could make about nursing care to those engaged in various aspects of nursing service as a means of improving service wherever it is given; to allied professions because nursing care is only a part of the total health provided by many groups, whose ability to work together improves the mutual understanding; and to consumers of nursing service who, as members of the community, share the responsibility for seeing that the care necessary for regaining and maintaining health is made available to themselves and to their families. The following are the basic assumptions:[12]

1. Nursing care encompasses health promotion, the care and prevention of disease or disability, rehabilitation, teaching, counselling, and emotional support as well as the care of illness.
2. Nursing care is an integral part of total health care and is planned and administered in combination with related medical, educational, and welfare services.
3. Nursing personnel respect individuality, dignity, and rights of every person; regardless of race, color, creed, national origin, social or economic status.

The nursing service is organized similarly to any other large service in the hospital. There is at its head a Director of Nursing who is generally an experienced nurse with administrative talent. The administrative nursing services carries ultimate administrative authority and responsibility in one or more health facilities for the nursing services provided individuals and families. As a member of the administrative staff, the administrative nursing service participates in formulating policy, and devising procedures essential to the achievement of objectives, and in developing and evaluating programs and services.

In some institutions, the Director of Nursing service is also responsible for the administration and operation of the School of Nursing. However, the modern trend is to separate the responsibility and assign it to an individual specifically trained in the educational aspect of nursing. In those institutions where the school of nursing has been separated from the nursing service, the individual heading the school assumes a position of responsibility similar to that of the Director of the Nursing Service and is responsible directly to the Chief Executive Officer of the hospital.

Dietetic Services

An essential service of each institution is that of the dietary department. The JCAH requires that the dietetic service be organized in such a manner that it shall effectively apply the principles of the science of nutrition to the preparation of palatable and appropriate food. The services are generally directed by a qualified person and staffed by adequate numbers of dietitians and technical and clerical personnel. Qualified personnel in the dietary division are generally considered to be individuals who are registered by the American Dietetic Association or has met that Association's standards for qualification.

In addition to the purchasing, planning and preparation of menus, both for patients and employees, the dietitian is generally responsible for recording dietary histories of patients such as those with food allergies and those unable to accept a limited diet regimen; interviewing patients regarding their food habits; counselling patients and their families concerning normal or modified regimens, and encouraging patients to participate in planning their own normal or modified regimens; and participating in appropriate ward rounds and conferences.

Medical Records Services

Every hospital is required by law to maintain adequate medical records on their patients. These must be accurately documented, readily accessible and can be easily used for retrieving and compiling information.[13]

The purposes of the medical record are:

1. To serve as a basis for planning and for continuity of patient care;
2. To provide a means of communication among the physician and any professionals contributing to the patient's care;
3. To furnish documentary evidence for the course of the patient's illness and treatment during each hospital stay;
4. To serve as a basis for review, study and evaluation of the care rendered to the patient;
5. To assist in protecting the legal interest of the patient, hospital and responsible practitioner;
6. To provide data for use in research education.

The medical record must contain all significant clinical information and should be sufficiently detailed to enable another practitioner to assume the care of the patient at any time, a consultant to give an opinion after his examination of the patient and the practitioner to to give effective continuing care to the patient.

A complete medical record is one which includes identification and sociological data, personal family history, history of present illness, physical examination, special examination such as consultations, clinical laboratory data, x-ray and other examinations, provisional or working diagnosis, medical or surgical treatment, gross and microscopical pathological findings, progress notes, final diagnosis, conditions on discharge, follow-up, and autopsy findings.

Identification data in the medical record is generally provided on what is known as the admission sheet. This sheet generally contains such pertinent information as the unit record number, the patient's name, address, name of the patient's spouse, home telephone number, business telephone number, sex, date of birth, birth place, marital status, occupation, referring family physician's name and address, staff physician's name and address, admission diagnosis, date and time of admission, and destination within the hospital. Attached to the admission sheet, one may generally find consent forms for the authorization for medical or surgical treatment, authorization for the release of information to insurance companies, and a general authorization for the release of information to other physicians or attorneys.

The admission history sheet usually provides space for recording the name of the informant as well as the name of the individual taking the history. The purpose of the admission history is to record the patient's chief complaint and a description of his present illness. In addition, it provides the opportunity of protecting the provisional or admitting diagnosis which is usually made on every patient at the time of admission.

The history and physical examination sheet provides the physician with such information as hospital admissions that have taken place in the past with their subsequent diagnosis, operations and major injuries that have been experienced by the patient, the history of childhood and adult infectious diseases, if applicable, pregnancies with dates, outcome and complications, immunization data, a history of transfusion with dates, reactions and complications, current medications, sociological data covering habits with alcohol or tobacco, diets, height, weight, date of birth, country of birth, education, military history, occupational history, marital status, health of spouse, family history.

The physical examination sheet consists of a routine systematic review of skin, head and neck, cardiorespiratory, breast, gastrointestinal, urinary, genitalia, endocrine-metabolic, lymph nodes and hematological, muscular skeletal and extremities, urological, psychiatric, and allergy.

Once the physician has obtained all of this information, he then proceeds to record in the medical record a suggested program to be followed during the hospitalization of the patient.

Signed laboratory sheets are entered into the patient's medical record. The laboratory reports include those obtained from chemistry, hematology, microbiology, serology, pathology as well as radiology. For this purpose, hospitals have preprinted form which permits for the recording of the data under each of the specific sections. However, some hospitals find it practical to paste the original laboratory reports into the medical record.

All treatment procedures performed upon the patient are recorded in the medical record. Operative notes are also included in the record and usually contain both a description of the findings as well as a detailed account of the technique used and the tissue removed.

Progress notes are made in the medical record for the purpose of providing the physician with a chronological picture and analysis of the clinical course of the patient.

Upon the completion of all of the diagnostic procedures to be performed, it is mandatory that the physician enter into the medical record a definitive final diagnosis which is based on the terms specified in the standard nomenclature of diseases and operations.

Upon discharge from the hospital, the patient's record will have entered into it a discharge summary. The purpose of this is to provide a recapitulation of the patient's hospitalization. In some hospitals, a copy of this discharge summary is forwarded with the patient whenever he is transferred either to another hospital or to an extended care facility or nursing home. Some of the items contained within the discharge summary include a brief history, results of the physical examination, laboratory data, a description of the patient's hospital course, the diagnosis, the present condition, medications that have been sent home with the patient, a listing of the operations performed, complications, disposition, and an estimated length of disability.

If the patient has died while in the hospital, and an autopsy has been performed, the medical record will contain a complete protocol of the findings that have resulted from the autopsy.

Pathology Services

The JCAH requires that the pathology services shall be directed by a physician who is qualified to assume professional, organizational and administrative responsibility for the facilities and for the services rendered and there shall be sufficient personnel who have had adequate training and experience to supervise and conduct the work of the laboratory. The Director of the Pathology Service is a member of the medical staff and has undertaken special training in pathology. Generally, he is certified by the American Board of Pathology or its equivalent. In addition to the cytological and gross anatomical analysis performed within the department of pathology, most hospitals group clinical laboratories within this division. Laboratories such as clinical chemistry, microbiology, clinical microscopy, hematology, and serology are but a few examples.

Blood Bank

Because of the essential nature of blood as a therapeutic agent, most hospitals operate a blood bank. This service is generally under the supervision of a licensed physician who has a basic interest in hematology. However, some hospitals assign the blood bank to the department of pathology because of its laboratory-like operation. Most hospital's blood banks operate as an adjunct to the local Red Cross Blood Program.

Radiology

One of the most important of the scientific and therapeutic facilities of the hospital is the department of radiology. Radiology is that branch of medicine which deals with the diagnostic and therapeutic application of radiant energy, chiefly in the form of roentgen rays and radium. The department is under the supervision of a qualified physician who has also obtained adequate training and experience in general radiology.

Radiology services are performed only upon the written order of a member of the medical staff who has been granted clinical privileges in the hospital. The therapeutic use of radium or sealed radioactive sources in the hospital is limited to physicians, who have been granted this privilege, after consultation with, and consideration of, the recommendations of the radiologist and/or a radiation safety committee. Only persons who have suitable training and experience are permitted to handle radioactive materials.

The department of radiology generally consists of physicians who are trained as radiologists, physicists, technicians, radiotherapists, isotopepharmacists, nurses, orderlies, and secretarial personnel.

Medical Social Service Department

The Medical Social Service Department is a very important liaison between the hospital and the patient and his community. The qualified social worker represents a discipline whose professional focus is on the social aspects of the patient and his family. Social service personnel generally provide information relating to medical social study of appropriate patients; social therapy and rehabilitation of patients; home environmental investigations for attending physician; cooperative activities with community agencies; social service summaries; and follow-up reports of discharged patients, confirming disposition, when obtained.

Anesthesia Service

The Anesthesia Service of a hospital is generally directed by a physician member of the medical staff who has had special training and is responsible for the following: quality of anesthesia care rendered by anesthetist in the surgical and obstetrical areas; availability of equipment necessary for administering anesthesia and for related resuscitative efforts; development of regulations concerning anesthetic safety; and retrospective evaluation of all anesthesia care.

Anesthesia care is usually provided by anesthesiologists, other qualified physician anesthetist, qualified nurse anesthetist, or appropriately supervised trainees in an approved educational program. Whenever nurse anesthetists are employed, they generally provide general anesthesia under the overall direction of the departmental director or his designee.

Central Service Department

The Central Service Department furnishes all supplies required for the nursing units. These supplies include sterile linen, sterile kits, operating room packs, needles, syringes, and other medical surgical supplies. In addition the personnel in this department clean, inspect, repair, assemble, wrap, and sterilize special treatment trays for the various nursing units. Reference to Chapter 22 will provide the student with a greater insight as to the functions of this department.

Pharmacy's Role in the Hospital

Reference to the Administrative Organization Charts (Figs. 1 and 2) will quickly support the claim that a hospital is truly a "city within a city." Within its four walls there is in operation: a hotel which manifests itself by the patient's room accommodations; a dormitory for the student nurses, residents and interns; a school for the training of nurses, technicians, dietitians; laboratories; a pharmacy; food vending operations; a laundry and linen service; housekeeping services; engineering and power generating services; delivery services; a post office; a massive internal and external communications system; blood bank; accounting and credit services; a public relations department; a motor service and security patrols.

Although the pharmacy department is only one of the many divisions of a hospital, it exerts a great deal of influence on the professional stature of the hospital as well as upon the economics of the total operational costs of the institution because of its inter-relation with and the inter-dependency of these other services upon it.

In the community practice of pharmacy, the pharmacist is keenly aware of the doctor-patient-pharmacist triad. In this setting, the doctor diagnoses and prescribes, the pharmacist dispenses the medication and the patient administers the prescribed drug to himself or at most it is administered to him, under ordinary circumstances, by a member of his family.

This is not true in the hospital or in an extended care facility. In this setting we find interjected into the doctor-pharmacist-patient triad the professional nurse who assumes the major responsibility of administering all medications to the patient (unless the patient is on a self-medication regimen).

Clearly then, the pharmacist who practices his profession in an institutional environment must be aware of the forces operating around him, and he must learn not only to understand them, but to assist in marshalling them towards the ultimate goal of better patient care.

Hospital Finances

All too often, the hospital pharmacist lacks a thorough knowledge of the ways and means by which the operation of a hospital is financed. This situation is brought about by the pharmacist's lack of interest or his belief that it is a subject which does not concern him or his department. In reality, the finances of the hospital affect every patient, employee, staff member, trustee and the community at large.

Accordingly, the following is a brief resumé of the sources from which income may be derived to meet operating expenses.

The primary source of revenue is derived from the billing of patients for services rendered. A patient receiving such a statement may either pay it in full himself or he may have *third party coverage* which may pay the bill in full or pay a specified portion with the patient serving as co-insurer. Since the phraseology "third party coverage" or third party payor" is non-specific in definition the student is reminded that it may mean that the bill, either in full or in part, will be paid by someone other than the patient. These "third party payors" may include agencies such as Welfare, Vocational Rehabilitation Services, Aid to Families of Dependent Children, Blue Cross, Medicare, Medicaid or private insurance carriers. Some of these payors pay charges as billed, while others reimburse the hospital on a fixed all-inclusive per diem rate.

Another source of income to the hospital is derived from overhead charged on research projects carried on in hospital property.

A fourth source of income to the hospital will be the income from its invested endowment funds. In many institutions, these earnings are referred to as "treasurer's income."

Still other sources of income are gifts and contributions towards general operating expenses by friends, staff, industry, charitable foundations and the local United Fund.

All of these monies, when pooled together, constitute the general category of *income* against which are applied the cost of operating the institution or "expenses." In well-managed non-profit hospitals income equals expenses. However, with today's spiraling costs the reverse is usually true thereby causing the hospital to either relinquish some of its capital assets in order to meet the deficit or attempting to underwrite it through charitable appeals.

Knowles[4] in a guest editorial entitled *On Hospital Costs and Care,* has stated that 80 per cent of the cost of operating his large university teaching hospital was represented by the professional services, whereas only 12 per cent represents those "general services" or "hotel costs." In addition, he observed that the professional services have been responsible for the skyrocketing hospital costs over the last decade. In support of this observation, the following "pie charts" were presented. For contrast the 1970 "pie chart" is presented.

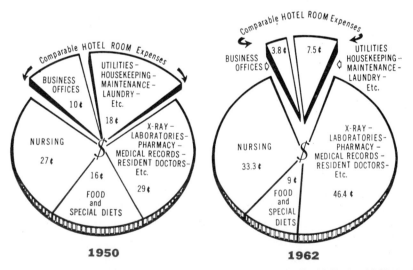

Fig. 4.   "Pie chart" showing the subdivision of the costs in 1950 vs. 1962 at the Massachusetts General Hospital in Boston. (Courtesy of *Resident Physician.*)

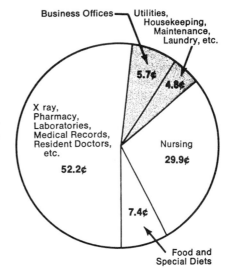

FIG. 5. "Pie chart" showing the subdivision of costs in 1970 at the Massachusetts General Hospital in Boston.

SELECTED REFERENCES

GEORGOPOULOS, BASIL S.: Hospital Organization and Administration: Prospects and Perspectives. Hospital Administration, 9:23, 1964.

DORNBLASER, BRIGHT M.: The Hospital Administrator—His Emerging Role. Hospital Administration, 11:6, 1966.

ROBERTSON, ROBERT L.: The Functions of a University Hospital, Hospital Administration, 11:70, 1966.

Chart of Accounts for Hospitals, 1966, American Hospital Association, Chicago, Ill.

Guidelines for the Formulation of Medical Staff Bylaws, Rules and Regulations, 1971, Joint Commission on Accreditation of Hospitals, Chicago, Ill.

Commission on Nursing Services Statement on Position, Role and Qualifications of the Administrator of Nursing Service, 1969, American Nurses' Association, New York.

Standards for Organized Nursing Services, 1965, American Nurses' Association, New York.

Food Service Manual for Health Care Institutions, 1966, American Hospital Association, Chicago, Ill.

Code of Federal Regulations, Title 42, Subchapter F, Part 74, U.S. Gov. Printing Office, Washington, D.C.

BIBLIOGRAPHY

1. *Job Descriptions and Organizational Analysis for Hospitals and Related Health Services,* U.S. Government Printing Office, Washington, 1952.
2. McGIBONY, JOHN R.: *Principles of Hospital Administration,* 2nd Ed., New York, G. P. Putnam's Sons, 1969.
3. MacEACHERN, MALCOLM T.: *Hospital Organization and Management,* 3rd Ed., Chicago, Physicians' Record Co., 1957.
4. *Accreditation Manual for Hospitals 1970,* Hospital Accreditation Program, Joint Commission on Accreditation of Hospitals, Chicago, Ill., 1970, page 1.

48 The Hospital and Its Organization

5. Ibid. page 19.
6. Ibid. page 31.
7. Ibid. pages 24-28.
8. CORDES, D. W.: Radius of Administrative Responsibility, Hospitals, *38*:44, June 16, 1964.
9. *The Hospital Administrator,* The Association of University Programs in Hospital Administration, Chicago, Ill.
10. Definition of a Teaching Hospital, American Hospital Association Memorandum, November 11-15, 1967.
11. HASSAN, WM. E.: The Teaching Hospital, Drug Topics, *112*:16:20, Aug. 5, 1968.
12. In Pursuit of Quality-Hospital Nursing Service, National League for Nursing, New York, 1964.
13. HASSAN, WM. E.: Clinical Pharmacy—The Medical Record, Drug Topics, *114*:9:16, April 27, 1970.

Chapter

3

The Pharmacy—Its Organization and Personnel

A number of years ago, Francke *et al.*[1] stated:

> "The dispensing function of the pharmacist, while important and even vital, is essentially a superficial practice of the profession which, by itself, does not require knowledge or skills basic to merit professional recognition to the depth that lies within the grasp of hospital pharmacists."

Clearly, the above observation was a forecast of pharmacy's future new role for, less than a decade later, pharmacists have assumed important new roles—those of clinical pharmacist and drug consultant. To be able to assume these positions, it has become necessary to alter the pharmacist's educational program and work habits.

The *Task Force on Prescription Drugs*[2] made the following comments on the new role of pharmacy:

> "The pharmacy profession currently faces a dilemma which is partly though not entirely of its own making. Many other aspects of health care—the practice of medicine and surgery, hospital operations and particularly drug manufacture—have developed and adopted new devices and techniques which have remarkably improved the provision of health services. In contrast, the number of important new methods introduced to enhance the efficiency of retail pharmacy operations, at least during the past two or three decades, has not been noteworthy . . ."

The role of the pharmacist is viewed by many people as simply transferring pills from a large bottle to a small one—counting tablets, typing labels and calculating the price. Much of his time is seen as devoted to routine merchandising of cosmetics, shaving supplies, stationery and other commodities which have little or no relationship to health care.

This has raised doubts concerning the relevance of modern pharmacy education. As with other members of health professions, on the one hand, it would seem that much of the traditional education is not utilized, since a nonprofessional pharmacist—working under the supervision of a licensed pharmacist—can effectively perform many of the routine tasks of counting, labeling and pricing. At the same time, many pharmacists are seeking a new role as drug information specialists, and thus it would appear that their formal educacation has not taken this into account.

Pharmacist Aides

Experience in numerous pharmacies—military and hospitals and others—has demonstrated that individuals without formal pharmacy education can effectively undertake many of the routine activities of pharmacists, under the supervision of a licensed pharmacist.

Such activities offer the possibility of developing the career of pharmacist aide, comparable to the nursing aide, the orthopedic aide, the pediatric aide, the obstetrical aide and similar paramedical positions.

Drug Information Specialists

At the other end of the spectrum, it is also becoming evident that appropriately trained pharmacists may become new and vital members of the total health team by serving as drug information specialists. Some hospitals—especially teaching institutions and those in major medical center complexes—are already using pharmacists as consultants on drug therapy. They serve not only as drug distributors, but also as sources of drug data for physicians, interns, residents and nurses. They may participate in ward rounds with the staff, providing valuable drug information on both old and new drug products. Although they do not prescribe for patients, they enable the physicians who do prescribe to keep up more effectively with drug information. While some pharmacists are already serving as drug information specialists, and others are probably competent to do so, not all pharmacists have adequate competency in this field. Some licensed pharmacists have received five or even six years of formal college training, but about 15 per cent of those now in practice have received two years or less of formal pharmacy education, and nearly half of these have had courses lasting only about six months.

Pharmacy Education

The manner in which pharmacists, pharmacy associations, pharmacy schools and the pertinent state pharmacy agencies respond to increasing demands for pharmaceutical services will unquestionably determine in large measure how the pharmacy profession will evolve during the years to come. As a guide to the responses which should be made, there is a clear need for a broad study of pharmacy education similar to the famed Flexner study of medical education made half a century ago.

The Task Force therefore recommends that the Bureau of Health Manpower should support—

(a) The development of a pharmacist aide curriculum in junior colleges and other educational institutions.

(b) The development of appropriate curricula in medical and pharmacy schools for training pharmacists to serve as drug information specialists on the health team.

(c) A broad study of present and future requirements in pharmacy, adequacy of current pharmacy education, and the educational changes which must be made.

The department of pharmacy is typical of the majority of other departments in the hospital in that, depending upon its size and services rendered, it employs both professional and lay personnel. Therefore, it behooves the administrator or his pharmacist to ascertain the necessary number of employees in each category which will be required to render safe and prompt service. In addition, due to legal criteria the duties and responsibilities of each category of employee must be quite clearly defined.

Job Descriptions

The federal government, in a 1952 publication,[3] has clearly and adequately provided us with job descriptions for the positions of "Chief Pharmacist," "Pharmacist" and Pharmacy Helper." Accordingly, the following is a direct excerpt of the job summary and performance requirements for the position of chief pharmacist.

> "Compounds and dispenses medicines and preparations according to prescriptions written by physicians, dentists, and other practitioners authorized by law to prescribe: Prepares and sterilizes injectable medication manufactured in hospital, and manufactures pharmaceuticals. Furnishes information concerning medications to physicians, interns, and nurses. Plans, organizes, and directs pharmacy policies and procedures in accordance with established policies of hospital. Implements decisions of pharmacy and therapeutics committee of which he is a member. Performs related duties.

> PERFORMANCE REQUIREMENTS

> "RESPONSIBILITY FOR: Preparation and sterilization of injectable medication manufactured in hospital; manufacture of

pharmaceuticals; dispensing of drugs, chemicals, and pharmaceutical preparations; filling and labeling of all drug containers issued to services; inspection of all pharmaceutical supplies on all services; maintenance of an approved stock of antidotes and other emergency drugs; dispensing of all narcotic drugs and alcohol and maintenance of a perpetual inventory of them; specifications for purchase of all drugs, chemicals, antibiotics, biologicals, and pharmaceutical preparations used in treatment of patients; furnishing information concerning medications to physicians, interns, and nurses; establishment and maintenance, in cooperation with accounting department, of a system of records and bookkeeping in accordance with policies of hospital for charges to patients, and control over requisitioning and dispensing of drugs and pharmaceutical supplies; planning, organizing, and directing pharmacy policies and procedures in accordance with established policies of hospital; cooperation in teaching courses to students in school of nursing and in medical intern training program; implementing decisions of pharmacy and therapeutics committee; and preparation of periodic reports on progress of department.

"Accuracy in use of chemical and pharmaceutical equipment for compounding and dispensing drugs and medicines. Follows prescriptions in detail, and is accurate in labeling of containers and indicating directions for use."

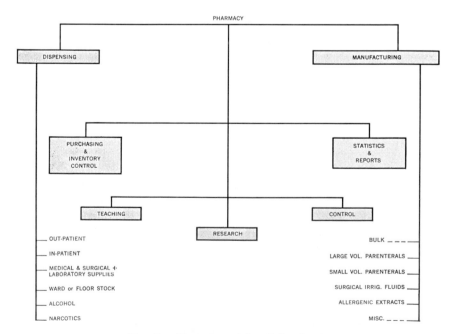

FIG. 6.   Departmental activity chart.

Determining the Departmental Staff—Professional

The number of professional and lay employees necessary cannot be determined until some thought has been given to the scope of service to be rendered. Is the department to serve in-patients only? How many? Is there to be any out-patient service? If so, how many patients per day? Is there to be a manufacturing section of the pharmacy? Is the pharmacy going to stock and dispense surgical and laboratory supplies?

Once these questions are answered, the pharmacist must then determine which of the duties must, by law, be assigned to pharmacists and those which are within the scope of reasonably intelligent lay personnel who are herein referred to as pharmacy helpers.

In order to understand and to ascertain the personnel requirements,

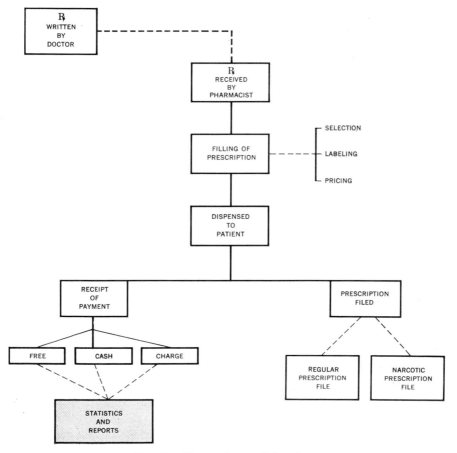

Fig. 7.   Out-patient activity chart.

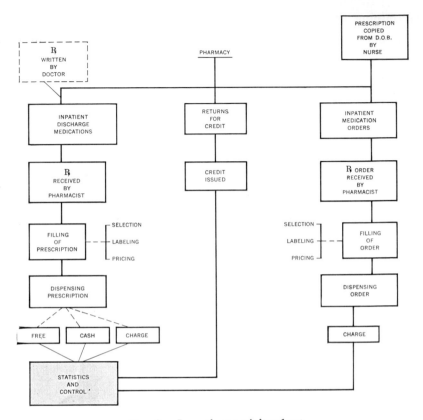

FIG. 8.   In-patient activity chart.

it is recommended that the department's major activities be dia-
grammed. Examples of such a process are provided in Figure 6 which
represents the over-all functions of a department of pharmacy in a
university teaching hospital, Figure 7 which briefly presents the activity
involved in the dispensing of an out-patient's prescription and Figure
8 which provides a diagrammatic representation of the various processes involved in accommodating in-patient drug needs.

Once these charts are prepared, the hospital pharmacist is
ready to evaluate the job, so diagramed, through the preparation of a
Flow Process Chart, Figure 9. By so doing, the pharmacist will be
able to evaluate the time and motion involved in the performance of
each job in the department. In addition, he will have a unique opportunity to utilize more efficiently the time of his personnel through the
simplification of the job by applying to it the various interrogatories
of work simplification, namely:

What is its purpose?
Why is it necessary?
Where should it be done?
When should it be done?
Who should do it?
How should it be done?

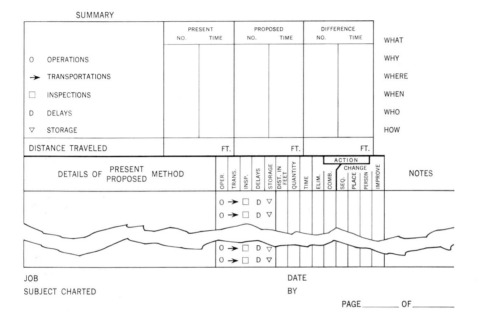

FIG. 9.   Flow process chart.

Once each detail involved in the performance of a particular job has been challenged, each job will become sufficiently streamlined so as to require a minimal expenditure of the employee's time, motion, and energy thereby providing for maximal production without any increase in the labor force on hand.

As a result of the preparation of these flow charts, the pharmacist should be in a better position to visualize the volume of activity in each category as well as the number of assistants necessary to dispense the medications and supplies to the correct area in the hospital.

There are no standard rules for the staffing of a hospital pharmacy which can be quoted. However, in the publication *Mirror to Hospital Pharmacy* the following reference to staffing is made[4]:

". . . in hospitals with from 100 to 500 beds and over, about 100 to 150 prescriptions or orders are processed daily for each full-time pharmacist employed. While it is difficult to make precise comparison of this workload with those reported by others, the number of prescriptions and requisitions filled falls within the range of those handled in pharmacies of the Public Health Service. For example, a report by Archambault (Division of Hospitals Bulletin No. 60–86 [1960]), states that the Pharmacy Branch considers a daily measurable workload of from 125 to 190 units plus a normal amount of non-measurable activities as reasonable for a pharmacist working with adequate non-professional assistance in hospitals utilizing six (6) or less pharmacists. A daily range of 126 to 158 units per pharmacist is considered normal by Archambault for the one- or two-man pharmacies, while 168-181 units per man is considered normal in pharmacies employing three (3) to five (5) pharmacists."

Those individuals who are desirous of using the above quoted standards are reminded that the work units employed in the Public Health Service include a number of bulk compounded and pre-packaged items, as well as prescriptions and requisitions. In addition, the authors point out that the above table omits consideration of a number of non-measurable workloads as well as the effect of non-professional assistance to the pharmacist.

Jeffries and Greenberg,[5] in their study on prescription pricing, state that the average time required for the proper dispensing of a non-compounded prescription is eight minutes and that fourteen minutes is required for a compounded prescription.

Because the dispensing pattern within the hospital differs from that employed in the retail practice of pharmacy, a personally conducted survey of the dispensing time in the hospital pharmacy of a 300-bed teaching hospital. The results showed that a pre-packaged medication could be dispensed in an average time of four minutes (which coincides with the arbitrarily selected time of four minutes referred to in the *Mirror to Hospital Pharmacy*).[4] Accordingly, it should not be too difficult to ascertain the workload within the pharmacy and thereby arrive at the approximate number of pharmacists required. If this system is used, the reader is again cautioned to take into consideration the fact that not all of the services rendered by the pharmacist are reflected in the prescription or order workload. Time must be provided for administrative work, purchasing, teaching, sick time, and vacation time, to mention a few.

The following table, which may serve as a guide to those contemplating using this method of ascertaining staff needs, is reproduced from the *Mirror to Hospital Pharmacy*.[4]

Daily In-Patient Workload per Pharmacist

Bed Capacity Short-Term	Prescriptions	Other Orders	Combined Work load
Under 50	10	10	20
50–99	45	17	62
100–199	96	44	140
200–299	101	50	151
300–399	100	52	152
400–499	89	38	127
500 and Over	61	35	96
Long-Term			
All sizes	39	38	77

Some investigators[6] have explored the applicability of the *queuing theory* as a mathematical tool in scheduling the pharmacist man-power needs of a hospital out-patient pharmacy. To apply this theory, it is necessary for the pharmacists to maintain time records to indicate "time in," "time start" and "time finish" of various types of prescriptions. The difference between "time in" and "time finish" is the waiting time (queue) of the patient.

Liebman *et al.*[7] suggest that the essential result of the use of the queuing theory is that the number of pharmacists on duty in the out-patient pharmacy should be synchronized to the fluctuations in the prescription order arrival rate.

Determining the Departmental Staff—Lay Personnel

Personnel falling into this category are secretarial or clerical workers, delivery men and hospital pharmacy technician-helpers.

The functions of secretarial or clerical workers would appear to be quite well defined and require no description here. Ascertaining the number of people required will depend on the amount of purchasing, inventory control and accounting procedures which are assigned to the pharmacy. Other factors which influence the need for secretarial assistance are the number of hospital committees upon which the pharmacist serves as secretary, the frequency of departmental publications such as pharmacy bulletins, frequency of updating the formulary, whether or not literature files are maintained and whether or not the pharmacist is active in teaching and research programs within the hospital.

Small hospital pharmacies usually have no need for delivery services or hospital pharmacy technician-helpers. The larger the unit, the more the need for this category of employee becomes. It can and has been argued that with modern means of communication, vertical conveyor

3

systems and pneumatic tube devices, the pharmacy has little or no need for a delivery service. This is a sound argument and may be perfectly valid in departments which are located in new buildings with all of the above refinements. But even in those departments, certain types and sizes of products must be transported by human beings. If the volume is not great, the pharmacist may arrange to share the services of one messenger with other departments or may utilize the services of the *central transport* and *messenger service* of the hospital, if one exists. If, on the other hand none of the above mentioned modern conveyance devices are available, then the need for human transporters becomes obvious. Because of the shortage of nurses, pharmacists, technicians and other specially trained personnel, they should be spared the inconvenience and waste of time of picking up and delivering supplies. Oftentimes hiring a delivery staff saves countless man-hours throughout the hospital.

Because of the acute shortage of pharmacists in many areas of the country, many hospitals have been forced to utilize hospital pharmacy technician-helpers. As this trend developed, it became evident that some standards for such a category of personnel was needed. Thus, the Joint Committee on Hospital Pharmacy of the American Society of Hospital Pharmacists and the American Association of Colleges of Pharmacy met and agreed upon the following:[8]

1. The worker classification of hospital pharmacy technician-helper exists in most hospitals today;
2. There may be a need for more formal methods of training to improve the quality and quantity of technician-helpers;
3. Recent publications stress the dilution of pharmaceutical talents resulting from the performance of non-professional duties by pharmacists;
4. Previous and current studies indicate the possibility of a grave shortage of professional manpower in the near future;
5. Attempts to establish similar programs in the past resulted in emotional outbursts which damaged professional unity.

It was also the consensus that the details of such a training program should be developed by the American Society of Hospital Pharmacists because of the unique need of this type of employee within the hospital.

The use of hospital pharmacy technician-helpers is strongly advocated only if they are properly trained and supervised. It should be clear that these people may not perform a "dispensing act" for this would be in violation of a majority of the state pharmacy codes.

As has been previously stated, there is in existence a need for supportive personnel in hospital pharmacy to assist in the newer programs of strip packaging, unit of use distribution systems and intravenous additive programs. However, no definitive guidelines for this type of personnel were available until the American Society of Hospital Pharmacists released its *Statement on Supportive Personnel in Hospital Pharmacy* which is reproduced[13] on page 63.

Beahm[9] in a recent study regarding the use of non-licensed personnel in pharmacy has reported that it is possible to ascertain which functions normally performed by a pharmacist may be done by a technician, those which may be done by a technician under supervision, and those which a technician is forbidden to do.

Among those which a non-licensed person is prohibited from doing are the following: take telephone orders for prescription refills from patients, weigh or measure ingredients to be used in compounding prescriptions, mix ingredients, already weighed or measured, to compound prescriptions, calculate percentages in prescription compounds, take telephone orders for new prescriptions, affix prescription labels to medication containers, provide information on use, precautions etc., to patients and professional personnel.

Those functions that may be done under supervision are as follows: type labels from prescription orders to be later attached to containers by pharmacist, assemble prescription ingredients immediately prior to pharmacist's filling of order, pre-package prescription drugs, print labels for pre-packaged drugs, affix pre-printed labels to containers of pre-packaged drugs, pre-package solid dosage forms in single unit packages, pre-package injectable dosage forms in single unit packages, pre-package all liquids in single unit packages, order and check in pharmaceuticals, calculate prices for prescriptions dispensed by pharmacists, maintain family prescription records, package finished dosage forms immediately prior to pharmacist's checking of prescription, weigh and measure ingredients in bulk compounding of pharmaceuticals, maintain narcotic drug inventory records, maintain drug inventory records.

Non-licensed personnel may perform the following duties independent of pharmacist's supervision: locate prescription order and file immediately prior to pharmacist's filling of prescription, routinely inventory supplies and re-stock prescription items, calculate the prices for prescriptions dispensed by pharmacists, clean bulk manufacturing and pre-packaging equipment, clean other prescription equipment, deliver prescription drugs to physicians and nurses in hospital or office for professional use, deliver prescriptions to patients but refer any questions to pharmacists, bill patients and/or third party and pay pharmacy accounts.

Although the foregoing classification is based upon responses from societies of hospital pharmacists, responses from colleges of pharmacy as well as boards of registration in pharmacy did not coincide with the entire breakdown. The variation in response relative to technician utilization in the various activities covered by the survey may have been due to the tradition of certain activities in hospital and/or community practice.

Unfortunately there are no reliable criteria whereby a formula may be arrived at which, when properly applied to a set of statistics, will reveal the magic number of pharmacy helpers required in any given situation. This, then, requires some serious planning and evaluation on the part of the pharmacist-in-chief.

Professional Services Rendered

The primary function of the hospital pharmacist is to dispense drugs to the in-patients and out-patients where hospital policy permits. However, there are a large number of important ancillary areas of pharmacy in which the pharmacist should exercise his skills. Again, depending upon the size of the hospital, the pharmacist may develop such areas as bulk compounding, sterile product manufacturing, control laboratory, distribution of laboratory and medical and surgical supplies, and expanding his role as a teacher and drug consultant. Another service worthy of consideration is the after-hour pharmacy service which will be discussed later under methods of drug distribution.

The bulk compounding and sterile manufacturing program are two areas which offer the hospital great financial savings and the pharmacist pride and prestige. These two areas are of such importance that they will be discussed in greater detail in a later chapter.

Charting of Pharmacy Organization

With the selection and categorizing of the employees, it now becomes essential to develop a chart showing the flow of administrative authority. Obviously, in the very small departments, this is usually generally understood and no problems arise. However, in the large units with assistant chief pharmacists, supervisors, and lay personnel, authority must be delegated by the chief pharmacist.

Sample distributions are depicted in Figures 10 and 11. Clearly this can and should be tailored to meet the specific requirements of the department and hospital. Once prepared and approved, it should be conspicuously posted for each of the departmental employees to read and adhere to.

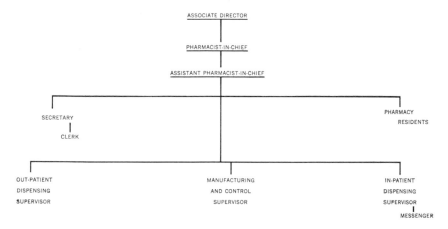

FIG. 10.   Departmental organization.

In large hospitals, departments of pharmacy have a more complex organization. For example, in 1969 the Ohio State University Hospitals Department of Pharmacy released an organizational chart similar to that shown in Figure 11. It should seem obvious to the student that each of the subdivisions of the department are assigned specific responsibilities. The following are some of the responsibilities of each division:

Administrative Services Division

1. Plan and coordinate departmental activities.
2. Develop policies.
3. Schedule personnel and provide supervision.
4. Coordinate administrative needs of the Pharmacy and Therapeutics Committee.
5. Supervise departmental office staff.

Education and Training Division

1. Coordinate programs of undergraduate and graduate pharmacy students.
2. Participate in hospital wide educational programs involving nurses, doctors etc.
3. Train newly employed pharmacy department personnel.

Pharmaceutical Research Division

1. Develop new formulations of drugs especially dosage forms not commercially available and of research drugs.
2. Improve formulations of existing products.
3. Cooperate with the medical research staff on projects involving drugs.

In-Patient Services Division

1. Provide medications for all in-patients of the hospital on a 24-hour per day basis.
2. Inspection and control of drugs on all treatment areas.
3. Cooperate with medical drug research. See Chapter 7.

Out-Patient Services Division

1. Compound and dispense out-patient prescriptions.
2. Inspect and control all clinic and emergency service medication stations.
3. Maintain prescription records.
4. Provide drug consultation services to staff and medical students.

Drug Information Services Division

1. Provide drug information on drugs and drug therapy to doctors, nurses, medical and nursing students and the house staff.
2. Maintain the drug information center.
3. Prepare the hospital's pharmacy newsletter.
4. Maintain literature files.

Departmental Services Division

1. Control and dispense intravenous fluids.
2. Control and dispense controlled substances.
3. Coordinate and control all drug delivery and distribution systems.

Purchasing and Inventory Control Division

1. Maintain drug inventory control.
2. Purchase all drugs.
3. Receive, store and distribute drugs.
4. Interview medical service representatives. See Chapter 10.

Central Supply Services Division

1. Develop and coordinate distribution of medical supplies and irrigating fluids. See Chapter 15.

Assay and Quality Control Division

1. Perform analyses on products manufactured and purchased.
2. Develop and revise assay procedures.
3. Assist research division in special formulations.

Manufacturing and Packaging Division

1. Manufacture wide variety of items in common use at the hospital.
2. Operate an overall drug packaging and prepackaging program.
3. Undertake program in product development.
4. Maintain a unit dose program.

Sterile Products Division

1. Produce small volume parenterals.
2. Manufacture sterile ophthalmologics, irrigating solutions etc.
3. Prepare aseptic dilution of lyophylizal and other "unstable" sterile injections for administration to patients.

Radiopharmaceutical Services Division

1. Centralize the procurement, storage and dispensing of radioisotopes used in clinical practice. See Chapter 23.

Intravenous Admixture Division

1. Centralize the preparation of intravenous solution admixture.
2. Review each I.V. admixture for physio-chemical incompatibilities.

Statement on Supportive Personnel in Hospital Pharmacy*

The increasing complexity of health care in the modern hospital is creating ever greater demands for the hospital pharmacy to broaden its scope of services. New health care legislation and rapid changes in health care technology are imposing new demands on hospital pharmacy which result in a need for increased manpower. These demands dictate for the hospital pharmacist a multifarious role which he can assume only when there is an adequate number of personnel within the pharmacy.

There is a growing concern about the present shortage of hospital pharmacists and an even greater concern about future shortages. The scope of pharmaceutical services being provided in most hospitals is limited largely by personnel shortages. Studies have indicated that many of the tasks performed in today's modern hospital pharmacy could be delegated to supportive personnel under the supervision of a pharmacist and, in fact, such personnel have long been used in most hospitals.

If the hospital pharmacist could be freed to a greater extent from performing routine tasks which could be delegated with supervision to trained supportive personnel, he would be able to direct more of his attention to professional tasks only, thereby expanding professional pharmacy service in the interest of patient care. Other professions—notably medicine, nursing, and dentistry—are in the process of delegating more and more functions to technicians and to other supportive personnel. Hospital pharmacy must do likewise if it is to keep pace with progress in the health field, meet the growing demand

* Approved by the Board of Directors, American Society of Hospital Pharmacists October 26-27, 1970. Approved by the AACP Executive Committee, December 1970.

for hospital pharmacy manpower, make maximum use of the hospital pharmacists' unique body of knowledge, and provide an opportunity for developing a scope of pharmaceutical services yet undefined and unrealized in the institutional setting.

Observations

Careful consideration of this subject by representatives of the American Association of Colleges of Pharmacy and the AMERICAN SOCIETY OF HOSPITAL PHARMACISTS has led to the following observations:

1. Previous and current studies indicate a growing shortage of professional hospital pharmacy manpower now and in the future.
2. The performance by pharmacists of duties which might appropriately be assigned to supportive personnel results in a dilution of pharmaceutical talents and limits the scope of pharmaceutical services provided.
3. Supportive hospital pharmacy personnel are used in most hospitals today.
4. The accelerating development of expanded professional services by the hospital pharmacy emphasizes the need for supportive personnel to assume many of the routine, nonjudgmental duties traditionally associated with the delivery of pharmaceutical services.
5. There is a need to recognize and define several different levels, or categories, of supportive hospital pharmacy personnel.
6. There is a need to define those functions and responsibilities which can be assigned to each category of supportive hospital pharmacy personnel, as differentiated from those which can be carried out only by the pharmacist.
7. There is a need to define training requirements and to develop training programs for each category of supportive hospital pharmacy personnel.
8. There is a need to standardize nomenclature used in referring to supportive personnel in hospital pharmacy.

Recommendations

Based on these observations and consistent with the developments of pharmacy practice in hospitals, it is recommended that:

1. The term "supportive personnel" be adopted as standard nomenclature to be used in referring collectively to all nonprofessional personnel.
2. The American Association of Colleges of Pharmacy and the AMERICAN SOCIETY OF HOSPITAL PHARMACISTS give priority considerations to adopting standard nomenclature to be used in referring to the different levels, or categories, of supportive personnel.

3. The American Association of Colleges of Pharmacy cooperate with the AMERICAN SOCIETY OF HOSPITAL PHARMACISTS in developing hospital-based training programs for hospital pharmacy supportive personnel with consideration being given to the potential role of academic institutions and to the experiences of existing training programs.
4. The American Association of Colleges of Pharmacy continue to provide consultation to the AMERICAN SOCIETY OF HOSPITAL PHARMACISTS in the development of training programs.
5. The American Association of Colleges of Pharmacy and the AMERICAN SOCIETY OF HOSPITAL PHARMACISTS support and participate in, where possible, projects defining the roles of, and the training requirements for, supportive personnel in hospital pharmacy.

Control of Personnel

This section is not intended as an invitation to the hospital pharmacist to subrogate the established personnel policies or procedures of his hospital. The purpose is to present a few relatively simple procedures whereby the pharmacist who is located in the smaller hospital and either functions alone or with lay help or who may be responsible for more than one department may maintain, in the absence of an

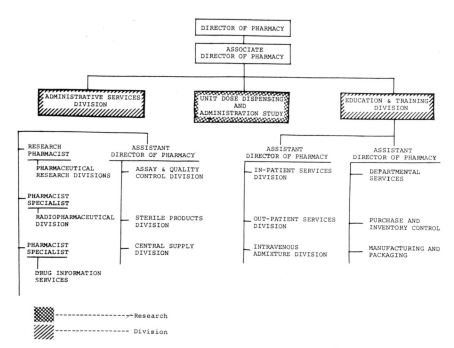

FIG. 11.   Departmental organization in a large university hospital pharmacy operation.

active personnel director, reasonable employee records for accounting and administrative purposes.

The *Application for Employment* should elicit from the prospective employee vital information relative to his personal history, education, military service, office skills when applicable, previous employment record, interviewer's comments and the employment contract. It would seem necessary to obtain all of the above information in order to make an intelligent decision whether or not the applicant has the necessary qualifications for the position which he seeks or for which he is being interviewed. Certainly, if the question ever arose as to whether or not due care was used in the selection of the employee, a record, such as the one illustrated, properly completed, would serve as *prima facie* evidence.

Figure 12, the *Performance Rating Form* can be used effectively in determining whether or not the employee is worthy of a pay increase. In addition, it can serve as a warning to the employee of his deficiency in certain areas. Many department heads in using this form assign a numerical value of 4 for each check mark under "excellent," 3 for "good," 2 for "fair" and 1 for "poor." A total is taken of the points and then divided by 10. The figure obtained determines where the category of "Overall Rating" is checked.

Figure 13, entitled *Paid Vacation,* is an example of a form which may be used within the department to keep an accurate record of those important fringe benefits due the employee, namely paid vacation or sick leave time. Improper records, particularly in the area of sick time, have been used to the detriment of the hospital in claims arising out of industrial accidents involving the employee or they may prove to be a great asset to him in his claim for insurance disability payments and income tax deductions.

Hiring of Pharmacists

The hiring of pharmacy personnel is an extremely important function of the director of pharmacy service and requires special consideration.[10]

The State Board of Registration in Pharmacy is empowered to make rules and regulations for the enforcement of administration of the pharmacy law. Such regulatory and enforcement procedures must be in accord with the expressed or implied purposes of the enabling statutes. In view of the fact that the Board is an administrative, not legislative agency, it may not exercise any power or authority not delegated to it, or which, by reasonable implication, is necessary to the proper functioning of the pharmacy law.

One of the clearly defined responsibilities of the State Board of

PERFORMANCE RATING FORM

Name   John Doe

Department   Pharmacy

Job Title   Staff Pharmacist   12 Months' Review

Rated by Wm. Roe   Title   Pharmacist-in-Chief Date January 1965

	Excellent	Good	Fair	Poor
Quality of Work	X			
Quantity of Work		X		
Knowledge of Position	X			
Initiative		X		
Dependability	X			
Attendance	X			
Attitude		X		
Appearance	X			
Ability to get along with Fellow Workers	X			
Leadership Qualities		X		
Overall Rating		X		

REMARKS: Please write one or two brief sentences about the employee describing his overall performance.

_____

_____

Employee's Signature   John Doe   Date January 1965

Employee's Comments _____

_____

Administrative Head_____

FIG. 12.

PAID VACATION

Date of Employment _____

              Name _____

Credit Balance 2/1/65
Starting 2/1/65
Period

	Added Credit	Paid Vac. Hours	Hours Balance
1 2/ 1/65– 3/ 7/65			
2 3/ 8/65– 4/11/65			
3 4/12/65– 5/16/65			
4 5/17/65– 6/20/65			
5 6/21/65– 7/25/65			
6 7/26/65– 8/30/65			
7 8/31/65–10/ 3/65			
8 10/ 4/65–11/ 7/65			
9 11/ 8/65–12/12/65			
10 12/13/65– 1/31/66			

VACATION DAYS

DATE TAKEN	HRS.	DATE TAKEN	HRS.	DATE TAKEN	HRS.

FIG. 13.

Registration in Pharmacy is to establish the educational and experience qualifications which individuals must meet at the time of examination or registration.

Once an individual has successfully qualified for practice he is generally awarded a certificate of registration which enables him to practice pharmacy in the setting of his choice—community or institutional.

The American Society of Hospital Pharmacists through its Minimum Standard for Pharmacies in Hospitals prescribes that the department be under the direction of a "—professionally competent, legally qualified pharmacist—he shall be well trained in the specialized functions of hospital pharmacy and shall be a graduate of an accredited college of pharmacy or meet an equivalent standard of training or experience—."

Because of the fact that many of the approximately 7000 hospitals registered by the American Hospital Association are minus the services of a trained pharmacist, too many administrators are prone to overlook or ignore the mandates of good hiring procedure. The same applies to the overworked pharmacist in the larger hospital who is anxious to hire "another pair of hands" for peak periods in the operation of the department. Both of these "short-cuts" may prove to be disastrous from a legal point of view.

In practice, the hospital administrator, personnel director or director of pharmacy services, should insist that applicants for pharmacist positions should show—

> Proof of graduation from an accredited college/school of pharmacy.
>
> Proof of licensure in the state in which the individual desires to practice.
>
> Proof of professional competency.
>
> Proof of good moral character.

In addition, a six-month probationary period satisfactorily completed would be further evidence of the quality of the hiring procedures of the hospital in the selection of the pharmacist.

Should an unfortunate accident then occur, a charge of negligence might be defended successfully in some states.

State pharmacy laws, hospital licensing acts, Food and Drug laws, and state public health laws and agency regulations are clear on the issue that the use, as pharmacists, of those not skilled and experienced in the practice of pharmacy, as evidenced by state registration, is a criminal offense. In this connection, it should be borne in mind that neither the hospital administrator nor the director of pharmacy services are relieved by law of their responsibility where pharmacists are employed yet the work-load is so great that non-registered personnel must perform duties that the law limits to the registered practitioner of pharmacy.

As reasonable and prudent individuals, the hospital administrator and the director of pharmacy services know or should know the relationship between the work-load and the number of qualified staff necessary to handle it—expertly and on schedule.

Also of serious import is the civil liability that attaches to the institution in malpractice or negligence suits arising from injuries or deaths resulting from medication errors committed by a non-pharmacist acting in the capacity of a licensed pharmacist with the consent, implied or expressed, of the hospital management.

Accordingly, it behooves all pharmacists who are delegated the responsibility of managing the institution's pharmacy to exercise due care in the selection and hiring of personnel as well as the determination of acceptable work-loads and work assignments for the employees.

Salaries

At nearly every meeting of hospital pharmacists, the subject of salaries is discussed. Many of the state associations have conducted surveys amongst their membership in an attempt to determine the wage levels within the area and, when possible, to promote higher salaries.

The instigators of the salary survey movement are usually those individuals within the lower salary brackets. Some of these pharmacists may be doing an exceptionally fine job within their institutions but are harnessed by an unrealistic wage range within the hospital or even governmental salary structure.

On the other hand, there is a small segment of the profession which is continually advocating higher personal recompense even though they offer very little in return for the higher salary.

Because the hospital pharmacist is a highly trained professional member of the health team, his salary requirements should not be arrived at in the same manner as other members of the hospital staff. Neither should his salary be restricted by what other institutions in the area are paying.

It is generally agreed that no two hospitals are alike in their operation. By the same token, no two hospital pharmacists can be evaluated by what they do in neighboring institutions. They must be evaluated on their own performance standard within the particular institution they serve.

In order that the administrator may determine how well his pharmacist has performed, it is recommended that he refer to the *Minimum Standard for Pharmacies in Hospitals.*

In the *Mirror to Hospital Pharmacy*[11] there appears the result of a survey of hospital pharmacists' salaries for the year 1957. The figures indicate that 50 per cent of the chief pharmacists in the United States were earning less than the estimated usual rate paid in a community pharmacy. It was further revealed that the median salaries are highest in the Pacific states and lowest in the New England states. The study further indicated that 17 per cent of chief pharmacists supplement their hospital salary by working on a part-time basis in retail pharmacies; that 1 out of 5 chief pharmacists has sources of income other than his hospital salary; that 4 per cent of the chief pharmacists receive a bonus in addition to their hospital salary, that 2 per cent receive consulting fees and 3 per cent receive additional funds from teaching activities.

Kahn[12] has conducted a comprehensive two-year survey of personal financial remuneration of hospital pharmacists throughout the nation. The survey disclosed a range in median salary for all areas of $11,500 (area 10) to $8,740 (area 1) with a national median of $9,780.

As a result of the economic pressures that are being exerted upon the hospital, many members of the professional staff are being subjected to unionization activities. Many pharmacists would prefer not to become involved with organizations whose sole goal is economic security but would demonstrate interest in a group combining both professional and economic goals.

Thus, the *Economic Status Program of the American Society of Hospital Pharmacists* came into being and is hereinafter reproduced.[14]

Economic Status Program of the American Society of Hospital Pharmacists* †

Policy on Economic Status

The professional and economic goals of the professional person are closely interrelated. Only in attainment of these goals can he assume the leadership role expected of him in the community by his colleagues, and by other health professions. When satisfactory economic status is achieved, the professional can realize his maximum potential and apply his full energies to the needs of society.

The American Society of Hospital Pharmacists has, since its inception, concentrated on the professional responsibilities of hospital pharmacists through promotion of high standards of professional ethics,

* Approved by the Board of Directors on January 11, 1970.
† Approved by the House of Delegates on March 29, 1971.

education and attainments. Nevertheless, the economic interests of members of the Society were acknowledged several years ago when the *Mirror to Hospital Pharmacy* and the Society's Commission on Goals counselled the ASHP to involve itself in activities dealing with the economic status of hospital pharmacists. Indeed one of the goals of the Society's statement, "Goals for Hospital Pharmacy," adopted in 1964 is to "Promote payment of realistic salaries to hospital pharmacists in both staff and managerial positions in order to attract and retain the services of career personnel." More recently, the Society conducted a salary survey to obtain factual data on the economic status of pharmacists in institutional practice.

The Society's concern for the economic welfare of its members complements the professional and scientific objectives presently set forth in the Constitution of the American Society of Hospital Pharmacists. Involvement by the Society in the economic well-being of its members is in the public interest since assurance of economic satisfaction tends to attract highly qualified pharmacists to institutional practice.

Salaries, working hours and fringe benefits of hospital pharmacists should be commensurate with professional education, responsibility and status and with the increased participation by hospital pharmacists in the actual planning and administration of pharmacy service and in the determination of policies which directly affect them. Both employers and employed pharmacists have an obligation to resolve employment issues fairly and in good faith.

The responsibility of the individual is primary. However, as institutions and the delivery of health care grow in size and complexity, collective effort may be necessary to solve group economic problems. With this view, the Society must meet the needs of its members by embarking on a broad program of economic status which may include such activities as the compilation of statistical data, the preparation of model contracts and, when necessary, mediation, conciliation and arbitration. When economic problems of employment cannot be resolved by the individual practitioner or the pharmacy staff of a hospital, the Society's Affiliated Chapters, with the legal and financial assistance of the ASHP, may find it necessary to engage in collective bargaining.

The Board of Directors of the American Society of Hospital Pharmacists, at its meeting of January 10-11, 1970 voted:

> To engage in collective bargaining by assisting Affiliated Chapters, upon request, in accordance with policies and guidelines as established by the House of Delegates of the AMERICAN SOCIETY OF HOSPITAL PHARMACISTS; further,
> To adopt the statement, "Economic Status Program of the American Society of Hospital Pharmacists."

In accordance with this action, the following are guidelines for individual members, Affiliated Chapters and the ASHP.

Guidelines for Collective Bargaining

Individual Members

1. Hospital pharmacists must recognize their obligation to the patient, the institution, the profession, the allied health professions and society.
2. Hospital pharmacists shall not deprive patients of pharmaceutical services by withholding their services in any form, including strikes, in support of economic demands.

Affiliated Chapters

1. Affiliated Chapters may engage in collective bargaining, preferably through the statewide Affiliated Chapter. Any such activity shall be conducted solely in the name of, and by, the Affiliated Chapter.
2. Affiliated Chapters may engage in collective bargaining when:
   a. Professional prerogatives of the pharmacists are endangered by the lack of effective representation; or
   b. wages or conditions of employment are below acceptable levels; or
   c. the environment in which the profession is practiced is not conducive to good patient care; and
   d. good faith attempts have failed to remedy the above situation(s).
3. Affiliated Chapters will make available the services of negotiating contracts to active ASHP members. All hospital pharmacists who practice at the contracting institution may be represented. Hospital pharmacists being represented who are not members of the Affiliated Chapter and the AMERICAN SOCIETY OF HOSPITAL PHARMACISTS must become members, if permitted by all applicable laws.
4. Affiliated Chapters will accept or reject contracts as determined by a majority of the members in the bargaining unit.
5. Affiliated Chapters will assess each hospital pharmacist a service fee for each contract negotiated, as determined by and paid to the ASHP, to the extent permitted by applicable laws.
6. Affiliated Chapters must follow procedures outlined by the ASHP.

American Society of Hospital Pharmacists

The SOCIETY will coordinate collective bargaining activities of Affiliated Chapters by providing:
a. statistical information and research assistance;
b. legal assistance; and
c. financial assistance when necessary.

SELECTED REFERENCES

FISCHELIS, R. P.: Pharmacist Helpers, J. Am. Pharm. Assoc. Pract. Pharm. Ed., *20*:1:23, 1959.

JOEL, L.: Composite Method for Estimating Drug and Personnel Needs, Hospitals, *33*:56, Aug. 1, 1959.

SPERANDIO, G. J.: How to Merit a Salary Increase, Tile and Till, *46*:72, 1960.

Anon.: Duties, Salaries of Pharmacists Surveyed, Hospitals, *34*:64, Jan. 1, 1960.

BAKER, NORMAN N.: Applying Work Simplification to Hospital Pharmacy, The Bulletin, A.S.H.P., *14*:6:670, 1957.

KRESNICKA, R. D. and KENNA, F. R.: Effective Use of Nonprofessionals Helps Pharmacists Expand Services: Hosp. Topics, *44*:11:98, 1966.

LUND, ROBERT S.: Hospital Pharmacy Service—An Administrator's View Point, Am. J. Hosp. Pharm., *26*:12:686, 1969.

HASSAN, WM. E.: An Administrator's View of the Future of Hospital Pharmacy, Hospital Pharmacy, *3*:10:15, Oct. 1968.

SUMNER, EDWARD D., MARETT, RALPH K., ROMAN, PAUL M. and WARE, GLENN O.: Pharmacy Technicians' Attitudes Towards Professionalization, Am. J. Hosp. Pharm., *28*:1:43, Jan. 1971.

PHAFF, HARRY: Proposal: A Formalized Pharmacy Technician Training Program, Hosp. Pharm., *4*:5:5, May 1969.

KASSEM, M. SAMI and DEJUTE, ANTHONY M.: Hiring Medical Personnel: The Team Approach, Hospital Administration *16*:2:15, Spring 1971.

BALDWIN, H. JOHN and McMAHON, J. LEO: The Use of Nonprofessional Personnel in the Dispensing Process, J. A.Ph.A. NS *12*:2:60, February 1972.

TINDALL, WILLIAM N. and McEVILLA, JOSEPH D.: Pharmacy Technicians— Findings in Ten Community Pharmacies, J. APh.A NS *12*:2:62 February 1972.

BIBLIOGRAPHY

1. FRANCKE, D. E., LATOLAIS, C. J., FRANCKE, G. N. and Ho, N. F. H.: *Mirror to Hospital Pharmacy,* American Society of Hospital Pharmacists, Washington, D.C., 1964, p. 6.

2. Task Force on Prescription Drugs, U.S. Dept. of Health, Education and Welfare, Washington, D.C., 1968, pp. 54-58.

3. Descriptions and Organizational Analysis for Hospitals and Related Health Services, U.S. Government Printing Office, Washington, D.C., 1952.

4. FRANCKE, D. E., LATOLAIS, C. J., FRANCKE, G. N. and Ho, N. F. H.: *Mirror to Hospital Pharmacy,* Easton, Mack Printing Co., 1964, p. 103.

5. JEFFRIES, S. B. and GREENBERG, J.: Prescription Pricing, J. Am. Pharm., Assoc. Pract. Pharm. Ed., *17*:383, June, 1956.

6. LAMY, PETER P., KITLER, MARYELLEN, LIEBMAN, JUDITH S., LESAGE, PAUL J., HORN, SUSAN M. and BOLLING, THOMAS V.: Predicting Manpower Needs for Outpatient Pharmacy, Am. J. Hosp. Pharm., *27*:4:300, Apr. 1970.

7. LIEBMAN, JUDITH S., LAMY, PETER P. and KITLER, MARYELLEN: Further Investigation of the Use of Queuing Theory To Predict Manpower Requirements in an Outpatient Pharmacy, Am. J. Hosp. Pharm., *27*:6:480, June 1970.

8. Report of Joint Commission on Hospital Pharmacy: Hospital Pharmacy Technician-Helpers, Hospital Pharmacy, *1*:7:9, 1966.
9. BEAHM, MICHAEL R.: A Survey of Opinion and Law Regarding the Use of Non-Licensed Personnel in Pharmacy, Am. J. Hosp. Pharm., *27*:9:713, Sept. 1970.
10. HASSAN, WM. E.: Hiring of Pharmacy Personnel, Drug Topics, *112*:24: 11, Nov. 25, 1968.
11. FRANCKE, D. E., LATOLAIS, C. J., FRANCKE, G. N. and HO, N. F. H.: *Mirror to Hospital Pharmacy*, Easton, Mack Printing Co., pp. 77-78, 1964.
12. KAHN, SIDNEY: Financial Status of American Hospital Pharmacists, 1968, Hospital Pharmacy, *3*:10:5, Oct. 1968.
13. Statement on Supportive Personnel in Hospital Pharmacy, Am. J. Hosp. Pharm., *28*:7:516, July 1971.
14. Economic Status Program of the American Society of Hospital Pharmacists, Am. J. Hosp. Pharm., *28*:7:517, July, 1971.

Chapter

4

The Pharmacy and Therapeutics Committee

Introduction

In these days of modern medicine when numerous agents are available for the treatment of disease, the judicious selection of drugs for use in the hospital has become an important administrative and therapeutic tool. During the last half century, there has been a dynamic change in the medical profession's attitude toward therapeutic agents. Fifty years ago there were few really worthwhile medicinal substances available; however, if one examines the formularies of that period, it is amazing to see the hundreds of preparations that were recommended. Perhaps one of the finest things that Sir William Osler did was to lead the endeavor to rid the profession of such valueless items.

Following Osler's period of clinical evaluation, there came a period of near therapeutic nihilism when most physicians were skeptical about nearly all therapeutic measures. As a consequence, it was difficult to get individuals deeply interested in the problems of reliable therapeutics. If an examination were made of the texts on therapy between 1920 to 1940, one notes that there was a definite lack of interest in therapeutics, and to a great extent, the use of various prescriptions and preparations was curtailed. Many of the medical graduates of this period had little idea about good therapy and received poor instruction in the subject during their clinical training in the hospital.

However, during this period, definite standards for improving drug therapy were established. Rules to guide manufacturers, as well as physicians, were established by the American Medical Association which did much to put drug therapy in a more desirable position. The Council on Pharmacy and Chemistry of the American Medical Association had been well established and was successfully operating when we were suddenly thrust into the modern era of therapeutics. This came about as a result of the discovery of the sulfa compounds and was quickly followed by the discovery of penicillin, streptomycin and the other antibiotics. In the 1950's, there was a flood of new sub-stances of high potency and activity in many fields of pathological physiology. This deluge of new therapeutic agents made it a nearly impossible task for the physician to become knowledgeable about more than a relatively few products.

Because of this profusion of agents, some excellent, some not so good, and some practically useless, it was necessary for the hospital to establish a system to bring the best medicinal agents to the attention of the staff, and thus assist them in the proper selection of therapeutic substances for the treatment of the hospitalized patient. This educa-tional program was best brought about through the formation of a good Pharmacy and Therapeutics Committee whose responsibility was to include the preparation of a hospital formulary, the publishing of a pharmacy educational bulletin, the establishment of automatic stop orders for dangerous drugs, the supervision of investigational use drugs, the development of a program for reporting and investigating adverse drug reactions and assisting in the preparation of emergency kits or carts for medical emergencies.

Despite the creation of these hospital oriented committees, there appeared to be a need for a systematic evaluation of the entire drug system in the country. Thus, in May of 1967, acting upon a direc-tive from the President, John W. Gardner—then Secretary of Health, Education, and Welfare—established the Task Force on Prescription Drugs. The charge to the Task Force was—

> "Undertake a comprehensive study of the problems of including
> the cost of prescription drugs under medicare."

To achieve the goal set by the charge, the Task Force was obliged to seek objective data on the health needs of the elderly; the present patterns of drug use; the nature of drug research, production and dis-tribution; current drug insurance programs in the United States and abroad; reimbursement methods and administrative approaches; legal and fiscal aspects; and the pharmacological and clinical aspects, in-cluding the intricate problem of chemical and clinical equivalency of generic products.[5]

In addition, a more drastic approach was taken. Under the author-ity granted to the Secretary of HEW by the Drug Amendments of 1962, the *National Academy of Sciences-National Research Council* (NAS-NRC) in 1966, at the request of the FDA, initiated a study to evaluate the effectiveness of new drugs marketed between 1938 and 1962. During that period of time, the law required only that a new drug be demonstrated to be safe. The requirement that a new drug be effective, as well as safe, was added by the Drug Amend-ments of 1962.

An advisory committee of the NAS-NRC created 27 panels of non-government experts to evaluate the efficacy of approximately 3000 drugs. On the basis of its findings, the *Drug Efficacy Study Group* classified the drugs as: *effective, probably effective, possibly effective, effective but,* or *ineffective.*

It has been stated[1] that the hospital Pharmacy and Therapeutics Committee is a tool for maintaining medical staff self-government. It is responsible to the medical staff as a whole and its recommendations are subject to medical staff approval. The Pharmacy and Therapeutics Committee is a mandatory committee under the **Conditions** of **Participation** of the Hospital Insurance Program—Medicare. Composed of physicians and the pharmacist, it serves as the organizational line of communication or liaison between the medical staff and the Pharmacy Department. This committee assists in the formulation of broad professional policies regarding the evaluation, selection, procurement, distribution, use, safety procedures and other matters relating to drugs in hospitals.

In 1959, the American Hospital Association and the American Society of Hospital Pharmacists approved a **Statement on the Pharmacy and Therapeutics Committee** which states[2]:

Preamble

HOSPITALS ORGANIZE AND MARSHAL the best professional skills and judgment available to provide care and treatment of patients The treatment of these patients in many cases is dependent upon the effective use of drugs. The multiplicity of drugs available today makes it mandatory that an organized sound program of activity be developed within the hospital to insure that patients receive the best care and protection possible.

One of the most effective ways of providing this kind of care and protection is by organizing a Pharmacy and Therapeutics Committee. This committee is designed to make maximum use of available professional skills and judgment. The establishment of a Pharmacy and Therapeutics Committee is strongly recommended to all hospitals. It is a measure which supports and enhances the principle of self-government in the area of high drug standards and practices for the medical staff connected with a hospital. Ultimate benefits accrue to the patient in improved patient care and treatment as established voluntarily by the medical staff.

The Pharmacy and Therapeutics Committee

The Pharmacy and Therapeutics Committee is an advisory group of the medical staff and serves as the organizational line of communication or liaison between the medical staff and the pharmacy department. This committee is composed primarily of physicians and the pharmacist and is selected under the guidance of the medical staff. It is also a policy-recommending body to the medical staff and to the administration of the hospital on all matters related to the use of drugs. (This committee does not have intrinsic authority or power of action unless specifically granted such authority.)

PURPOSES

The primary purposes of the Pharmacy and Therapeutics Committee are:

A. *Advisory.* The committee recommends the adoption or assists in the formulation of broad professional policies regarding evaluation, selection, procurement, distribution, use, safe practices, and other matters pertinent to drugs in hospitals.

B. *Educational.* The committee recommends or assists in the formulation of programs designed to meet the needs of the professional staff (doctors, nurses and the pharmacist) for complete current knowledge on matters related to drugs and drug practices.

ORGANIZATION

While the composition of the Pharmacy and Therapeutics Committee may vary from hospital to hospital, the following is offered as a guide:

A. The Pharmacy and Therapeutics Committee of the medical staff should be composed of no less than three physicians and the pharmacist, appointed by a governing unit or elected official of the organized medical staff. The hospital administrator or his designated representative should be an ex officio member of the committee.

B. A chairman from the physician representatives should be appointed. The pharmacist is generally designated secretary.

C. The Pharmacy and Therapeutics Committee should meet regularly, no less frequently than twice per year and should meet on call when necessary.

D. The committee should feel free to invite to its meetings persons within or without the hospital who can contribute from their specialized knowledge or experience.

E. An agenda is desirable and should be prepared and submitted to members of the committee in sufficient time before the meeting.

F. Minutes should be kept by the secretary and should be maintained in the permanent records of the hospital.

G. Recommendations of the Pharmacy and Therapeutics Committee shall be presented to the medical staff or its appropriate committee for adoption or recommendation.

FUNCTIONS AND SCOPE

The basic organization of the hospital and medical staffs will determine the functions and scope of the Pharmacy and Therapeutics Committee. The following list, which is not necessarily comprehensive, is offered as a guide:

A. To serve in an advisory capacity to the medical staff and hospital administration in all matters pertaining to the use of drugs.

B. To serve in an advisory capacity to the medical staff and the pharmacist in the selection or choice of drugs which meet the most effective therapeutic quality standards.

C. To evaluate objectively clinical data regarding new drugs or agents proposed for use in the hospital.

D. To prevent unnecessary duplication of the same basic drug or its combinations.

E. To recommend additions and deletions from the list of drugs accepted for use in the hospital.

F. To develop a basic drug list or formulary of accepted drugs for use in the hospital and to provide for its constant revision.

G. To make recommendations concerning drugs to be stocked in hospital patient units or services.

H. To establish or plan suitable educational programs for the professional staff on pertinent matters related to drugs and their use.

I. To recommend policies regarding the safe use of drugs in hospitals, including a study of such matters as investigational drugs, hazardous drugs, and others.

J. To study problems involved in proper distribution and labeling of medications for inpatients and outpatients.

K. To study problems related to the administration of medications.

L. To review reported adverse reactions to drugs administered.

M. To evaluate periodically medical records in terms of drug therapy.

Committee Name

The actual name given to this type of committee is irrelevant. For the sake of clarification, the following nomenclature has been applied to that committee acting in an advisory capacity to the hospital and its staff on all matters pertaining to drugs and pharmaceuticals: **Pharmacy Committee; Formulary Committee; Therapeutics Committee** and **Pharmacy and Therapeutics Committee.**

Committee Membership

Although the approved statement by the American Hospital Association and the American Society of Hospital Pharmacists provides for a membership of not less than three physicians and the pharmacist, the majority of the larger hospitals list committees which often include representatives of the following groups:

Surgery	*Medicine*
Anesthesiologist	Allergist
Urologist	Cardiologist
General Surgeon	Dermatologist
	Endocrinologist
	Gastroenterologist
Pharmacist	Pharmacologist
Administrator	Psychiatrist
Nurse	Internist

It is admitted that this constitutes a large committee; however, this is justifiable since no single individual is competent to rule on all categories of drugs which are being developed. A committee of these specialists can certainly provide a learned opinion as to the merit of any pharmaceutical agent.

Flack[6] has observed that too many hospitals had pharmacy and therapeutics committees with only two or three physician members and that such committees were not truly representative of all medical staff services. In describing the Pharmacy Committee of the attending medical staff at the Jefferson Medical College Hospital, it was shown to consist of three physicians, all of whom were department heads. However, there existed an Advisory Sub-committee to the Pharmacy Committee consisting of the head of each of the divisions of the department of medicine. Such an arrangement is beneficial in that it provides the parent committee with advisory input derived from a broad base of clinical expertise.

On occasion, the issue is raised as to whether or not the pharmacist should serve as a full voting member of the committee or to serve in an *ex officio* capacity. The pharmacist should serve as a full voting member of the committee. Furthermore, he should serve as the secretary of the group and should, therefore, be fully responsible for developing the agenda and the preparation and distribution of the minutes of the meetings.

The Committee Agenda

A successful meeting depends upon the preparation of an interesting agenda which is made available to the committee members reasonably far in advance of the scheduled meeting. Because of the broad scope enjoyed by this committee, many interesting subjects may, rightfully, be placed upon the agenda for discussion.

A typical agenda may consist of the following general categories:

1. Minutes of the previous meeting.
2. Review of a specified section of the Formulary for up-dating and deletion of products.

3. New drugs which have become commercially available.
4. Investigational use drugs currently in use in the hospital.
5. Review of adverse drug reactions reported in the hospital since the last meeting.
6. Drug safety in the hospital.

Generic vs. Brand Named Drugs[3]—A Committee Dilemma

A quarter century ago, approximately 75 per cent of all prescriptions were extemporaneously compounded by pharmacists. Today the reverse is true: nearly 90 per cent are written for manufactured entities which usually bear a brand name. During this same twenty-five-year period, material, labor and operational costs have steadily risen and industry has spent many millions of dollars in research for new drugs. Because of this increasing cost spiral, each newly released prefabricated brand name medication appeared to be closely associated with high prices. Thus the concept of brand name prescribing and dispensing has been erroneously linked with such descriptive adjectives as "expensive," "highly priced" and "exorbitantly priced" in comparison to generic prescribing and dispensing which is supposedly "inexpensive" and "money saving."

The advocates of generic prescribing and dispensing have been vociferous and have commanded much space in our drug journals. In addition, they have monopolized administrative and legislative sessions at both the federal and state levels. Their lobbyists have proposed that the government require generic prescribing and dispensing in all welfare programs. Others contend that the federal government offer the States a bonus payment with its Federal welfare payments whenever generic drugs are dispensed in state-operated programs. Still others suggest that the Federal government approach the issue by penalizing the State through lower welfare reimbursement rates if the State advocated the use of brand named drugs in its welfare programs. Some welfare departments have already succumbed to the pressure thus forcing pharmacists to become involved with the purchasing and dispensing of generic drugs.

Because hospitals with large active clinics usually carry a high welfare census in order to maintain an adequate resource of teaching cases, the hospital pharmacist will be faced with the problem of generic vs. brand name drug. Furthermore, the hospital administrator and many members of the medical staff will advocate generic prescribing and dispensing. They will do this in good faith and with good intentions. They want the clinic patients and the welfare agencies to pay as little as possible for medications.

At each meeting of the Pharmacy and Therapeutics Committee

the hospital pharmacist will be, and in many institutions already has been, faced with the allegation that if several medications made by different companies conform to the standards of the U.S.P., then all of those medications will have identical effects on patients and the least expensive one will be just as good as the most expensive.

Hospital pharmacists know that this is not wholly true. Two preparations each labeled with the generic name and the symbol U.S.P. may be generic equivalents from a chemical point of view but the important question is whether the two products are *clinically effective equivalents.*

It should be noted at this point that clinicians advocate a comparison of the clinical effectiveness of a drug. Too often this is confused with a drug's pharmacologic activity which manifests itself by means of a specific physiologic response, whereas the clinical effectiveness of a drug includes not only its pharmacologic activity, but also such criteria as ease of application or removal, flavor and odor, allergic manifestations, tissue irritation, caloric values, disintegration and absorption rate to mention a few.

It should be common professional knowledge that the active ingredient alone does not make a medication. This chemical entity must be made into one of the accepted medicinal forms—tablet, capsule, injection, cream, ointment, elixir, syrup, a sustained release form or a suppository. This then means that other materials must be used to produce the pharmaceutical form desired. The choice of ingredients and method of combining is left to the judgment and experience of the manufacturer. The U.S.P. itself states that the actual formulating processes, by which the active ingredient becomes a medication, "are in general, beyond the scope of the Pharmacopeia."

Reference to any pharmacy textbook will show that the producer of a medication must concern himself with such things as potency, strength, purity, compatability, solubility, particle size, choice of vehicle or base, pH tonicity, melting point, surface tension, viscosity, storage factors, packaging and control. Deviation from accepted standards or omission of any of these may result in a product which because of its active chemical component is a generic equivalent but not a clinically effective equivalent.

By the same token, two products may both meet U.S.P. standards but, because of differences in composition or the way they are compounded, may not be clinically effective equivalents.

It should be emphasized at this point that all generic drugs are not being condemned. An observation is being made to the extent that if a manufacturer applies all of the standards of high quality ingredients, rigid manufacturing and control procedures, adequate packaging and supports medical research and development programs, the final product will be a generic equivalent with clinical effectiveness. However, its production cost will probably be the same as that of the brand name equivalent and therefore it will have the same retail price to the consumer.

Some hospital pharmacists operating in large metropolitan teaching and research hospitals may well be in a position to purchase generic products from manufacturers who are unfamiliar to them, because they have adequately staffed and equipped control laboratories and clinical testing programs in which they are able to make the assays necessary to ascertain the quality and effectiveness of the product purchased. It should be noted here that oftentimes when the cost of the hospital conducted analyses are added to the purchase price of the product, little financial advantage remains.

Pharmacists certainly realize that there are both high and poor quality pharmaceuticals available under both generic names and brand names.

The hospital pharmacist by virtue of his educational background and general familiarity with the reputation, integrity and facilities of pharmaceutical manufacturers is in an excellent position to evaluate the merits of brand name drugs vs. their generic equivalents. He should not relinquish this position of professional authority and competence to any administrator, physician, politician or welfare agency commissioner. He should, on the other hand, make himself available to all of these people to advise and teach them that the quality of a drug and its subsequent clinical effectiveness are quite independent of its name.

The hospital pharmacist can carry on his teaching program in a number of ways. As a member of the Pharmacy and Therapeutics Committee, he can make available to the Committee membership various articles dealing with the therapeutic implications of brand interchange, publications pertaining to clinical ineffectiveness of drugs due to faulty formulation and the various reports of the F.D.A. in which they describe drug seizures due to faulty labeling or improper strengths.

As the editor of the hospital pharmacy newsletter, the hospital pharmacist should avail himself of the opportunity to editorialize his views on the subject.

As a lecturer in pharmacology in the school of nursing and as a lecturer in the in-service training programs for nurses and interns, the hospital pharmacist should deliver knowledgeable lectures on the subject in order that the doctors and nurses—and particularly those in training—may keep in clear perspective the relationship between quality pharmaceuticals and therapeutic efficacy.

The Committee's Role in Drug Safety

With the advent of each new class of therapeutic agents, the scope, knowledge and responsibility of the hospital pharmacist increases commensurately. Hand-in-hand with this increased responsibility goes the moral, legal, and professional obligation of insuring safety in the handling and administration of drugs.

Unfortunately, too many pharmacists and physicians take drug safety for granted. They are lulled into a false state of complacency by the fact that pharmacy "accidents" resulting in serious injury to or death of patients are relatively infrequent.

However, with the first press release describing a tragic drug "accident" in a neighboring hospital, every trustee, administrator, physician, and pharmacist suddenly awakens to the fact that their policies governing the pharmacy ought to be reviewed in the light of modern dispensing and prescribing trends.

This function could well be the responsibility of the Pharmacy and Therapeutics Committee and should be an on-going program. The following may serve as a guide to this Committee in ascertaining the safeness of the hospital pharmacy:[4]

1. Does the hospital employ a qualified registered pharmacist to supervise the pharmacy?
2. Does the hospital permit non-pharmacist personnel to dispense drugs and allied materials?
3. Does the hospital employ a sufficient number of qualified personnel to allow for adequate coverage of the pharmacy seven days per week?
4. Does the hospital employ personnel commensurate with the pharmacy work load?
5. Does the hospital provide adequate, safe work space, and safe storage facilities for the pharmacy?
6. Does the pharmacy have the equipment necessary to safely and adequately carry out the modern practice of pharmacy?
7. Does the hospital have an automatic stop order regulation for dangerous drugs such as narcotics, hypnotics and anticoagulants?
8. Does the hospital have a firm policy regarding the use of research drugs in the hospital and its clinics?
9. Does the hospital have a drug formulary? If so, is it periodically revised and kept up-to-date?
10. Does the hospital permit anybody other than a licensed pharmacist into the pharmacy "after hours"?
11. Are poisonous materials adequately segregated from non-

poisonous materials in the pharmacy and on the nursing stations?

12. Are external use preparations separated from internal use medications in the pharmacy and on the nursing stations?

13. Does the pharmacy manufacture products for patient's use? If so, are these products checked for accuracy and asepsis by chemical and bacteriologic means?

14. Does the hospital allow the pharmacist sufficient help to permit him to engage in a teaching program to acquaint the nursing and resident staff with new drugs and to teach the student nurses the basic courses of pharmaceutical mathematics and pharmacology?

15. Are all nursing drug stations periodically inspected for the purpose of removing deteriorated and outdated drugs as well as to check all labels for legibility?

16. Does the pharmacy have an adequate reference library which contains texts on pharmacology, toxicology and posology?

The Committee's Role in the Adverse Drug Reaction Program

A consequence of recent advances in drug therapy is the proportionate increase in drug reactions. In order to gain an understanding of these problems and to formulate competent opinions as to the best type of prevention and treatment, the Pharmacy and Therapeutics Committee must assume the responsibility for developing and instituting a procedure for the prompt reporting of an adverse drug reaction.

An adverse drug reaction has been defined by the Food and Drug Administration as follows:[7]

"An adverse drug reaction includes any pathological condition precipitated by a drug regardless of its nature or the circumstances of its occurrence, *i.e.,* toxicity caused by overdosage (therapeutic, accidental, suicidal, homicidal); hypersensitivity; allergy; or injury from improper technique of administration, use of the wrong drug, error in compounding, labeling, or packaging, or from other error in the manufacture of the drug, or in its preparation for use in the hospital. Reactions caused by blood and plasma products need not be reported unless a chemical agent other than the basic substance is responsible."

An *Adverse Drug Reaction Report Form,* such as that shown in Figure 14, should be prepared by the Committee and made available on every nursing station.

A simple yet effective reporting program may be established by adopting the following criteria:

Every case of adverse drug reaction must be reported by the attending physician to the clinical pharmacologist, if one is available on the

Addressograph

ADVERSE DRUG
REACTION REPORT

Directions:

Every case of drug reaction (unusual or unexpected reactions), including acute poisonings by narcotics, barbiturates and amphetamines and industrial poisonings is to be reported by the attending physician to the Division of Pharmacology at the Peter Bent Brigham Hospital. The physician in charge of the patient is also responsible for notifying the allergist, dermatologist and others interested in the problem. Diagnostic procedures and therapy when such exist, will be instituted.

1. Drug or agent involved:

2. Type of reaction:

3. Therapy and Results:

4. Age	5. Sex:	6. Source of drug:
__Under 20	__M. __F.	__Prescription
__21–30		__Over the counter
__31–40	5A. Color:	__Other
__41–50	__Negro	
__51–60	__White	
__61 and Over	__Other	

Attending Physician

FIG. 14.

staff, otherwise to the Chairman of the Pharmacy and Therapeutics Committee. The attending physician should complete an *Adverse Drug Reaction Report Form* on any patient having an adverse reaction. The Medical Record Room will, upon the patient's discharge, remove the *Adverse Drug Reaction Report Form* from the medical record and forward it to the clinical pharmacologist or to the Chairman of the Pharmacy and Therapeutics Committee who, in turn, will periodically forward essential data to the Central Committee on Adverse Drug Reactions of the American Medical Association. Adverse drug reactions should be listed in the medical record as a diagnosis whenever such applies.

Drug Product Defect Reporting Program

In 1971, the ASHP, the USP and the FDA initiated a drug product defect reporting program. Since then, the program has been expanded to include, in addition to ASHP members who were in active practice, community pharmacists, the American Nurses' Association and hospital pharmacists who are not members of the ASHP.

Reporting forms (Fig. 15) are automatically sent to all those participating in the program. Reportable defects include inadequate packaging; confusing or inadequate labels or labeling; deteriorated, contaminated, or defective dosage forms; inaccurate fill or count of a drug product; faulty drug delivering apparatus etc. Obviously, the participants should report anything which, in their professional opinion, is considered to be defective or undesirably associated with the product.

The completed report forms are sent directly to the USP. The staff of the USP then forwards copies of the reports to the FDA and to the manufacturer or distributor involved for their information and use.

The Automatic Stop Order for Dangerous Drugs

The Pharmacy and Therapeutics Committee should develop a means whereby dangerous drugs may be properly administered under reasonable medical staff control.

The questionnaire for accreditation by the Joint Commission on Accreditation of Hospitals specifically determines whether or not the hospital has an automatic stop order in force.

The way two hospitals handle this matter is shown below. Either may be copied in principle by any hospital desiring to do so:

> "All drug orders for narcotics, sedatives, hypnotics, anticoagulants, and antibiotics (administered orally or parenterally) shall

be automatically discontinued after 48 hours, unless (1) the order indicates an exact number of doses to be administered, (2) an exact period of time for the medication is specified, or (3) the attending physician reorders the medication."

The second example of an automatic stop order is:

"All orders for narcotics, sedatives and hypnotics must be re-written every 24 hours.

"All P.R.N. (pro re nata) and standing orders for all medications except narcotics, sedatives and hypnotics shall expire at 10:00 a.m. on the seventh day unless renewed."

Form Approved; OMB No. 57-R0059

HOSPITAL PHARMACIST'S DRUG DEFECT REPORT

| DO NOT USE THIS SPACE |
| DATE RECEIVED |
| REFERENCE NO. |

1. TRADE NAME, DOSAGE FORM, STRENGTH

2. LOT NUMBER(s)

3. DATE PURCHASED (If known)

4. SOURCE OF PRODUCT (Where purchased, if known)

5. NAME AND ADDRESS OF DRUG MANUFACTURER

6. REPORTING PHARMACIST'S NAME

7. NAME AND ADDRESS OF HOSPITAL (Include ZIP Code) 1/

8. PHONE NUMBER OF HOSPITAL (Include Area Code)

9. DEFECTS NOTED OR SUSPECTED

1/ Additional forms and postage-paid envelopes will be mailed to you automatically at this address when this report is received.

| RETURN TO | United States Pharmacopeia
12601 Twinbrook Parkway
Rockville, Maryland 20852
Attention: Dr. Joseph G. Valentino |

FD FORM 2519 (2 '72)

FIG. 15.   Hospital Pharmacist's Drug Defect Report Form.

Committee's Role in Developing Emergency Drug Lists

Because in most true emergencies time is of the essence, it is imperative that emergency drug or "Stat" boxes containing drugs and supplies be readily available for use by the bedside. The Pharmacy and Therapeutics Committee should develop a list of supplies and drugs which ought to be in an emergency box and instruct the pharmacist and nursing service supervisors of their joint responsibility to have the box ready for use at all times.

Once the content of the box has been established and the responsibility for its stocking assigned, the units should be prepared and placed on each pavilion, in the clinic, in the emergency ward and in the special procedures room of the department of radiology.

After the emergency boxes have been placed on the wards, it is mandatory that a program be developed whereby they are checked daily either by the hospital pharmacist or by the nursing supervisor responsible for the ward.

The following list of contents is provided to serve as a guide:

Supplies to be Maintained in Emergency Box:

Syringes:
4– 2 ml.
4– 5 ml.
1–20 ml.
1 insulin

Needles:
2 #16
2 #18
2 #20
2 #23
2 cardiac, #20, 4″

Files, ampul.
Airway
Tourniquets

Drugs for the Emergency Box:

Aminophylline 0.25 Gm./10 ml.
Amphetamine Sulfate 20 mg./ml.
Amyl Nitrite Inhalation
Atropine Sulfate 0.4 mg./ml.
Caffeine Sodium Benzoate 0.5 Gm./2 ml.
Calcium Gluconate 1 Gm./10 ml.
Chloroprophenpyrimadine Maleate 50 mg./ml.
Digoxin 0.25 mg./ml.
Diphenylhydantoin Sodium 50 mg./ml.
Epinephrine HCl. 1 : 1000
Heparin 10,000 Units/ml.
Hydrocortisone 100 mg.
Isoproterenol 1 : 100
Magnesium Sulfate Injection 10% and 50%
Metaraminol Bitartrate 10 mg./ml.

Mannitol Injection 25%
Nalorphine HCl 10 mg./2 ml.
Neostigmine Methylsulfate 0.25 mg./ml.
Nor-epinephrine Injection 0.2%
Pentobarbital 50 mg./ml.
Pentylenetetrazol Injection 0.1 Gm./ml.
Phenobarbital 120 mg./ml.
Phenylephrine HCl 10 mg./ml.
Phytonadione Injection 50 mg./ml.
Picrotoxin Injection 3 mg./ml.
Procaine Amide 100 mg./ml.
Protamine Sulfate 10 mg./ml.
Saline for Injection 30 ml.
Sodium Molar Lactate Solution
Water for Injection 50 ml.

Supplies for Cabinet or Pavilion Utility Room:

1 Venous cannulization set	3 Sterile suction catheters
2 each—#14 and #17 venous catheters	1 Sengstachen-Blakemore tube
	1 Razor with blades
2 6″ shock blocks	1 pkg. sterile gelatin sponge
2 Oxygen catheters	1 Resuscitation tube

Other Emergency Supplies:

Resuscitation carts	Tracheostomy sets
Phlebotomy sets	Dextran and tubing
Oxygen equipment	Burn sheets

Drug Utilization Review

Drug utilization has been defined as the prescribing, dispensing, administering, and ingesting of prescription drugs.[8] Clearly, the magnitude of the problems associated with drug utilization is of great public concern and warrants the attention of health care practitioners. Yet, as a result of this study of the problem Brodie[8] concluded that "there is no organized mechanism for what can properly be called drug utilization review in the private sector of medical care."

Within the hospital, the Pharmacy and Therapeutics Committee provides the institutional authority for the formulary system of drug-use control as well as the mechanism for the continuing education of physicians, nurses and pharmacists. Thus, some institutions have initiated *patient drug utilization profiles* and medication history taking as part of their clinical pharmacy programs thereby enabling the pharmacists to monitor drug utilization within the hospital.

Medication histories are taken by pharmacists of every patient admitted to the hospital or seen in the ambulatory care section. These may be accomplished by personal interview or via a computerized questionnaire specifically designed for the purpose. In addition to personal identification and general diagnosis, the following information is elicited:

1. Medications being taken at time of admission.
2. Medications taken during the recent past. (Including antibiotics.)
3. Home remedies (OTC Drugs) used.
4. Drug allergies.
5. Laboratory tests performed out of the hospital during which diagnostic agents were ingested.
6. Idiosyncrasy towards food products.

The Patient Medication Profile (Fig. 16) is developed by the pharmacist for the following purposes.[9]

1. To help improve drug prescribing practices by promoting the safe and rational use of drugs.
2. To detect and help prevent potential drug interactions.
3. To help detect and prevent adverse drug reactions in sensitive patients.
4. To detect and prevent IV additive incompatibilities.
5. To detect drug-induced laboratory test abnormalities.
6. To detect possible drug-induced diseases.
7. To help detect and prevent potential drug toxicities.

PATIENT MEDICATION PROFILE

Name_____Location_____Physician_____

Admitted_____Source of Admission_____Home_____Other hospital

_____Nursing   _____Emergency
         Home   Service

Admission Diagnosis_____

Other Pathology_____

Operative Procedure Required_____

Pre-Op Medications Used_____

_____

_____

DRUG PROFILE
(includes I.V.'s)

DATE	MEDICATION	DOSE, ROUTE FREQUENCY	DISCONT. DATE	LAB. TESTS	PHARM. NOTE

DISCHARGED_____   PHARMACIST_____

FIG. 16.   Patient Medication Profile for use by clinical pharmacists.

When the Patient Medication Profile, Patient History and Laboratory Procedure Profile are compared, the pharmacist is in an excellent position to monitor proper drug utilization.

It should be obvious to the student that the compilation of drug utilization is a tedious responsibility that can be automated. A computer-based system provides for the entry of the information into the computer through the use of punch cards, magnetic tape, scanning device, or an electronic input terminal device. In the National Center for Health Services Research and Development Study[8] it was pointed out that the ideal system should provide for both retrospective and prospective review.

Retrospective analysis is provided through the use of the punch cards and magnetic tapes whereas when electronic terminal devices are employed, both retrospective and prospective analyses are possible. Control of drug utilization by prospective review is possible when a computer read-out station is located on the patient pavilion. This device can display the profile of a patient's drug regimen (and others if desired) at the time a new drug is prescribed or when changes are made in therapy. In either case, the entry to the computer is made through an input station utilizing a typewriter keyboard, thereby making an instant entry into the on-line system.

Generally, the input information for an electronic data processing system is taken in a codified form the source documents which, in this instance, are the prescription, medication order or doctor's order book. The following provides an idea of the type and scope of information utilized: patient's name, age, sex, ethnic background, diagnosis, drug product, manufacturer, therapeutic class, dosage form, strength, route of administration, directions for use, amount dispensed, days of therapy, drug effectiveness, toxicity, adverse reactions, reasons for termination of therapy, prescriber's name and specialty, etc.[8]

In those hospitals and nursing homes where it is not possible to develop patient drug profiles for the continuing surveillance of drug utilization, it may be advisable for the pharmacist to become a member of the Utilization Review Committee. Membership on this committee of a pharmacist is possible because it is required to be broadly representative of the entire scope of professional practice carried out in the institution. The pharmacist's training and experience in drug problems uniquely qualifies him to sit on such a committee and review patient drug utilization while physicians review clinical utilization of hospital services.

A search of the hospital literature did not reveal methods for a drug utilization review as part of the general medical utilization review procedure. Accordingly, the following is offered as a starting point for the pharmacist to review the patient's drug therapy record in order to ascertain whether or not his stay was affected by drug therapy. Obviously, good therapy coupled with good clinical care can reduce the patient's length of stay whereas poor therapy, which leads to complications, may increase the patient's hospital stay.

I. Proper Choice of Therapeutic Agent
   1. Was the drug employed one with a specific effect upon the diagnosed ailment? If not, why was it prescribed? If the medication prescribed was of multiple composition, was there contained therein a sufficient amount of the principal ingredient to produce a therapeutic effect?
   2. If the drug employed was a sulfonamide or antibiotic, were cultures of the infecting organism taken for the purpose of identification? Were sensitivities performed?
   3. Was any effort made to ascertain the patient's sensitivity to the drug?
   4. Did administration of the drug have any effect upon subsequent laboratory analyses essential to the diagnosis of the ailment?

II. Proper Choice of Dosage Form
   1. Did the patient receive his therapy via the parenteral route when the enteral route should have been employed or vice versa?
   2. Were enteric coated tablets used when indicated?
   3. If time disintegrating dosage forms were employed, was there any evidence to indicate that the medication was being properly released?
   4. If intravenous fluids were employed, what drugs were administered simultaneously? Were they compatible with each other? With the intravenous vehicle?

III. Proper Route of Administration
   1. Was the route of administration preferable to another?
   2. If the oral route was selected, was the medication prescribed for administration at the recommended times *i.e.* pre- or post-prandially?

IV. Drug Allergy
   1. Were there any manifestations of drug allergy?
   2. Were tests for predicting drug allergies done on patients with a suspicious history?

3. Were the drug allergies subsequently managed adequately?

V. Drug Idiosyncrasy and Pharmacogenetics
   1. If there was an abnormally prolonged drug effect, were steps taken to reduce dosage frequency?
   2. If there was evidence of increased drug sensitivity, were steps taken to reduce dosage?
   3. Were any novel or unusual drug effects noted?
   4. If there was evidence of decreased responsiveness to the drugs employed, were counter measures taken?
   5. Was there any evidence of the development of physical dependence upon the drug?

VI. Effect upon Utilization of Hospital Facilities
   1. As a result of improper drug therapy, was the length of stay increased? How many days? At how much additional cost?
   2. What additional laboratory tests were necessary? At how much additional cost?
   3. What additional diagnostic and therapeutic measures were necessary due to the improper therapy? At what additional cost?
   4. What additional medication was necessitated? At what additional cost?

VII. Follow-up and Discharge Medications
   1. Were discharge medications prescribed?
   2. Were they necessary? If yes, were the label instructions adequate to insure proper administration to the patient by lay or semi-professional personnel?
   3. If a follow-up visit is scheduled, were sufficient drug doses prescribed to carry the patient until the visit date? If not, does the prescription order indicate that a refill is permissible?

SELECTED REFERENCES

LOVELL, R. F.:   How a Pharmacy and Therapeutics Committee Improves Pharmacy Service, Hospitals, *34*:71, Dec. 1, 1960.

HELLER, E. M.:   The Doctor's Point of View of the Pharmacy and Therapeutics Committee, Hosp. Pharm. (Canada), *13*:18, 1960.

BOWLES, G. C.:   Pharmacy Committee Agenda, Modern Hosp., *93*:1:104, 1959.

KOLINS, NATHAN S.:   The Pharmacy and Therapeutics Committee in the Community Hospital, Hosp. Formulary Management, *1*:25 (Sept.), 1966.

NELSON, K. R., LETOURNEAU, C. U., and HIMMELSBACH, C. K.: The Pharmacy and Therapeutics Committee, Hosp. Formulary Management, *1*:25 (Feb.), 1966.

DAVIS, NEIL M.:   Emergency Drug Boxes, Hospital Pharmacy, *1*:8:11, 1966.

DAVIS, NEIL M.: Stability of Common Emergency Box Pharmaceuticals, Hospital Pharmacy, *1*:8:15, 1966.

ERICKSON, JAMES C.: Drugs Found in Hospital Emergency Boxes, Hospital Pharmacy, *1*:8:18, 1966.

————Current American and Foreign Programs.

————The Drug Makers and The Drug Distributors.

————The Drug Users.

————The Drug Prescribers, Task Force on Prescription Drugs, U.S. Department of Health, Education and Welfare, Washington, D.C. 20201, Dec. 1968.

DEREWICZ, H. J.: The Minutes of the Pharmacy and Therapeutics Committee, Drug-Intelligence and Clin. Pharm., *3*:258-259, Sept. 1969.

RUCKER, T. DONALD: Drug Insurance, Formularies, and Pharmacy, Medical Marketing & Media, *6*:10:11, October 1971.

LINKEWICH, JOSEPH A.: Guidelines on the Operation of the Pharmacy and Therapeutics Committee—Hospital of the University of Pennsylvania, Hosp. Form. Mgt., *7*:2:16, March-April 1972.

KOSSLER, ALBERT S.: Guidelines on the Operation of the Pharmacy and Therapeutics Committee—University of Arkansas Medical Center, Hosp. Form. Mgt., *7*:2:25, March-April 1972.

BIBLIOGRAPHY

1. *Hospital Accreditation References,* Chicago, American Hospital Association, p. 120, 1964.

2. Statement on the Pharmacy and Therapeutics Committee, Am. J. Hosp. Pharm., *16*:122, 1959.

3. HASSAN, WILLIAM E., JR.: There is no Generic Equivalent for Quality, Drug Topics, *110*:30 (Oct.), 1966.

4. HASSAN, WILLIAM E., JR.: Ensuring Safety in Drug Administration, Hospital Management, *84*:108, 1957.

5. ————: The Drug Prescribers, Task Force on Prescription Drugs, U.S. Department of Health, Education and Welfare, Washington, D.C. 20201, Dec. 1968.

6. FLACK, HERBERT L.: Goals for Hospital Pharmacists, Am. J. Hosp. Pharm., *18*:17:383, July 1961.

7. FRANCKE, DON E.: The Reporting of Adverse Drug Reactions as a Function of the Pharmacy and Therapeutics Committee, Am. J. Hosp. Pharm., *19*:10:533, Oct. 1962.

8. BRODIE, DONALD C.: Drug Utilization and Drug Utilization Review and Control, D.H.E.W. Publication No. (HSM) 72-3002, Dept. Health, Education, and Welfare, 5600 Fishers Lane, Rockville, Maryland, 20852, May 1971.

9. GOLDMAN, LAURENCE: The Pharmacist's Role in Monitoring Drug Therapy, Hospital Pharmacy, *6*:6:5, June 1971.

Chapter

5

The Hospital Formulary

American hospital and pharmaceutical literature is replete with both favorable and unfavorable comments and views on the use of the formulary system in hospitals. This chaotic state has been brought about because of the complete misunderstanding by certain minority groups, of the purpose, scope and function of the hospital formulary system.

Those who denounce the system often cite the following reasons to make valid their claims:

(a) The hospital formulary system deprives the physician of his prerogative to prescribe and obtain the brand of his choice.

(b) The hospital formulary system, in many instances, permits the pharmacist to act as the sole judge of which brand of drug is to be purchased and dispensed.

(c) The hospital formulary system allows for the purchase of inferior quality drugs, particularly in institutions where there is no staff pharmacist.

(d) The hospital formulary system does not reduce the cost of drugs to the patient or to the third party payor because most institutions purchase large volumes of drugs at reduced rates but do not pass on to the patient any reductions in their cost.

Needless to say, in an institution with an active Pharmacy and Therapeutics Committee, none of the above citations will prove to be valid because a well-formed Committee will consist of interested persons whose primary interest in serving on the committee is to assist in the selection of the most therapeutically beneficial drugs at the most economical cost to the hospital and the patient. This philosophy combined with the inherent integrity of physician and pharmacist goes a long way to protect the rights and interests of all concerned.

With the advent of Medicare, the hospital formulary system has taken on a new measure of importance in the hospital's economy. This is due to the fact that the Federal government will reimburse hospitals for the drugs administered or dispensed to a Medicare covered patient if the drugs were approved and listed in certain specified compendia or the hospital's formulary.

Statement of Guiding Principles on the Operation of the Hospital Formulary System

In August of 1960 the Board of Trustees of the American Hospital Association and the Executive Committee of the American Society of Hospital Pharmacists jointly issued a statement of guiding principles on the operation of the hospital formulary system.

Shortly thereafter, the American Medical Association attacked the statement's legality as well as the right of the physician to give prior consent to a pharmacist to dispense a generic drug in place of the brand-named product indicated on the clinician's prescription.

In order to avoid a recurrence of this embarrassing situation, a series of combined meetings of representatives of the American Medical Association, American Pharmaceutical Association, American Hospital Association and the American Society of Hospital Pharmacists were called for the purpose of modifying the original set of guiding principles.[1]

As a result of these meetings a new set of guiding principles was issued in early 1964[2] and are hereinafter set forth in detail.

Statement of Guiding Principles on the Operation of the Hospital Formulary System*

Approved by American Hospital Association, American Medical Association, American Pharmaceutical Association and
AMERICAN SOCIETY OF HOSPITAL PHARMACISTS†

Preamble

THE TREATMENT OF PATIENTS IN HOSPITALS in many cases is dependent upon the effective use of drugs. The multiplicity of drugs available makes it mandatory that a sound program of drug usage be developed within the hospital to ensure that patients receive the best care and protection possible.

In the interest of better patient care, there should be a program of objective evaluation, selection and use of medicinal agents in the hospital. This program is the basis of rational drug therapy. The hospital formulary concept is a method for providing such a program in hospitals and has been utilized as such over the years.

The hospital formulary system is based upon its approval by the organized medical staff, the concurrence of individual staff members and the functioning of a properly organized Pharmacy

*Reprinted from: American Journal of Hospital Pharmacy, 21:40, 1964.
†Action approving the above Statement was taken by the ASHP Board of Directors, meeting in Washington, January 10, 1964.

and Therapeutics Committee‡ of the medical staff. The basic policies and procedures governing the hospital formulary system should be incorporated in the medical staff bylaws, or in the medical staff rules and regulations.

The Pharmacy and Therapeutics Committee, composed of physicians and pharmacists, selected under the guidance of the medical staff, represents the official organizational line of communication and liaison between the medical staff and the pharmacy. The Committee is responsible to the medical staff as a whole and its recommendations are subject to approval by the organized medical staff, as well as to the normal process of administrative approval.

This Committee assists in the formulation of broad professional policies relating to drugs in hospitals, including their evaluation or appraisal, selection, procurement, storage, distribution, use and safety procedures.

Definition of Hospital Formulary and Hospital Formulary System

The hospital formulary is a continually revised compilation of pharmaceuticals which reflects the current clinical judgment of the medical staff.

The hospital formulary system is a method whereby the medical staff of a hospital, working through a Pharmacy and Therapeutics Committee, evaluates, appraises and selects from among numerous available medicinal agents and dosage forms those that are considered most useful in patient care.

The hospital formulary system provides for the procuring, prescribing, dispensing and administering of drugs under either their nonproprietary or proprietary names in instances where drugs have both names.

Guiding Principles

The following principles may serve as a guide to physicians, pharmacists and administrators in hospitals utilizing the hospital formulary system:

1. The medical staff shall appoint a Pharmacy and Therapeutics Committee composed of physicians, and pharmacists and outline its purposes, organization, function and scope.

2. The hospital formulary system shall be sponsored by the medical staff based upon the recommendations of the Pharmacy and Therapeutics Committee. The medical staff should adapt the principles of the hospital formulary system to the needs of the particular hospital.

‡For recommendations of AHA and ASHP, see Statement of Pharmacy and Therapeutics Committee, adopted by the Board of Trustees of the American Hospital Association and the Executive Committee of the AMERICAN SOCIETY OF HOSPITAL PHARMACISTS in February 1959.

3. The medical staff shall adopt written policies and procedures governing the hospital formulary system as developed by the Pharmacy and Therapeutics Committee. Action of the medical staff is subject to the normal process of administrative approval.

These policies and procedures shall afford guidance in the evaluation or appraisal, selection, procurement, storage, distribution, use, safety procedures, and other matters relating to drugs in the hospital and shall be published in the hospital's formulary or other media available to all members of the medical staff.

4. To insure the maintenance of the responsibility and prerogatives of the physician in the exercise of his professional judgment, the hospital formulary system shall not contain any policies or procedures which, prior to the time of prescribing, provide for consent by the physician to the dispensing of a nonproprietary drug or to the dispensing of a proprietary brand different from the brand which he prescribed. However, it shall be within his discretion at the time of prescribing to approve or disapprove the dispensing of a nonproprietary drug or the dispensing of a different proprietary brand.

5. The medical staff shall adopt the policy of, and formulate the procedure for, including drugs in the formulary by their nonproprietary names, even though proprietary names are and will continue to be in common use in the hospital. Physicians may be encouraged to prescribe drugs under their nonproprietary names, although the nomenclature used is entirely a matter of the individual medical practitioner's discretion.

6. In the absence of written policies approved by the medical staff relative to the operation of the hospital formulary system, and authorization from the prescribing physician, the pharmacist must dispense the brand prescribed, bearing in mind his professional prerogative to confer with the physician should the prescribed brand be unavailable.

7. A hospital shall make certain that its nursing personnel are informed in writing (through its established means of communication) about the existence of the formulary system in the hospital and the procedures governing its operation.

8. In the formulation of policies and procedures, the terms "substitute" and "substitution" should be avoided, since these terms have been used to imply the unauthorized dispensing of a brand different from that prescribed or the dispensing of an entirely different drug, neither of which takes place under a properly operated hospital formulary system.

9. Provision shall be made to apprise the medical staff of changes in the working of the hospital formulary system or in the content of the hospital formulary.

10. Provision shall be made for the appraisal and use by members of the medical staff:

a. of drugs not included in the formulary.

b. of investigational drugs.*

11. The pharmacist, with the advice and guidance of the Pharmacy and Therapeutics Committee, shall be responsible for specifications as to quality, quantity, and source of supply of all drugs, chemicals, biologicals and pharmaceutical preparations used in the diagnosis and treatment of patients, and for assuring that quality is not compromised for economic considerations. When applicable, such products shall meet the standards of quality of the *United States Pharmacopeia* or *National Formulary*.

12. The labeling of a medication container with the nonproprietary name of the contents is always proper. The use of a proprietary name other than that describing the actual contents is improper if it is used in a manner that can be taken as descriptive of the contents, even though personnel familiar with the hospital formulary system may understand that it is not descriptive. The following format is recommended for labeling individual patient's containers used within hospitals:

(Nonproprietary Name)
(Name of Manufacturer or Distributor)

Note for information of staff:

Prescription or order for
(Proprietary Name)
dispensed as per formulary policy; contents are same basic drug as prescribed but may be of another brand.

Recommendation

A hospital formulary system, based upon these guiding principles, is considered to be important in drug therapy in hospitals. In the interest of better patient care, its adoption by hospital medical staffs is recommended.

The Legal Basis of the Formulary System

A written and signed prescription or a written and signed medication order in the Doctor's Order Book constitutes the only legal permit to dispense or administer a prescription legend drug. If the physician in writing the prescription or medication order uses a generic or chemical name for the desired preparation, the pharmacist may then dispense the brand which, in his professional judgment, meets the therapeutic

*For recommendations of AHA and ASHP, see Statement of Principles Involved in the Use of Investigational Drugs in Hospitals, adopted by the Board of Trustees of the American Hospital Association in September 1957, and approved by the Executive Committee of the AMERICAN SOCIETY OF HOSPITAL PHARMACISTS in June 1958.

need, and there will arise no legal problems irrespective of whether or not the hospital has adopted a formulary system.

The problem usually arises when the hospital has in effect a formulary system yet the prescriber continues to use a proprietary name for the drug desired. In many instances, the prescriber is aware of the fact that the hospital is operating under the formulary system but, through habit, writes for brand-named drugs. Under these circumstances, if the prescriber had previously agreed to the policy that all prescriptions and medication orders will be dispensed without reference to brand identity, then the pharmacist may so dispense. On the other hand, if there had been no previous consent to the policy by the physician, the pharmacist is professionally and morally duty bound to honor the prescriber's wishes as to brand.

In general, this system of prior **blanket consent** is no longer recommended because it is established upon unsound legal principles.

In order to avoid such situations, hospitals have devised many ways of obtaining the prescriber's consent to the hospital formulary system of dispensing.

One common method is the use of a suitably worded imprint on the prescription form. Examples of such wording are: *"Generic Equivalent Permitted"* or *"Dispensed in accord with the hospital formulary system."* Any physician not desirous of the generic equivalent may obtain the selected brand merely by drawing a line through the permissive statement. In some hospitals, the consent statement is often followed by a check box with a "Yes" or "No," thereby giving the physician an option each time he prescribes. Although both methods are acceptable, I prefer the former since it takes the positive permissive approach and places the responsibility upon the physician of giving notice to the pharmacist of the deviation from accepted policy.

The second method of obtaining prior medical consent to the operation of a hospital formulary system is to incorporate the basic policy and procedures governing its use in the medical staff by-laws or in the rules and regulations. Therefore, as each physician accepts appointment or reappointment, he accepts the formulary system. It is strongly recommended that the acceptance of the appointment and the willingness to abide by the by-laws or the rules and regulations be executed in writing. Members of the intern and resident staffs who normally do not sign documents to abide by the by-laws or rules and regulations of the medical staff should be requested to execute separate consent agreements. Since this method is a modification of the blanket prior consent policy, it should be used with caution.

The third method of obtaining prior medical consent to the operation of a hospital formulary system is to express the policy and procedures governing the formulary system in a separate document and request that all physicians sign it.

The second and third methods have long been criticized on the basis that they abrogate the professional prerogatives of the clinician. This is no longer a valid argument since the adoption of the Statement of Guiding Principles on the Operation of the Hospital Formulary System which provides a means whereby a physician who, for clinical reasons, desires the brand-named product may still obtain it for his patient.

It is the opinion of some attorneys[3] that whenever a physician accepts an appointment to a hospital staff, he "commonly yields to the medical staff as a whole, so far as his practice in that hospital is concerned, certain professional decisions which he is otherwise free to make for himself." It should be quite clear that if the physician does not wish to conform to all of the rules of the particular hospital, he is free to take his patients elsewhere and practice as he chooses. However, so long as he admits to and treats patients in the hospital, he may not disregard or willfully circumvent the accepted by-laws of the staff or the institution.

Preparation of the Formulary

The preparation of the hospital formulary, although the prime responsibility of the Pharmacy and Therapeutics Committee, rests upon the Pharmacist-in-Chief. This is desirable for the sake of expediency. The Committee is here free to make the necessary decisions relative to the materials to be included in the formulary and the pharmacist undertakes the production aspects of preparation.

The initial step in the development of a formulary for any hospital, irrespective of size, specialty, or control, is the selection of a competent Pharmacy and Therapeutics Committee. Because of the importance of this Committee, a separate chapter has been devoted to its organization, membership and functions. Suffice it to say here that, once established, this Committee must take the initial step in the preparation of the formulary.

Some of the decisions which must be reached by this Committee concern themselves with the following:
- *a.* What type of publication will best suit the needs of the hospital?
  1. A hospital owned formulary?
  2. A simple drug list or catalogue?
  3. A purchased formulary service?
- *b.* Irrespective of what decision is reached in the above, it will be necessary to promulgate a series of rules or guides which the

Committee may use to evaluate drugs for admission to the formulary or drug list.

c. If the desirable end product is to be a formulary, a decision must be reached as to possible contents other than the sections on various therapeutic agents.
1. Section on prescription writing?
2. Section governing the use of drugs?
3. Tables of metric weights and apothecary and household equivalents?
4. Tables of common laboratory values?
5. Section on the calculation of dosages for children based on established rules and by use of the body surface method?
6. Pharmacological index?
7. Section on reagents?

d. What type of format should the formulary take?
1. Size?
2. Loose leaf or bound?
3. Printed or mimeographed?
4. Categorizing and indexing—to what extent?

Once answers to the above have been provided the Pharmacist-in-Chief, the preparation of the formulary becomes a routine matter requiring diligence to detail, accuracy and perseverance.

Formulary vs. Drug Catalogue or List

Unfortunately, too many people use the terms *formulary* and *drug list* interchangeably. This is erroneous in view of the fact that there exists a vast difference in the scope and preparation of a formulary over a drug list.

A formulary usually consists of a listing of therapeutic agents by their generic names followed by information on strength, form, posology, toxicology, use, and recommended quantity to be dispensed, whereas a drug list usually consists of a listing of therapeutic agents by their generic names followed by data on strength and form. There may or may not be any additional information although some drug lists may provide the prescriber with recommended quantities to be dispensed.

Clearly then, the formulary is the more informative type of publication and may exert an influential role in the educational aspects of drug therapy particularly in hospitals with an active intern and residency training programs and a school of nursing.

If a formulary type of publication is desirable, then the Committee has the option of either preparing a private formulary for the hospital or to subscribe to a perpetual drug monograph service such as the

American Hospital Formulary Service, a publication of the American Society of Hospital Pharmacists.

Either a well-prepared private formulary or the *American Hospital Formulary Service* will provide the hospital with adequate information concerning drugs. Each has its own merits.

Some of the advantages of the private formulary are that it is prepared locally by the hospital's own clinical staff and thereby engenders in them a sense of pride and loyalty as well as a determination to make the system succeed; its contents with respect to the amount of information provided under each monograph is subject to local needs and desires; it may include sections on related clinical matters which are characteristic to the local hospital; it may be published in a more convenient size and format; drugs may be added or deleted with greater frequency; and finally certain drugs may be added to the formulary before they have attained sufficient stature to be considered on a national level.

Some of the advantages of the *American Hospital Formulary Service* are that it is a continuing drug monograph subscription service published by a national professional society of means; it has the official approval of the American Pharmaceutical Association, the Catholic Hospital Association and the American Hospital Association; it is prepared by a reference panel of the nation's outstanding clinicians, pharmacologists and pharmacists; each monograph contains a complete run-down on drugs including physical and chemical properties, pharmacologic responses, uses, toxicology, contraindications, posology and preparations; and the drugs are classified and coded according to pharmacologic action and therapeutic indications by a system of numbers which can be adapted to the filing of all informative drug literature in the pharmacy library.

Selection of Guiding Principles for Admission or Deletion of Drugs

Of all the tasks which face the Pharmacy and Therapeutics Committee, the selection of criteria by which to gauge the worthiness of a drug for admission to the formulary is the most difficult and troublesome. This is due to the fact that no single member of the Committee is qualified to evaluate the therapeutic efficacy of every drug in every area of clinical specialization. Accordingly, from the outset, the Committee should feel free to invite staff specialists to attend specific committee meetings for the purpose of evaluating preparations commonly used in his specialized practice for inclusion into the formulary.

Thus one of the first criteria to be established is whether or not the local general and specialty staff consider the drug to be of proven clinical value based upon their experience with it.

A second may be that the drug must be recognized by the *United States Pharmacopeia,* the *National Formulary,* or their supplements.

A third may be that the manufacturer of the drug must be one of proven integrity and dependability as well as having the reputation of initiating and supporting research activities of merit.

A fourth criterion may be that no preparation of secret composition will be considered or admitted to the formulary.

A fifth criterion may deal with products of multiple composition. Some hospitals have adopted the policy that no preparation of multiple composition may be admitted if the same therapeutic effect can be achieved through the use of a single drug entity.

On the same subject, the **Drug Efficacy Study** considered questions of efficacy peculiar to combination drug products and in its 1969 Final Report to the F.D.A., the National Academy of Sciences stated:[5]

> "It is a basic principle of medical practice that more than one drug should be administered for the treatment of a given condition only if the physician is persuaded that there is substantial reason to believe that each drug will make a positive contribution to the effect he seeks. Risks of adverse drug reasons should not be multiplied unless there be overriding benefit. Moreover, each drug should be given at the dose level that may be expected to make its optimal contribution to the total effect, taking into account the status of the individual patient and any synergistic or antagonistic effects that one drug may be known to have on the safety or efficacy of the other.
> On these grounds, multiple therapy using fixed dose ratios determined by the manufacturer and not by the physician is, in general, poor practice."

This general opinion of combination drugs is shared by other expert bodies. The Council on Drugs of the American Medical Association in a letter accompanying the recent first edition of AMA Drug Evaluation says:[5]

> "The effects of drugs are intrinsically so complex that it is generally advisable to administer multiple agents separately in order that the dosage and frequency of administration of the individual drugs may be varied in accordance with a patient's requirements. Therefore, most fixed-ratio combinations listed are not recommended. This reflects a long-standing policy of the Council."

The FDA is not opposed to combination drug products; it recognizes that many are safe and effective and provide important advantages to patient and physician.

For a combination to be approved under the law there must be substantial evidence that each active component contributes to the claimed effect of the product, a requirement since 1962. If this requirement is satisfied, two or more drugs may be combined in a single dosage form when, in good medical practice, they would be given concurrently and when putting them together in the same product in no way detracts from their safety and efficacy. Such a combination product should provide appropriate dosage for a significant patient population that can be defined in the labeling. A special case of this general rule is the addition of an ingredient that enhances the safety or effectiveness of the principal active component or minimizes its abuse potential.[5]

Obviously, the above criteria are merely presented as sample guides and should be either elaborated upon or restricted in their scope depending upon the requirements of the local committee and hospital.

Once the Pharmacy and Therapeutics Committee agrees upon a set of principles to guide them in their decisions relative to admissions or deletions from the hospital formulary, it is recommended that these principles be published and included in the finished formulary. In addition, it may be desirable to circulate these amongst the medical staff in order that they may have prior knowledge of them and therefore acquire an understanding of why a particular preparation may not have been included in the final publication.

Contents

The decision as to the contents of the private formulary rests with those responsible for its publication. There are no published requirements for such which are established by an accrediting agency or professional association.

It would, therefore, appear that the Pharmacy and Therapeutics Committee should be guided and influenced by the role which they foresee or expect the formulary to take. If the formulary is to function merely as a control of what drugs may be used in the hospital by the staff, then all that is required is a listing of the drugs with whatever ancillary information the Pharmacy and Therapeutics Committee deems desirable.

On the other hand, if it is the intent that the formulary in addition to its control value is to function as a useful helpful informative tool in the clinician's daily practice, then its contents should be expanded to meet this goal.[4]

Experience has demonstrated the fact that a section on prescription writing is a valuable asset to the young physician joining the intern staff, for throughout his medical school education this facet of his training is relatively skimpy. The section should be brief yet should cover the important parts of the prescription, the use of the metric system, a list of acceptable abbreviations, and the essentials of a narcotic prescription. The following is a briefly written section on prescription writing which may serve as a guide to those contemplating such a chapter in a hospital formulary.

PRESCRIPTION WRITING

All prescriptions must be written clearly and correctly. Every prescription must bear the following information:

Name and address of the patient.

The date.

The medication prescribed.

(This should be written for in the terminology listed in the formulary.)

The strength of the medication prescribed.

(This must be given in the metric system, *e.g.* milligrams [mg.], grams [Gm.], milliliters [ml.] or micrograms [μg. or mcg.].)

The total amount to be dispensed should be clearly indicated.

The signa, containing the instructions to the patient, should be in clear, concise and simple terminology. The physician should avoid mixing Latin and English abbreviations. The term, "As directed," should seldom, if ever, be used.

When refills are desired, the number wanted should be indicated. If this is not done, the prescription will not be refilled.

Prescriptions calling for a narcotic must have, in addition to all of the above information, the narcotic number of the prescribing physician and, in Massachusetts, the patient's age.

It is essential that all prescriptions be signed by the physician issuing them.

Other important data such as normal laboratory values; tables of heights and weights; tables for the calculation of percentages, milliequivalents and dosages; formulas of the various diagnostic stains and reagents in common use in the hospital as well as a myriad of other factual information may be considered for inclusion. Obviously, all of this material cannot be included without making the publication unwieldy and expensive. Therefore the judicious evaluation of each entry by the Pharmacy and Therapeutics Committee is vital.

The Format

The format is extremely important since it will determine the practicality of daily use of the formulary as well as the publishing costs.

Prior to commencing work on the development of the hospital formulary format, it is suggested that the hospital pharmacist gather formularies from various hospitals. The hospital pharmacist may also obtain a representative sample of formularies from many different types of hospitals merely by requesting same from the American Society of Hospital Pharmacists. Needless to say, once the local hospital formulary is published, two copies should be forwarded to the Society in order that their collection continue to expand and therefore be of assistance to other pharmacists seeking ideas.

Size

Experience has shown that a formulary which is sufficiently small in size to permit its being carried in a uniform or laboratory coat pocket will, in all probability, enjoy widespread use in the hospital. A small-sized book also can be carried in the doctor's bag along with his prescription blanks. Many physicians who have become accustomed to using the formulary in their hospital practice often use the hospital formulary in their private office practice.

No specific size can be recommended at the present time, and therefore this determination must be arrived at after careful study of the local need as well as the formularies gathered from the Society and local hospitals.

Loose-leaf vs. Bound

Whether or not the hospital formulary should be loose-leaf or bound will depend upon a number of factors. The most important of these is the ease by which a loose-leaf formulary can be kept current. A bound volume is difficult to keep up-to-date and therefore requires more frequent revision. In comparison, a loose-leaf formulary can be revised at will simply by printing, distributing and inserting the necessary page or pages.

The type of loose-leaf binder is immaterial and is left to the decision of the Pharmacy and Therapeutic Committee. The local stationer, if consulted, will be able to provide sample binders in all price ranges.

Those desiring a permanently bound volume also have many selections to choose from ranging from paper to cardboard to plastic to leather or its substitutes. The controlling factor here will, in all probability, be the cost involved.

Publication

A printed hospital formulary is obviously more esthetic in appearance, easier to read, and imparts to the user the impression that the hospital considers the formulary as an extremely important document and therefore worthy of the cost of printing. This does not mean that a mimeographed formulary will not be used or is not good. A study of a number of formularies will show that some of the better units are mimeographed. However, where it is possible, it is recommended that printing be the selection of choice.

Some formularies appear to have been developed by individuals with a flair for public relations or advertising. Drawings, colored ink, and colored paper should be avoided. The formulary is a professional publication and should reflect the high ethical standards of the hospital and its staff. Therefore, a white or slightly off-white paper should be used. Black ink is always in good taste.

Many authors have been concerned about the use of electronic data processing equipment in preparing and publishing the hospital formulary.[6-8] Reasons generally given for the utilization of the computer for this task are (*a*) to take advantage of the computer process to lower the cost of producing the formulary and (*b*) to adopt the formulary information for future applications resulting from computerized hospital information systems.[8]

Generally, the program has two phases. Phase-I produces the drug information file which is maintained on magnetic tape. Punched cards prepared from the source documents are used as the input to the drug information file. Phase-II produces the printed formulary using the magnetic tape drug information file.

A coding technique must be either developed or adopted for the purpose, as well as data concerning choice of paper, printing technique and photoreduction if necessary.

The American Society of Hospital Pharmacists has developed a computer-processable *Drug Products Information File* which is available to hospitals and nursing homes and from which a hospital formulary can be prepared. Because of the comprehensive nature of the Drug Products Information File (DPIF) it also may be used in drug-drug interaction and drug-laboratory interaction programs.

Formulary Drug Listing Service

"FDLS" refers to the Formulary Drug Listing Service of the American Society of Hospital Pharmacists (ASHP). The service provides reproducible copy of a hospital's drugs in two parts: a Drug Listing Section and a Pharmacologic-Therapeutic Index. The hospital uses the printout to reproduce as many copies of its formulary drug list as are required for distribution to the hospital's professional staff, nursing units, out-patient clinics and libraries.

The Drug Listing Section contains each of the drug products selected by the subscriber, including the nonproprietary name of the drug; selected trade names, synonyms and/or abbreviations; the therapeutic category of the drug; and the specific dosage forms and strengths of the drug selected by the hospital. Package sizes are included for injectable preparations. The ingredients of combination products are listed in tabular form. The section is alphabetically arranged by non-proprietary drug names. Trade names and synonyms are cross-referenced in alphabetical sequence. The Pharmacologic-Therapeutic Index consists of the nonproprietary drug names categorized according to the classification system of the American Hospital Formulary Service (AHFS). Only those drugs and categories included in the Drug Listing Section are included in the index.

All hospitals should have a list of drugs which the medical staff considers acceptable for use in the hospital (i.e., a formulary). Both the Conditions of Participation for "Medicare," and the Standards for Pharmaceutical Services of the Joint Commission on Accreditation of Hospitals (JCAH) stipulate the existence or development of a formulary or drug list.

Since the development of a formulary drug list requires a substantial investment in professional personnel time and because of limited budgets or staff shortages, many hospitals have not prepared a formulary drug list or have not revised an out-of-date edition. The amount of professional personnel time required, annually, to revise a formulary drug list can easily exceed 300 hours!

Under these circumstances, it behooves the hospital administration to approve a subscription to the ASHP'S Formulary Drug Listing Service. By so doing, a substantial reduction in cost of personnel time can be realized by the hospital thereby permitting this valuable professional time to be allocated to other hospital programs.

Formulary Drug Listing Service Preparations

The ASHP sends to the hospital a checklist, containing about 3,000 "core" drugs—those found to be the most frequently approved by Pharmacy and Therapeutics Committees for use within the nation's hospitals. The description of these core drugs on the checklist includes nonproprietary name, trade name, route of administration, dosage form and strength. The format of the checklist includes an access number for ASHP use and a "check" column for use by the subscribing hospital. The checklist is arranged alphabetically by nonproprietary name.

The hospital pharmacist reviews and marks the checklist. Checks on the appropriate lines assure that the products so identified will be included in the drug list for that individual hospital.

The subscribing hospital writes in those additional drug products to be listed in its formulary drug list which do not appear on the checklist.

The checklist, with individual additions, is returned to the ASHP where the input codes for the products designated by the hospital are punched into machine readable form. The input data for a number of uniquely identified hospitals are rung against the ASHP's computerized Drug Products Information File and individualized formulary drug lists are output.

Each subscribing hospital receives a listing of only those drugs it has selected. The hospital receives a single computer printout of its formulary drug list.

The hospital then reproduces the desired number of copies required for distribution within the institution.

The reproduction masters (printout) provided by FDLS can be reproduced in any desirable page size. The masters can be reproduced at exact size (*e.g.*, xerography) on standard 8½″ × 11″ pages. If necessary the masters can be photo-reduced for the printing of pocket-sized lists.

Categorizing and Indexing

The ease by which a physician may locate an item in the formulary will have an impact upon its usability. Too often, the formulary contains all of the desired information, but due to poor indexing data are not readily found. Therefore, since the index is the key to a good formulary, it behooves the pharmacist to expend effort on it.

Most formularies have a general index located at the end of the text. This index is usually alphabetical by generic name and is cross-indexed with brand names of drugs used in the text portion of the formulary. Although the general index is an essential and integral part of any text and cannot be eliminated, it presumes that the user knows what he is looking for. In a formulary, this presumption is not always valid. Here the physician knows that he has need for an anticholinergic drug and he obviously has knowledge of the generic or brand names of a number of drugs which bear this pharmacologic classification. This now means that he must search the index to find a familiar anticholinergic agent. Because this is a burdensome and time-consuming procedure, it is strongly suggested that the general index be implemented with a pharmacological index which will alleviate similar occurrences.

A Sample Pharmacological Index

The following pharmacological classification represents main headings only and the pharmacist in conjunction with the Pharmacy and Therapeutics Committee should classify the drugs which are to be listed in the hospital formulary under each heading. This complete index should then be placed in the front or rear of the formulary.

Amebicides
Analgesics
  1. Narcotic
  2. Non-narcotic
Anesthetics
  1. General
  2. Local
Anthelmintics
Antiallergenics
Antibacterials
  1. Antibiotic
  2. Chemotherapeutic
Antiepileptics
Antihistaminics
Antihypertensives
Antimalarials
Antiparkinsonism Agents
Antisyphilitics
Antituberculous Agents
Cardiovascular Agents
  1. Cardiac Drugs
    a. Accelerators
    b. Depressants
    c. Glycosides
  2. Vascular Drugs
    a. Constrictors
    b. Dilators
    c. Sclerosing Agents
Central Nervous System Drugs
  1. Depressants
    a. Analgesics
    b. Anesthetics
    c. Antispasmodics
    d. Hypnotics
    e. Sedatives
  2. Stimulants
  3. Tranquilizers
Dermatological Agents
  1. Anhydrotics
  2. Antipruritics
  3. Antiseborrheics
  4. Antiseptics
  5. Astringents
  6. Bactericides
  7. Caustics
  8. Cleansers
  9. Emollients
  10. Fungicides
  11. Keratolytics

12. Parasiticides
    a. Lice
    b. Scabies
13. Protectives
Deterrent Therapy
Diuretics
  1. Mercurial
  2. Thiazide Derivatives
  3. Other
Gastrointestinal Agents
  1. Anorexogenics
  2. Antacids
  3. Antidiarrheals
  4. Antinauseants
  5. Antispasmodics
  6. Cathartics
  7. Choleretics
  8. Digestives
  9. Emetics
  10. Emulsifiers
  11. Spasmogenics
Genitourinary Agents
  1. Antibacterials
    a. Antibiotic
    b. Chemotherapeutic
  2. Antiseptics
  3. Antispasmodics
  4. Diuretics
  5. Oxytocics
  6. Spasmogenics
Hematics
  1. Antianemics
  2. Anticoagulants
  3. Coagulants
  4. Expanders
  5. Hemostatics
  6. Neoplastics
Hormones and Synthetic Substitutes
  1. Adrenal hormones
  2. Ovarian hormones
  3. Pancreas hormones
  4. Parathyroid hormones
  5. Pituitary hormones
  6. Placental hormones
  7. Testicular hormones
  8. Thyroid hormones
    a. Depressants
    b. Stimulants
Muscular Relaxants

Nutritional Aids
1. Albumin preparations
2. Amino acid preparations
3. Carbohydrate preparations
4. Choline preparations
5. Fat preparations
6. Gustatory aids
7. Mineral preparations
8. Nutritives
9. Protein hydrolysates

Parasiticides—Internal
1. Amebicides
2. Malaria Therapy
3. Spirochete
4. Trichomoniasis
5. Worms

Respiratory Agents
1. Antihistaminics
2. Bronchial dilators
3. Cough preparations
   a. Depressants
   b. Expectorants
4. Respiratory stimulants

Sedatives and Hypnotics
1. Barbiturates
   a. Short duration
   b. Moderate duration
   c. Long duration
2. Non-barbiturates

Serums and Vaccines
Vitamin and Vitamin Mixtures

In addition to the general and pharmacological index, the formulary may be divided into specific sections with each section segregated by a divider. A suggested subdivision of the formulary is as follows:

Ear
Eye
Nose
Rectal
Throat

Vaginal
Skin
Nutritional Aids
Oral and Injectable

By such a subdivision, the clinician can easily refer to the agents specifically used for either the anatomical entity or to the broad category of drugs used orally or by injection.

The Text

Finally, the selection of the scope of the text material under each generic named drug should be given serious consideration. The amount of material published will depend upon the goals established by the Pharmacy and Therapeutic Committee. The membership of the committee is hereby cautioned that insufficient information does not enhance the use and acceptance of the formulary by the staff. On the other hand, the busy practitioner will also shy away from the formulary if it develops into a miniature text on pharmacology. The ideal situation obviously lies somewhere in between these extremes. As an aid to the hospital pharmacist, three examples are presented.

Figure 17 represents a sample page from the American Hospital Formulary Service. The important point to notice here is the detailed nature of the text material.

SEDATIVES AND HYPNOTICS *28:24*

Aprobarbital   **Alurate®**

Aprobarbital, 5-allyl-5-isopropylbarbituric acid, is classified as a short-acting barbiturate. It occurs as a bitter, white, crystalline powder and is very slightly soluble in water and soluble in alcohol.

Aprobarbital is useful as a hypnotic and for the treatment of conditions in which mild sedation is desirable, as in hypertension, preoperative apprehension, functional gastrointestinal disorders, anxiety neuroses, and coronary artery disease.

For the mode of action, cautions, and contraindications in therapy with aprobarbital, and for the treatment of acute or chronic toxic reactions, see the general statement on The Barbiturates 28:24.

Dosage

Aprobarbital is administered orally. The recommended sedative dosage for adults is 20 to 40 mg. three times daily. The adult hypnotic dose is usually 80 to 160 mg. Dosage for children has not been established but, as for adults, the smallest effective dose should be used.

Preparations

APROBARBITAL
  Elixir, 40 mg. per 5 ml.
  Tablets, 20 mg. and 40 mg.

Only those Preparations underlined or checked above are included in the Formulary of this hospital.
© *Copyright, December 1963, American Society of Hospital Pharmacists*

FIG. 17. Sample page from the American Hospital Formulary Service.

Figure 18 represents a sample page from the Formulary of the Peter Bent Brigham Hospital. Note here the fact that although brief in nature, the practitioner is provided with all of the necessary information.

Figure 19 represents a sample page from the Formulary of the Massachusetts General Hospital. Note here the interesting presentation of each drug in the form of an individual prescription.

Figure 20 represents a sample page from the Formulary of the Newton-Wellesley Hospital. This presentation is of interest due to the fact that it combines the brevity of a drug list with a pharmacological classification and the routes of administration for injectable preparations.

Figure 21 represents a sample page from the Commonwealth of Massachusetts' formulary entitled *The Massachusetts Drug Formulary*. This formulary was prepared by a state drug formulary commission consisting of physicians, nurses and pharmacists and must be used for the prescribing of medications for patients on state welfare plans.

NICOTINIC ACID
(Niacin)

> FORMS AVAILABLE:
>   Tablet: 50 mg.
>   100 mg.
>   Injection: 100 mg./10 ml.
>   USUAL DOSE: 25 mg. to 50 mg.
>   DAILY DOSE: 50 mg. to 100 mg.
>   ROUTE: Orally.
>   Intravenously.
>   Intramuscularly.
>   CAUTION: High doses produce a flushing of the skin.
>   PRESCRIBE: 25 Tablets (1) either strength.
>   1 Ampul (1).
>   USE: Vasodilator, correct nicotinic acid deficiency.

NITROFURANTOIN
(Furadantin)

> FORM AVAILABLE:
>   Tablet: 100 mg.
>   USUAL DOSE: 5 to 10 mg. per Kg. of body weight per 24 hours;
>   given in 4 doses with meals and at bedtime.
>   PRESCRIBE: 25 Tablets (6).
>   USE: Urinary antibacterial.

FIG. 18.   Sample page from the Formulary of the Peter Bent Brigham Hospital, Boston, Massachusetts.

AUTONOMIC DRUGS

SYMPATHOMIMETIC DRUGS
(Adrenergic)

Ephedrine Sulfate Injection
  1 ml. contains 50 mg.
Disp.: 1 ml.
Route: Subcutaneous, intramuscular
Dose: 25 to 50 mg. every 4 hours

Epinephrine Injection
  1 ml. contains 1 mg.
Disp.: 1 ml.
Route: Subcutaneous
Dose: 0.2 to 1 mg. every 4 hours

Epinephrine in Oil Injection, Suspension
  1 ml. contains 2 mg.
Disp.: 1 ml.
Route: Intramuscular, only
Dose: 2 mg. every 8 or 12 hours.

Levarterenol Bitartrate Injection
  4 ml. contains 4 mg. Levarterenol
Disp.: 4 ml.
Route: Intravenous only, by infusion
Dose: 4 mg. is added to 1000 ml. 5% Dextrose solution. Each 1 ml. of this
    dilution contains 4 mcg. Levarterenol.

Metaraminol Bitartrate Injection
  1 ml. contains 10 mg.
Disp.: 10 ml.
Route: Intramuscular, intravenous, not subcutaneous
Dose: Intramuscular 2 to 10 mg. Intravenous 15 to 100 mg. added to 200 ml.
    isotonic sodium chloride solution or 5% dextrose in water. Administered
    by drip.

Phenylephrine Hydrochloride Injection
  1 ml. contains 10 mg.
Disp.: 1 ml.
Route: Subcutaneous
Dose: 1 to 10 mg. every 8 hours.

FIG. 19.   Sample page from the Formulary of the Massachusetts General
Hospital, Boston, Massachusetts.

CARDIOVASCULAR DRUGS

Vasodilators

Amyl Nitrite Pearles

Glyceryl Trinitrate
 (Nitroglycerin)
   .3 mg H.T.
   .6 mg H.T.
   .4 mg H.T.

Mannitol Hexanitrate
  30 mg. Tablets

Paveril Phosphate
  .1 Gm Tablets

Papaverine HCl
  30 mg Tablets
  30 mg Ampuls
  30 mg = 1 cc   For subcutaneous or intravenous use

Pentaerythritol Tetranitrate (Peritrate)
  10 mg Tablets

Priscoline Hydrochloride
  25 mg Tablets
  10 cc vials 25 mg/cc   For subcutaneous, intramuscular, or
                                   intravenous use

FIG. 20.   Sample page from a Formulary (Drug List) of the Newton-
Wellesley Hospital, Newton, Massachusetts.

THE MASSACHUSETTS DRUG FORMULARY

Brand Name	Generic Name
Acidulin OTC	Glutamic Acid Hydrochloride
Acon OTC	Vitamin A Water Soluble USP
Acthar	Corticotropin USP
Acthar Gel	Corticotropin Gel USP
Adrenalin OTC	Epinephrine Hydrochloride USP
Adrenalin Injection	Epinephrine Hydrochloride USP
Adrenotrate	Epinephrine Bitartrate USP
Albolene OTC	Mineral Oil, Light NF
Alcon-Efrin OTC	Phenylephrine Hydrochloride USP
Almocarpine	Pilocarpine Hydrochloride USP
Alphalin OTC	Vitamin A USP
Alurate	Aprobarbital NF
Ambodryl	Bromodiphenhydramine Hydrochloride NF
Amnestrogen	Esterified Estrogens USP
Amphicol	Chloramphenicol USP

FIG. 21. Sample page from the Massachusetts Drug Formulary of 1972.

SELECTED REFERENCES

BRODIE, DONALD C.: The ASHP-AHA Formulary System—a Critique, Am. J. Hosp. Pharm., 20:6:286, 1963.

Editorial, Hospital Formulary System, J. Am. Med. Assoc., 185:534, 1963.

LAWSON, ROBERT E.: Understanding The Hospital Formulary System, Am. J. Hosp. Pharm., 19:5:222, 1962.

GOOCH, JOHN M.: Important Elements of Quality Control Under the Formulary System, Am. J. Hosp. Pharm., 19:2:58, 1962.

LAMY, PETER B., BOURN, IVAN F. and FLACK, HERBERT L.: Application of Data Processing Equipment to the Hospital Formulary, Am. J. Hosp. Pharm., 18:11:642, 1961.

ANDERSON, B. J.: Legal Aspects of the Hospital Formulary, Hosp. Form. Mgt., 6:8:18, August 1971.

RUCKER, T. DONALD: The Role of Computers in Drug Utilization Review, Am. J. Hosp. Pharm., 29:2:128, Feb. 1972.

WERTHEIMER, ALBERT I. and EVANSON, ROBERT V.: A Community Formulary? J. A. Ph. A. NS 11:10:549, October 1971.

SHAW, CLAYTON T.: A Sociological Evaluation of Commercialism and Incon-
sistencies in Pharmacy, J. A.Ph. A. NS *11*:10:539, October 1971.
RAYBURN, J. MICHAEL: Professionalism and Pharmacy Unionism, J. A.Ph.A.
NS *11*:10:541, October 1971.

BIBLIOGRAPHY

1. A.H.A.-A.S.H.P. Statement of Guiding Principles on the Operation of the
   Hospital Formulary System, Hospitals, J.A.H.A., *34*:54, Oct. 16, 1960.
2. Statement of Guiding Principles on the Operation of the Hospital Formulary
   System, Am. J. Hosp. Pharm., *21*:1:40, 1964.
3. WILLCOX, ALANSON W.:   The Legal Basis of the Hospital Formulary System,
   Hospitals, J.A.H.A., *34*:55, Oct. 16, 1960.
4. PELLEGRINO, E. D.: A Physician Appraises the Formulary System, Hospitals, J.A.H.A., *39*:1:77, 1965.
5. Fixed Combination Prescription Drugs, FDA Bulletin, June 1971, U.S.
   Dept. HEW, Food and Drug Administration, 5600 Fishers Lane, Rockville,
   Md. 20852.
6. LAMY, P. P., BOURN, I. F. and FLACK, H. L.: Applications of Data Processing Equipment to the Hospital Formulary, Am. J. Hosp. Pharm., 18:11:
   642, Nov. 1961.
7. FLACK, H. L., DOWNS, G. E. and LANNING, L. E.: Electronic Data Processing and the Hospital Formulary, Am. J. Hosp. Pharm., *24*:1:5, Jan. 1967.
8. FRANKENFELD, F. M., BLACK, H. J. and DICK, R. W.: Automated Formulary Printing from a Computerized Drug Information File, Am. J. Hosp.
   Pharm., *28*:3:154, March 1971.

Chapter

6

The Pharmacy Bulletin*

IT is a well-documented fact that the majority of the hospitals in this country lack a good method of communicating with the staff. The methods employed to disseminate interdepartmental information are usually well prototyped, namely, bulletins, memoranda, bulletin board notices and committee meetings. In most instances, this form of communication is adequate even though it is limited in its scope.

The department of pharmacy, because its method of operation brings it into close contact with the major hospital services, departments and the entire medical staff, is in a position to alleviate that portion of the problem that relates to the dissemination of data concerning drugs and related supplies.

As has been stated earlier, one of the duties of the Pharmacy and Therapeutics Committee is to assist the pharmacist in conducting a teaching program within the hospital via a pharmacy publication. The membership of this committee can be extremely helpful by preparing brief lead articles concerning the latest therapeutic advances in their specialty and by reviewing the materials gathered by the pharmacist for publication.

The preparation of a worthwhile pharmacy publication requires a great deal of time and forethought. The purpose of this chapter is to provide some ideas relative to possible contents, format, duplication, and distribution of such an educational and informative medium.

Selection of a Title

The title selected for the publication should be specific, short and of such a nature that it identifies the publication as well as its contents.

Too often, a title is selected which imparts the impression that the publication is a collegiate gossip paper rather than a professional journal.

*This chapter adapted from an article appearing in the Am. J. Hosp. Pharm., 16:4:154, 1959 by William E. Hassan, Jr. and Ernest S. Lentini.

5

Examples of good titles are: Pharmacy Bulletin, Pharmacy News, Pharmacy Review, and Pharmacy Newsletter.

Examples of titles which are not acceptable are: The Mortar and Pestle, The Pill Roller News, Drug Store News, News Capsules, etc.

Contents

Since the purpose of this publication is to educate as well as to inform, it is imperative that its contents be of such a nature.

In general, the publication should be divided into five categories. They are as follows:

A. Editorial.
B. New Drug Section.
C. Abstract of the Pharmacy Committee Meeting.
D. Lead articles by prominent members of the medical staff.
E. General.

The *editorial,* prepared by the Pharmacist-in-Chief or other interested member of the Pharmacy and Therapeutics Committee, should be a means whereby new procedures relative to ordering, prescribing, storage or administration of drugs within the hospital are introduced and publicized. It may also be used to focus attention on infractions of established procedures and to editorialize therapeutic trends and opinions. For example, the following lead article appeared in one issue of a pharmacy bulletin.[1]

TO LABEL OR NOT TO LABEL

"The professional as well as the lay press is replete with articles relative to the labeling of prescriptions with the name of the drug prescribed.

"The American Medical Association's Council on Drugs has recently passed a resolution approving such a move.

In the resolution, the Council stated—

It is recommended that prescription pads contain boxes for a "yes" or "no" on whether to label; if these boxes are not filled in by the physician, the prescription will be labeled.

"At the Brigham, the general policy is not to label the prescription with its contents. Every prescription blank has boxes for a "yes" or "no" on whether to label. A "yes" checked off means that the pharmacist will, in addition to the directions, place upon the label the name of the ingredient. If neither box is checked, only the directions for use will appear on the label.

"Some advantages to identifying the active ingredient of each prescription are:

1. It helps when a patient changes doctors, moves to another location, or calls a doctor when records are not available.

2. It may save crucial minutes in cases of accidental poisoning or suicide attempts.
3. It helps prevent mix-ups between a patient's drugs and those of other members of the family.
4. The patient would be more likely to cooperate with physicians by reporting side effects and quickly reporting complications.

"We all recognize the fact that some drugs should not be labeled particularly if the physician feels that the patient might use them for self-destruction. Examples of these products are barbiturates, tranquilizers and narcotics.

"The next time you write a prescription, give some careful thought to the desired labeling and check the appropriate box on the prescription blank."

The *new drug section* should contain the major data on each new drug accepted for use within the hospital by the Pharmacy Committee. Major information in this instance includes a brief description of the drug, its range of usefulness, indications, side effects, administration and dosage and how supplied by the pharmacy. The format employed in the presentation of this information may be in a number of forms, therefore, the following is presented as an example of only one.

VINCRISTINE SULFATE
ONCOVIN

"Vincristine Sulfate (ONCOVIN—Lilly) is an alkaloid obtained from the periwinkle plant. It was formerly known as leurocristine and has been referred to as LCR and VCR. It is an antineoplastic agent chemically related to vinblastine sulfate (Velban) but with a different anti-tumor spectra than the latter.

"Vincristine sulfate is recommended only for the treatment of acute leukemia in children. In this condition, the drug may be effective from the standpoint of palliation and survival time in patients who have become resistant to other agents.

"Side effects from the drug include some degree of alopecia, and in some cases neuromuscular disturbances.

"Vincristine sulfate is supplied in either 1 mg. per 10 ml. or 5 mg. per 10 ml. ampoules for intravenous use only. The diluent is sodium chloride 0.9 per cent with benzyl alcohol as a preservative."

The *abstract of the minutes* of the Pharmacy Committee meeting is a worthy inclusion in the publication in that it keeps the entire staff aware of the constantly changing trend of therapeutics within the institution. In addition, it allows those members of the staff who have had reason to communicate with the Pharmacy Committee to note that their recommendations have received attention.

Each issue should have a *lead article* by a prominent member of the staff. The article should not be lengthy and should be restricted to an evaluation of current pharmaceuticals or trends of therapy within the author's field of specialization or to topics of current interest to the staff.

The following is an example of a lead article which was of interest to the staff. Note that the article was co-authored by the chairman of the Pharmacy and Therapeutics Committee and the pharmacist.[2]

YOUR ROLE IN DRUG CONTROL

"During the past ten to fifteen years, medicine has witnessed the development of more new therapeutic agents than at any other period in its history. As each of these drugs has been developed, industry, federal agencies, and clinicians the world over have worked diligently to screen those products which may have an adverse effect upon living tissue. Unfortunately, the results obtained from the wide clinical use of an already screened product do not always parallel the results obtained from an original testing under carefully controlled conditions. Kerlan* states that, "with wider use there may be a shift in the incidence or pattern of side effects or nature of toxicity from that associated initially with the drug's use." An excellent example of this observation is the recent Thalidomide episode."

"Because the initial clinical evaluation and subsequent large scale use of a new drug usually takes place in a hospital, members of the medical and nursing staff as well as the hospital pharmacist are in a key position to observe, record, and disseminate vital information concerning a drug's adverse reaction. These three members of the health team must function as a unit in order to make the effort a successful one."

"The role which each member of the above triad must play is carefully outlined in our present Current Practice Bulletins. No. 4 (Drug Classification) and No. 75 (Reporting Adverse Reactions)."

The section categorized as "General" may include anything the editor feels is of interest to the medical staff, nursing service or laboratory staff. Samples of the type of information that might well be placed in this category are abstracts of releases from the state department of public health, abstracts of articles of interest on current situations such as the recurrence of an outbreak of Asian influenza and abstracts from the various journals relative to unusual sources of poisoning in humans, drug research news or drug warnings.

Format and Duplication

The format of the publication will vary with the originality of the pharmacist; therefore, the following description is provided as a basis for further development by the individual concerned.

*Kerlan, Irvin: The Bulletin of the American Society of Hospital Pharmacists, *13*:4:311, 1956.

PHARMACY

R   **BULLETIN**   R

PETER BENT BRIGHAM HOSPITAL   BOSTON, MASS.

FIG. 22.

The paper should be a good quality mimeograph paper measuring 8½″ × 11″. In view of the fact that the first page should be inviting to the potential reader, it is recommended that the heading be pre-printed. By so doing, you will have the advantage of being able to use stock cuts of pharmaceutical symbols which the printer can obtain for you in order to decorate the publication. In addition, you will be able to have the heading of each issue printed in a different colored ink on the white or colored paper stock. Neither of the above sugges-tions would cost much, but would serve to draw the attention of the potential reader (see Fig. 22).

In cutting the stencil, some authors have suggested that the page be longitudinally split in half and the data typed in columns. The advantage of this being that many of the readers like to clip out the data on a new drug and affix it to a page in their Formulary or, in the case of the nursing service, 3″ × 5″ cards in their new drug file.

The method of duplication will vary with the availability of equip-ment within the institution. Either mimeograph, multigraph, or multi-lith will reproduce a neat and attractive publication whose individual pages can be collated and stapled together.

Distribution

The completed issue should be distributed to the following areas and individuals, provided they exist in the particular hospital:

A. Every member of the medical staff and to the staff library.
B. Administration.
C. Nursing Service.
    1. A copy to each station
    2. Several copies to Nursing School Office
    3. Nursing School Faculty
    4. Nurses' Library
D. Laboratories.

Advantages

The preparation of a pharmacy publication requires the time, effort and imagination of the pharmacist who undertakes such a project. On the other hand, a well-prepared issue can save the pharmacy a great deal of time by reducing the number of telephone calls concerning new drugs or newly instituted procedures.

In addition, it will add to the professional stature of the pharmacist within the institution and give him the satisfaction of having made a contribution towards better communication between his department and the professional staff.

SELECTED REFERENCES

JEFFREY, L. P.: The Pharmacy Newsletter—Voice of the Department, J.A.H.A. Hospitals, 34:57, Sept. 1, 1960.

Get Doctors to Write on Their Specialties in Hospital Bulletin, Am. Druggist, 129:68, 1954.

CHABACK, L. L.: Communications and Interdepartmental Relations—The Pharmacists' Viewpoint, Hosp. Pharm. (Canada), 11:293, 1958.

CLARK, J. S.: Communications and Interdepartmental Relations—The Nurses' Viewpoint, Hosp. Pharm. (Canada), 11:292, 1958.

HEGARTY, JOHN F. and KENNA, F. REGIS: Bulletins Improve, Broaden Hospital Pharmacy Service, Hosp. Topics, 44:81, 1966.

WILLIAMSON, ROBERT E. and KABAT, HUGH F.: Pharmacist-Physician Drug Communications, J. A. Ph. A. NS, 11:4:164, April 1971.

BIBLIOGRAPHY

1. HASSAN, W. E., JR.: To Label or Not to Label, Pharmacy Bulletin of the Peter Bent Brigham Hospital, 8, No. 3, 1963.
2. FRIEND, D. G. and HASSAN, W. E., JR.: Your Role in Drug Control, Pharmacy Bulletin of the Peter Bent Brigham Hospital, 7, No. 3, 1962.

Chapter

7

Investigational Use Drugs

By definition, research or investigational use drugs are those compounds or mixtures which have not been released by the Federal Food and Drug Administration for general distribution and use. These drugs usually bear the following statement on their labels:

> Caution: New Drug—Limited by Federal Law to Investigational Use

They are released only to physicians who sign the proper Federal Food and Drug Release form for the manufacturer.

With the increased use of the clinical facilities of teaching hospitals for the therapeutic evaluation of investigational use drugs, it has become necessary to define the responsibility for the use of these products and to centralize pertinent information concerning them.

A lack of control and information relative to investigational use drugs in a hospital obviously can lead to chaos. This can induce drug administration "accidents" as well as deter suit-conscious, yet competent, clinical investigators from carrying out this important phase of medicine within the hospital.

Prior to 1950, the literature describing methods of controlling this class of preparations was sparse. As the tempo for the clinical evaluation of new drugs increased, so too did the literature describing methods employed by various hospitals to control the drugs and disseminate information concerning them to the proper personnel.

The U. S. Public Health Service Policy

The U. S. Public Health Service now requires assurance that the rights, privacy and welfare of human beings involved as subjects in research or training activities are protected, and that their informed consent has been obtained before subjecting them to any research procedure, and that any protocol involving human subjects has received *a priori* review and approval by a committee of the staff of the hospital.[1]

Thus each hospital has found it necessary to establish a Committee on Human Use in Research.

The Committee on Human Use in Research, a standing committee of the hospital, is charged with the responsibility of considering the problems associated with the use of human subjects for clinical research and other biomedical (including psychological) investigations, to establish guiding principles with respect to these matters, and to advise the Administrative officers with respect to policy issues that may arise. In accordance with the recommendations of this Committee, mechanisms are established to assure that every proposal for clinical research or investigation involving human subjects will receive the best possible review and guidance.

Any investigation that proposes to apply to human subjects a procedure or protocol potentially hazardous or uncomfortable (or which may invade his rights of privacy) and it is not clearly for the individual's benefit, is to be reviewed prior to its initiation by the Committee on Human Use in Research at the hospital with reference to (1) the risks and potential medical benefits of the investigation, (2) the rights and welfare of the individuals involved, and (3) the appropriateness of the methods used to obtain informed consent. The committee's comments and any recommended changes in protocol or procedure should be reported to or discussed with the principal investigator and his chief of service. Appropriate written records should be maintained. A signed and dated report of the committee's recommendation on each application submitted by the hospital to outside sources of support for research or training should be forwarded to the proper administrative officer and kept on file.

All research involving the use of human subjects must be approved by the appropriate chief of service, who is responsible for maintaining oversight as the investigation proceeds. Any significant changes in protocol or emergent problems which would alter the experimental situation or adversely affect the rights or welfare of the subjects should be promptly referred to the Committee on Human Use in Research for review and advice.

In order to ensure continuing surveillance of the research project by the Committee on Human Use in Research, each principal investigator should prepare a Continuing Surveillance Report, on a quarterly basis, and forward it to the Secretary of the Committee on Use of Humans in Research.

FDA Amendments of 1966

The Federal Food, Drug and Cosmetic Act was amended in 1966 by the addition of a new statement of policy as follows:

Consent for use of investigational new drugs on humans; statement of policy.[2]

(a) Section 505(i) of the act provides that regulations on use of investigational new drugs on human beings shall impose the condition that investigators "obtain the consent of such human beings or their representatives, except where they deem it not feasible or, in their professional judgment, contrary to the best interest of such human beings."

(b) This means that the consent of such human beings (or the consent of their representatives) to whom investigational drugs are administered primarily for the accumulation of scientific knowledge, for such purposes as studying drug behavior, body processes, or the course of a disease, must be obtained in all cases and, in all but exceptional cases, the consent of patients under treatment with investigational drugs must be obtained.

(c) *"Under treatment"* applies when the administration of the investigational drug for either diagnostic or therapeutic purposes constitutes responsible medical judgment, taking into account the availability of other remedies or drugs and the individual circumstances pertaining to the person to whom the investigational drug is to be administered.

(d) *"Exceptional cases,"* as used in paragraph (b) of this section, which exceptions are to be strictly applied, are cases where it is not feasible to obtain the patient's consent or the consent of his representative, or where, as a matter of professional judgment exercised in the best interest of a particular patient under the investigator's care, it would be contrary to that patient's welfare to obtain his consent.

(e) "Patient" means a person under treatment.

(f) *"Not feasible"* is limited to cases where the investigator is not capable of obtaining consent because of inability to communicate with the patient or his representative; for example, where the patient is in a coma or is otherwise incapable of giving informed consent, his representative cannot be reached, and it is imperative to administer the drug without delay.

(g) *"Contrary to the best interest of such human beings"* applies when the communication of information to obtain consent would seriously affect the patient's disease status and the physician has exercised a professional judgment that under the particular circumstances of this patient's case, the patient's best interest would suffer if consent were sought.

(h) *"Consent"* or *"informed consent"* means that the person involved has legal capacity to give consent, is so situated as to be able to exercise free power of choice, and is provided with a fair explanation of all material information concerning the administration of the investigational drug, or his possible use as a control, as to enable him to make an understanding decision as to his willingness to receive said investigational drug. This latter element requires that before the acceptance of an affirmative decision by such person the investigator should make known to him the nature, duration, and purpose of the administration of said investigation drug; the method and means by which it is to be administered; all inconveniences and hazards reasonably to be expected, including the fact, where applicable, that the person may be used as a control; the existence of alternative forms of therapy, if any; and the effects upon his health or person that may possibly come from the administration of the investigational drug. Said patient's consent shall be obtained in writing by the investigator. (See Figure 28, p. 139, for a sample Consent Form.)

The Office of Grant Administration Policy

The Office of Grant Administration Policy, Department of Health, Education and Welfare has issued its Manual, Chapter 1-40, entitled "Protection of Human Subjects." The stated purpose of the new manual is to establish uniform policies for the protection of human subjects involved in research, demonstration and other activities supported by the Department's grants and contracts.

Chapter 1-40 attributes broad definitions to the terms "subject" and "at risk" to include anyone exposed to the possibility of physical, psychological, sociological, or other adverse effect as a consequence of any activity which goes beyond the application of standard and accepted methods to meet individual needs. The determination of when an individual is at risk is a matter of the application of common sense and sound professional judgment to the circumstances of the activity in question.[7]

Emphasized in the policy is the responsibility of the grantee or contractor to safeguard the rights and welfare of human subjects. To provide for the proper discharge of this responsibility, the Department of Health, Education and Welfare will now require the grantee or contractor to carry out initial and continuing committee review of all activities involving human subjects. The review must establish that the rights and welfare of the subject are adequately protected, that the risks to him are outweighed by the activity's potential benefit, and that informed consent is to be obtained by methods that are adequate and appropriate.[8]

This review is expected to take into consideration such matters as local standards of professional practice, applicable laws, practical aspects of community acceptability, and to benefit from the committee's knowledge of the personnel involved and of the conditions under which the study is to be carried out. The policy also requires a review of the grant application by a committee of the Department of Health, Education and Welfare.[8]

The manual chapter further spells out procedures for certifying institutional review of applications, for institutional review of cooperative activities, for documentation of institutional committee actions, and for Department of Health, Education and Welfare administration of policy. Responsibility for administration of the policy has been delegated to the Division of Research Grants, National Institute for Health because of its experience in the administration of a similar Public Health Service Policy.

Principles Involved in the Use of Investigational Drugs in Hospitals

The following *"Statement of Principles Involved in the Use of Investigational Drugs in Hospitals"* was approved by the American Hospital Association and the American Society of Hospital Pharmacists in 1957 and by the American Nurses' Association in 1962. It has been published in the October 1961 issue of the *Journal of the American Society of Hospital Pharmacists* and is reprinted here for convenient reference.[3]

HOSPITALS ARE THE PRIMARY CENTERS for clinical investigations on new drugs. By definition these are drugs which have not yet been released by the Federal Food and Drug Administration for general use.

Since investigational drugs have not been certified as being for general use and have not been cleared for sale in interstate commerce by the Federal Food and Drug Administration, hospitals and their medical staffs have an obligation to their patients to see that proper procedures for their use are established.

PROCEDURES for the control of investigational drugs should be based upon the following principles:

1. Investigational drugs should be used only under the direct supervision of the principal investigator who should be a member of the medical staff and who should assume the burden of securing the necessary consent.
2. The hospital should do all in its power to foster research consistent with adequate safeguard for the patient.
3. When nurses are called upon to administer investigational drugs, they should have available to them basic information concerning such drugs—including dosage forms, strengths available, actions and uses, side effects, and symptoms of toxicity, etc.
4. The hospital should establish, preferably through the pharmacy and therapeutics committee, a central unit where essential information on investigational drugs is maintained and whence it may be made available to authorized personnel.
5. The pharmacy department is the appropriate area for the storage of investigational drugs, as it is for all other drugs. This will also provide for the proper labeling and dispensing in accord with the investigator's written orders.

Classification of Drugs

Summarized, the *Statement of Principles Involved in the Use of Investigational Use Drugs in Hospital* espouses four distinct purposes:

1. To establish a drug classification.
2. To centralize pertinent information concerning drugs available for research use.
3. To define the availability of such drugs to staff members.
4. To establish a single stocking and dispensing unit within the hospital.

In order to attain the above goals, it is necessary for the Pharmacy and Therapeutics Committee to establish a drug classification system within the hospital. By establishing drug categories, a more definitive approach to the control, distribution and utilization of drugs, within each category, may be realized.

One simple classification which can be adapted to any hospital research program is to categorize all drugs in the institution into four classes: Classes A, B, C, and D.

Class A, should contain all investigational use drugs that are in a preliminary experimental stage. The use of drugs in this category is usually restricted to the principal investigator. With regard to the storage and dispensing of drugs in Class A, there are two schools of thought. One group believes that products in this category should be stocked and dispensed by the principal investigator; the other group firmly holds that all drugs should be stored and dispensed through the pharmacy by pharmacists. The advantages of the latter are obvious; however, both systems will work if the interested parties, the clinical investigator and the pharmacist, will cooperate in a united endeavor.

Class B should consists of investigational use drugs which have passed through the preliminary research stage. Usually, drugs in this category are supplied to the department of pharmacy by the principal investigator and are dispensed only upon his written prescription or those of his duly designated co-investigators.

Class C is limited to drugs approved by the United States Pharmacopeia, National Formulary, or passed by the Federal Food and Drug Administration for commercial distribution.

Drugs in this category may be used within the hospital or its clinics if the physician complies with the following procedure:

If the product is to be used by a single patient, the prescriber must obtain the consent of the Chief-of-Service or his duly designated alternate (usually the Chairman of the Pharmacy and Therapeutic Committee) before the product may be obtained by the pharmacist.

A Class C preparation, which various members of the Staff feel has therapeutic promise, may be introduced into the hospital on a six-month trial. A request for such drug must be made to the Pharmacy and Therapeutics Committee which may then authorize the pharmacist to purchase, stock, and dispense the product. Pertinent data, concerning this special drug, are to be gathered and filed in the pharmacy office. At the completion of the trial period, the clinical experience is reviewed by the Pharmacy and Therapeutics Committee along with the clinician. If the results are favorable, the product is accepted into the hospital formulary; if the evidence is not favorable, the product is barred from further use within the hospital.

Class D drugs are preparations which have been accepted for use in the hospital and are listed in the hospital formulary.

Information concerning these products is to be kept in the general literature file in the pharmacy library.

Preparations in this class may be prescribed routinely by any licensed physician on the hospital staff.

Control of Investigational Use Drugs

All investigational use drugs should be registered with the Pharmacy and Therapeutics Committee. This may be accomplished by a letter from the principal investigator which provides the following information on each drug:

1. New Drug Number	7. Pharmacology
2. Generic Name	8. Toxicology
3. Manufacturer	9. Dose Range
4. Proprietary Name (if any)	10. Method of Administration
5. Chemical Name	11. Antidote (if known)
6. General Chemistry	12. Therapeutic Uses

The above data are usually found in the brochure prepared by the manufacturer and supplied to each investigator. Therefore, the brochure may be sent to the Pharmacy and Therapeutics Committee with a letter indicating the investigator's intent to use such a product.

Many pharmacists have developed various forms which may be used to disseminate the above information on an investigational use drug to the various staff doctors and nurses. These forms are usually titled *"Physician's Data Sheet on Investigational Drugs," "Nurse's Data Sheet on Investigational Drugs"* and *"Pharmacist's Data Sheet on Investigational Drugs."* Figures 23, 24 and 25 illustrate these various data sheets which have been used by the Pharmacy Service of the Veterans Administration Hospital in Albany, New York.[4] Under this system, the pharmacist completes the necessary form or portion of a form and sends it to the appropriate physician or pavilion each time a new investigational drug is prescribed. Although this method does offer control and proper dissemination of information, it is burdensome upon the pharmacist since three different forms bearing similar information must be prepared.

PHYSICIAN'S DATA SHEET ON INVESTIGATIONAL DRUGS

1. Name of Investigational Drug _____

2. Manufacturer or Other Source _____

3. Strength and Form of Investigational Drug _____

4. Amount Received _____

        Date Received _____

        Control or Batch No. _____

5. *Pharmacologic and Therapeutic Properties, Dosage, Precautions:*

6. *Arrangements Which Have Been Made for its Administration:*

                                          _____

                                              Investigator

Registered:

      _____

          Date

FIG. 23

NURSE'S DATA SHEET ON INVESTIGATIONAL DRUGS

1. Name of Investigational Drug:_____

2. Manufacturer or Other Source:_____

3. Strength and Form of Investigational Drug:_____

4. Pharmacologic, Therapeutic Properties and Precautions to be Observed:

5. *Arrangements Which Have Been Made for its Administration:*

                                        _____

                                      Chief Pharmacist

FIG. 24

PHARMACIST'S DATA SHEET ON INVESTIGATIONAL DRUGS

Investigational Drug:_____ Manufacturer:_____

Chief Investigator:_____

DATE	PHYSICIAN	PATIENT	℞ No.	AMOUNT	WARD
___	_____	_____	_____	_____	_____
___	_____	_____	_____	_____	_____
___	_____	_____	_____	_____	_____
___	_____	_____	_____	_____	_____
___	_____	_____	_____	_____	_____

FIG. 25

Figure 26 illustrates a *New Drug Report Form* used at the Peter Bent Brigham Hospital in Boston, Massachusetts. This form, as designed, provides all of the data required for the proper handling of the investigational use drug by physician, pharmacist and nurse.

The *New Drug Report Form* may be placed on each pavilion, where it is readily available to any investigator. Each time a clinician desires to prescribe an investigational use drug, he must complete the *New Drug Report Form* in duplicate, place the original in the patient's medical record folder, and have the carbon copy sent to the pharmacy with the drug order slip appended. By so doing, the pharmacist is

PETER BENT BRIGHAM HOSPITAL

NEW DRUG FORM

Addressograph Use Only

New Drug No.:_____

Generic Name: _____   Date & Time of 1st Dose:_____

Trade Name (If Any):_____

Chemical Name: _____

Chemistry:

Pharmacological Action:

Dose: _____   Method of Administration:_____
_____   _____
_____   _____

Toxicity: Antidote(s):

Therapeutic Uses: Names of physicians from whom drug
                             is available:

FIG. 26

aware that the new drug is being used on a particular patient in a specific area, the nurses have the necessary information, and the physicians on the pavilion also have all the necessary data. This same procedure should be followed irrespective of the number of patients using the drug on the same pavilion. In order to save the clinician's time in such a situation, he may complete one form in detail and permit either the medication nurse or resident to complete similar forms for each of the other patients on the same pavilion.

In hospitals where the research load may not be quite so heavy, the pharmacist may undertake to complete each set of *New Drug Report Forms* each time he receives an order for an investigational use drug.

The fact that carbon copies are used saves time and provides the identical information to both clinician and nurse. A separate file for prescriptions for each investigational use drug readily serves the purpose of tracing the drug and accounting for each dose consumed.

Identification of Investigational Use Drugs

Whenever Class A or Class B drugs are dispensed from the pharmacy, they should be labeled in such a manner as to differentiate them from routine prescription drugs. In some hospitals, investigational use drug labels are printed in red ink on white paper stock. In addition to the commonly required label information of patient's name, date, prescription number, doctor's name and directions for use a space for the research drug number is provided. This double set of numbers, the prescription number and the manufacturer's research drug number, provides a two-way control relative to the identity of the product dispensed.

Charge Policy for Handling and Dispensing

Because it is usually difficult to convince drug investigators that investigational use drugs should be stored and dispensed from the pharmacy, many hospital pharmacists waive a charge for this service, the consensus being that it serves as an inducement to the investigator to avail himself of the pharmacist's service. In these institutions a charge is made when a special dosage form is prepared in the pharmacy. The basis of the charge is arrived at by determining the cost of materials and labor involved.

In hospitals where there is a potent Pharmacy and Therapeutics Committee, a routine nominal charge is made for handling and dispensing research drugs. This charge is usually passed on to the patient but, where sufficient funds are available to the investigator, he may wish to assume the total cost of the project and accordingly requests the pharmacy not to charge the patient but to bill his research grant or fund on a monthly basis.

Authorization for Treatment with Drug Under Clinical Investigation

The Law Department of the American Medical Association[5] states that drugs under clinical investigation should be administered only where:

1. the informed consent of the patient or his authorized representative has been obtained;
2. the physician is convinced of the reasonable accuracy of his diagnosis and, if necessary, has confirmed it by adequate consultation; and
3. existing methods of treatment have proven unsatisfactory.

AUTHORIZATION FOR TREATMENT WITH DRUG
UNDER CLINICAL INVESTIGATION

A.M.

Date_____Time_____P.M.

I authorize Dr. _____, the attending physician, to

treat_____with the drug presently
(Name of Patient)

identified as_____for the following condition:

_____

_____

_____

(Describe symptoms of disease to be treated)

It has been explained to me that the safety and usefulness of the drug in the treatment of patients for the above condition are now being investigated and that the manufacturer or distributor has supplied the drug for the purpose of providing further evidence of its safety and usefulness.

I voluntarily consent to treatment with the drug and release the attending physician from liability for any results that may occur.

Signed_____
(Patient or person authorized
to consent for patient)

Witness_____

FIG. 27

The voluntary participation of the patient will not excuse a deviation from the physician's obligation to exercise his best skill in rendering the care required of a reasonable practitioner. Furthermore, the physician is advised to confine his clinical investigations of new drugs to those furnished by reputable sources who have supplied him with comprehensive written information concerning:

1. animal experimentation;
2. previous clinical investigations, if any;
3. recommended dosages;
4. contraindications;
5. possible side effects to be watched for, and
6. the safety and possible usefulness of the drug from existing data.

Since oral consent is not sufficient, the American Medical Association has developed medicolegal form number 29 (Fig. 27).

Another example of a consent form which does not limit itself to the use of investigational use drugs is that used on the Clinical Center of the Harvard Medical School at the Peter Bent Brigham Hospital (Fig. 28).

Since this text material is not intended to offer legal advice due to the fact that state laws vary from state to state, the hospital pharmacist is urged to consult the hospital's legal counsel for the law applicable to the area in which the hospital is located.

Role of the Pharmacist in the Clinical Evaluation of a Drug

Once the pharmacologist has demonstrated a new compound to be effective and safe in animal tests, clinical trials are invariably commenced. These trials usually proceed in two steps—preliminary and extended.

During the preliminary stage, the principal investigator cautiously administers the drug to a limited number of selected patients and closely follows the results. After having gained experience and confidence in its use, the investigator is generally ready to conduct an extended comprehensive evaluation of its efficacy.

It is during this stage that the pharmacist can play an important role by assisting in the development of the protocol and the control of a double blind study. Such tests are devised by having the experimental drug and the placebo prepared in exactly the same dose form. The identified products are then entrusted to the pharmacist to dispense according to a predetermined pattern and to maintain an exact record of which patient received the true drug and which received the placebo. Neither the patient nor the physician is informed as to whether the placebo or potent article is being tried in any individual

CONSENT FORM

CLINICAL CENTER
OF THE
HARVARD MEDICAL SCHOOL
AT THE PETER BENT BRIGHAM HOSPITAL

Patient's Name:_____ Date:_____

Project Title:

Description of procedure to be undertaken:

I have fully explained to the patient_____
the nature and purpose of the procedure described above and such risks as
are involved in its performance.

_____

Physician's signature

I have been fully informed of the risks and possible consequences involved
in the performance of the procedure described above, have been advised
that unforeseen results may occur and, nevertheless, hereby authorize Dr.
_____and such assistants as he may designate
to perform the procedure upon me and hereby release and forever discharge
him, such assistants, the Peter Bent Brigham Hospital, its officers, agents and
employees, and all persons on its medical and surgical staff who are in any
way connected with the procedure from liability for any injury which may
result directly or indirectly from the performance of the procedure.

_____

Patient's signature

_____

Witness

Fig. 28

patient. All information for breaking double blind codes must be kept
in the pharmacy. Should an emergency arise requiring the breaking of
the code, the pharmacist on duty or on call is authorized to provide the
necessary information.

In addition to the above role, the hospital pharmacist can render
a valuable service to the new drug researcher by formulating new
dosage forms from the pure chemical. A word of caution should be
interjected at this point—since time is of the essence in a research
project, many investigators will attempt to speed up the pharmacist
by waiving certain control tests. The pharmacist should insist upon
the time necessary to develop a scientifically sound formulation as well

as for the performance of chemical and bacteriological tests for potency and sterility.

As the Colleges of Pharmacy train more and more clinical pharmacists, these individuals become available to participate in the clinical evaluation of new drug products. Because of their training in biopharmaceutics, pharmacokinetics and in the use of modern instrumentation techniques of analysis, clinical pharmacists can monitor the blood and tissue levels of the new drugs as well as their excretion rates and thereby advise the clinical pharmacologist relative to the need for dosage adjustment, mode of administration or product formulation.

A Brief Abstract of the New Food and Drug Administration Regulations[6]

The complete text of the regulations issued by the Food and Drug Administration, United States Department of Health, Education, and Welfare which require an industry-wide review of the safety and effectiveness of drugs was published in the *Federal Register* of Thursday, May 29, 1964.

The regulations apply to all drugs for human use that have been cleared prior to June 20, 1963, since drugs approved after that date are already subject to basic FDA regulations requiring periodic reporting and review.

Prior to the 1962 Kefauver-Harris Drug Amendments, the only basis for the clearing of new drugs was safety. It was not necessary to demonstrate therapeutic efficacy. Under the new law, all claims for therapeutic activity must have sound medical support.

Another strict requirement of the new law is that records of clinical and other experience with the drugs be maintained and that reports be submitted on a current basis so that the FDA's files can be kept current.

The following is an abbreviated outline of the steps which must be taken to comply with the regulations.

(1) Within *sixty days,* the pharmaceutical manufacturer must report to the FDA the approved new drugs which are still on the market and those which have been discontinued or never marketed. If the drug has been discontinued, the reasons for such action must be given.

(2) Within *one hundred twenty days* the pharmaceutical manufacturer must report on each drug previously cleared through the new drug and antibiotic certification provisions of the Federal Food, Drug and Cosmetic Act of 1938 and currently being marketed—

(*a*) Whether the label, package insert, and other promotional material currently in use offer the drug only for the conditions covered by the original new drug application, antibiotic submission, or any approved supplement.

(*b*) If claims are being made which were not in the original application, the firm must submit data to validate their claims.

(*c*) Whether any of the current promotional material includes any claims which are not clinically established, and whether the firm has learned of any side effects, contra-indications, or untoward reactions which may have been due to the drug and which are not adequately covered in the present labeling and advertising material.

(*d*) What the manufacturer plans to do about either discontinuing or obtaining acceptance of unapproved claims and revising any and all promotional literature to include any side effects, contraindications, and warnings that have been shown to be needed by clinical experience.

(*e*) Whether there have been any mix-ups in the preparation or labeling, or any bacteriological problem, or significant chemical, physical or other change, or failure of any batch to meet specifications during the last two years.

(3) Beginning in one year, annual reports are required to be filed on each approved new drug, listing any changes or additions to the information previously submitted. These reports shall be due on the anniversary date of approval of the drug. Willful or repeated failure to comply with this section may result in the suspending from the market any that should have been reported on.

Basically, what Congress intended with the passage of these regulations was a comprehensive review of all drugs on the market for the purpose of making certain that they are safe for their intended uses and that they be effective for the conditions for which they are prescribed.

Investigational Drug Circular

Because hospital pharmacists have great interest in investigational use drugs, it is suggested that they subscribe to the *Investigational Drug Circular*. This publication is issued by the Bureau of Medicine of the Food and Drug Administration. It is stated that the purpose of this *Circular* ". . . is to answer questions asked by drug sponsors and clinicians regarding requirements of the Food, Drug and Cosmetic Act . . ."

Advisory Committee on Investigational Drugs

This Committee was established in June 1963 to advise the Food and Drug Administration on the implementation of the Kefauver-Harris Drug Amendments of 1962 covering investigational use drugs.

The Committee is appointed by the Commissioner of the FDA and it consists of a number of eminent physicians and pharmacologists. The Committee reports to the Medical Director of the FDA.

SELECTED REFERENCES

TEPLITSKY, B.:   The Use of Investigational Drugs in Hospitals, Am. Profess. Pharmacist, 22:10:896, 1956.
————: A Method for Handling Investigational Drugs, Am. Profess. Pharmacist, 22:11:1018, 1956.
BUDAY, P. V. and MARTIN, E. W.:   Information Needs in Clinical Testing of Drugs, Am. J. Hosp. Pharm., 20:2:84, 1963.
SMITH, AUSTIN and HERRICK, ARTHUR D.:   Drug Research and Development, New York, Revere Publishing Co.
CASE, R. W.:   Pharmacy Control of Investigational Drugs, Am. J. Hosp. Pharm., 19:10:512, 1962.
D'AMBOLA, J. V.:   Projection and Plan and Practice = A Successful Method for Handling Research Drugs in the Hospital Pharmacy, Am. J. Hosp. Pharm., 19:10:520, 1962.
CURRAN, W. J.:   The Law and Human Experimentation, New Eng. J. Med., 275:323, 1966.
GILGORE, SHELDON G.:   Researching a New Drug in Man, Medical Marketing and Media, 4:5:15, 1969.
HASSAN, WILLIAM E., JR.:   Investigational Use Drugs in Humans—Chapter 8, p. 143, Law for the Pharmacy Student, Philadelphia, Lea & Febiger, 1971.

BIBLIOGRAPHY

1. Surgeon General's Memorandum of July 1, 1966, Policy and Procedure Order No. 129, Revised.
2. Title 21, Subchapter C, Part 130 Section 130–37 Federal Register, 31, No. 168, August 30, 1966.
3. Statement of Principles Involved in the Use of Investigational Drugs in Hospitals, Am. J. Hosp. Pharm., 19:10:509, 1962.
4. TEPLITSKY, B.:   American Professional Pharmacist, 22:11:1018, 1956.
5. Medicolegal Forms with Legal Analysis, Chicago, American Medical Association, 1961.
6. U.S. Department of Health, Education and Welfare, Food and Drug Administration, Press Release HEW-B33, 1964.
7. Manual Grants Administration 1-40-10B, Chapter 1-40, Protection of Human Subjects, Dept. Health, Education and Welfare, Washington, D.C.
8. DHEW Policy on Protection of Human Subjects, DRG Newsletter, p. 3, May 1971.

Chapter

8

Developing the Budget

ONE of the most important tasks in the fiscal operation of the department is the preparation of the annual budget. Too often, many administrators and chief pharmacists take the development of the budget too lightly and thereby arrive at a document which does not serve its true purpose.

Hahn[1] describes the budget as an instrument

". . . through which hospital administration, management at departmental levels, and the governing board can review the hospital's services in relationship to a prepared plan in a comprehensive and integrated form expressed in financial terms."

In order that the over-all hospital budget complies with the above definition, each and every departmental budget must be accurately prepared and submitted.

Hahn[1] further states that—

"A properly developed and used budget should have as its goals (1) development of standards of performance, (2) comparison of actual results with these standards thus identifying deviations, and (3) subsequent analysis of deviations to determine whether they are controllable or uncontrollable."

A budget is a short-range plan for future operations. The meaning and appropriate use of a budget must be clearly understood by those in managerial positions since their participation is required in its preparation and their cooperation is essential if it is to serve the function of a control device over operations. Prior to embarking upon a plan, management must first define the purpose of the unit, establish policies for its operation, and project the hospital's growth.

The plan should be reasonable and, through the conscientious efforts of all personnel, attainable. It should not forecast results that are not possible under current and anticipated conditions. Students must not be misled when first exposed to the jargon "estimated results" during a discussion of a budget. This does not mean guesswork but rather carefully determined values based upon a knowledge of current financial and operating conditions and their relationship to future periods. The budget must not be construed as a tool to restrict initiative or to be impervious to the effects of changing conditions.

Divisions of the Budget

Every budget consists of three separate parts, (*a*) Income Accounts, (*b*) Expense Accounts and (*c*) Capital Equipment Requests.

The Income Account

Insofar as the department of pharmacy is concerned, its income is the dollar value of the prescriptions and requisitions processed.

The *Uniform Chart of Accounts and Definitions for Hospitals*[2] provides that—

> "Records may be kept of the number of prescriptions compounded for in-patients and out-patients consistent with the classifications of nursing units, accommodations, finanical status or type of medical care received as maintained by the hospital. This information, however, will not disclose the amount of pharmaceuticals issued as routine medication to various patient classifications, nor will it indicate the amount of drugs requisitioned by special service departments such as the operating rooms, delivery rooms, radiology department, etc.

> "A special study might be made to determine the cost of preparing and issuing pharmacy items. These amounts could be added to the dollar value of the supplies used to reflect the total cost of processing requisitions and compounding prescriptions, or the requisitions and prescriptions may be priced for statistical purposes, at only the dollar value of the supplies used. If the pharmaceuticals issued as routine medication to patient services and requisitioned by special service departments are on a cost basis, then the dollar value of the prescriptions must be adjusted to a cost basis for this statistical purpose. Another possibility is to price the requisitions of routine medications to the various patient services and special service departments with the same percentage of markup as used on prescriptions. The amounts of the priced requisitions should be classified according to the routine and special services consistent with the designations maintained by the hospital."

Of the procedures outlined above, the method recommended is whereby either the department of pharmacy or the accounting department maintains a daily, weekly, monthly or annual total of the cost of the pharmaceuticals issued to the various patient services as well as to the special service departments. This total, when added to that obtained from the processing of patient prescriptions and requisitions, represents the true income of the department.

In addition, there are other statistics that are of value in assisting management to accurately predict the volume of activity of the department of pharmacy. They are:

a. Number of prescriptions according to subcategories.
b. Number of prescriptions dispensed per pharmacist.
c. Hours of service.
d. Prescription volume per hour of service.
e. Medication cost per patient day.
f. Medication cost per clinic visit.
g. Average drug cost per prescription.
h. Average salary cost per prescription.
i. Average supply cost per requisition.

Although, "income" is considered as a single figure by the beginner, it is important to understand the derivation of the figure. Generally, income in the hospital pharmacy is limited to the sale of drugs to in-patients, ambulatory patients and departments of the hospital. However, the sale of drugs to patients may be sub-divided further based upon the patient's ability to pay or to their employment status if they are employed by the hospital. The following sub-division is but one example:

a. Full pay.   d. Physicians.
b. Part pay.   e. General employee.
c. Non-pay.

If income is generated from a combination of the above, it is desirable to separate the data because it will lead to more accurate appraisal and evaluation.

In some hospitals, the Controller may choose to treat income from the sale of drugs to other hospital departments as a "deduction" from the Purchase Account rather than added to the Income Account on the premise that such a maneuver enables a better evaluation of drug purchase costs for patient use.

The Expense Accounts—General Information

The American Hospital Association[2] recommends that expense accounts be divided into four general categories—*Administration and General, Professional Care of Patients; Out-Patient and Emergency* and *Other Expenses.*

The department of pharmacy is listed under the category of Professional Care of Patients and is assigned code number 644. (This code need not be used by all hospitals.) Each subdivision under this expense code number is coded by the addition of a dot and another digit, *e.g.*, 644.1 is the code for Salaries and Wages; 644.2 for Supplies and Expenses.

Although the hospital pharmacist will not be involved with the establishing of expense codes for his department (this being the prerogative of the comptroller), he should have a general understanding of what expenses belong under each section of the American Hospital Association expense code or of whatever similar code is in use in his hospital.

Accordingly, the following is a direct quotation of the recommended codes and their contents[2]—

> *644.1 Salaries and Wages*
> "Salaries and wages of pharmacists, assistants, clerks, and others employed in the hospital pharmacy department."
>
> *644.2 Supplies and Expense*
>
> *644.2.1 Drugs and Pharmaceuticals*
> "Drugs and pharmaceuticals dispensed by prescription or otherwise from the hospital pharmacy department. Drugs and Pharmaceuticals used in the out-patient and emergency departments should be charged there and not to this account."
>
> *644.2.2 Purchased Services*
> "This account should include the cost of prescriptions (excluding those intended for out-patients) purchased from an outside pharmacy in the event the hospital does not have its own pharmacy."
>
> *644.2.3 Miscellaneous Supplies and Expense*
> "Bottles, labels, glassware, narcotic and alcoholic permit fees, printed forms and stationery, pharmacists' uniforms, reference books, etc. Parts required to repair and maintain equipment used by this department and repairs made by outside concerns to such equipment also should be charged to this account, to separate sub-accounts if significant in amount."

It should be clearly understood that the above codes and designations are not intended to provide the ideal system of segregating costs. At most, it is a guide and should be modified by the individual hospital to meet its particular need.

Expense Account—Salaries and Wages

In order to arrive at an accurate determination of the salaries and wages, it is recommended that the Pharmacist-in-Chief prepare a breakdown of the personnel in the department of pharmacy into the following categories:

a. Authorized permanent full-time positions—filled.
b. Authorized permanent full-time positions—vacant.
c. Authorized permanent part-time positions—filled.
d. Authorized permanent part-time positions—vacant.
e. Authorized temporary positions.
f. Proposed new positions.
g. Overtime requested.

It may also be of value to the Pharmacist-in-Chief if he further sub-divided the above positions into three sub-categories, *i.e.* administrative, professional and non-professional staff. It may be useful to prepare a table of all full-time administrative, professional and non-professional pharmacy staff and a similar table for the part-time employees in each category. Once the proposed annual salary for each employee is determined, the cost of new positions is added and finally any overtime which, according to past experience may be necessary, is also added. This, then, represents the total anticipated salary and wage expenditure for the next fiscal year.

Expense Account—Supplies and Materials

In developing the supplies and expense portion of the budget, it is important for the department head to have available the dollar amount budgeted for each expense code for the fiscal year. It is also necessary to have available the latest financial statement showing the present actual cost of materials and supplies. From this, it is a relatively simple mathematical process to estimate what the actual expense will be for the present fiscal year. If the budgeted figure and the estimated actual figure agree, then the previously prepared budget was well done. On the other hand, if these two figures are too far apart, it indicates that either there was an error in the calculation of the previous year's expense budget or something has occurred or is occurring in the present fiscal year which was not anticipated and, therefore, needs investigation and evaluation.

If the department is to be involved in an expansion program of service, *i.e.* dispensing to new clinics, opening of a new wing, etc., then the Pharmacist-in-Chief should ascertain the cost of the materials and supplies to be consumed by the new program and so provide for it in the new budget.

From the above discussion, it would appear that the department of pharmacy is required to keep rather detailed records in order to arrive at the figures requested by the budget. Although it is highly desirable to accumulate one's own statistical data, it is common practice for the pharmacist to rely upon the accounting department for many of his base figures. Therefore, there should be developed a close rapport between the Pharmacist-in-Chief and the Comptroller.

Equipment and Construction Budget

In hospitals where funding of the depreciation of physical plant and equipment is practiced, the actual cash for replacement or remodeling is usually readily available. In those hospitals where funding is not a policy, then construction and purchase of equipment creates a major financial burden requiring the development of a comprehensive and detailed budget.

However, irrespective of the policy with regard to funding, an equipment and construction budget must be prepared. Many hospitals require that any piece of equipment with a unit cost of $100 or more is considered to be "capital equipment" and must be included in this portion of the budget. By the same reasoning, any construction with a total cost which exceeds $100 is considered "major" and must also be included in this section of the budget. Although the figure of $100 appears to be quite low, it is usually intentionally set at this level in order to exert greater control.

For the convenience of the reader, the following is a check list of depreciable equipment commonly found in the department of pharmacy[4] and which provides an indication of the "life" of the item:

DEPRECIABLE EQUIPMENT CHECK LIST

Professional Equipment	Life in Years	Professional Equipment	Life in Years
Balances	10	Meters, conductivity	25
Cabinets		Mixers, electric	10
Metal	20	Prescription cases, cabinets	15
Wood	15	Pumps, vacuum and pressure	10
Capsule machines	15	Refrigerators	10
Chemical hoods	10	Rinsers	10
Cleaners, pressure	15	Safe, Narcotic	25
Distilling apparatus	15	Scales	15
Drum hoists	15	Sterilizers	20
Filters (except glass)	10	Tanks	15
Homogenizers	15	Typewriters	5
Hot plates	10	Worktables	10
Labels, cabinet	15		

Administrative Equipment	Life in Years		Life in Years
Adding machines	10	Clocks	15
Bookcases, metal	20	Desks, wood	15
Bulletin Boards	10	Filing cabinets, metal	20
Calculators	10	Lockers, metal	20
Cash registers	10	Worktables	10

SELECTED REFERENCES

MARTIN, T. LEROY: *Hospital Accounting Principles and Practice*, 2nd Ed., Chicago, Physicians' Record Co., 1952.
Chapter 3—Recording Income from Sales or Services
Chapter 9—Budgeting for Hospitals
Chapter 10—Capital *vs*. Revenue Expenditures
JENNINGS, LEE W. and BURNS, ALLAN L.: Hospital Cost Accounting, Management Controls, *15*:6:137, June, 1968.

BIBLIOGRAPHY

1. HAHN, JACK A. L.: Budgetary Reporting and Management Action, Hospitals J.A.H.A., *37*:46, Mar. 16, 1963.
2. _____: *Uniform Chart of Accounts and Definition for Hospitals*, Chicago, American Hospital Association, pp. 40-41.
3. Ibid. p. 117.
4. Ibid. pp. 163 and 168.
5. GRAESE, C. E.: Budgeting and Hospital Management, Management Controls, *15*:6:123, June, 1968.

Chapter

9

Purchasing and Inventory Control[1]

THE purchase and inventory control of pharmaceuticals is a special and important phase of the operation of a successful hospital pharmacy.

A portion of the purchases, controlled drugs and alcohol, is rigidly controlled by Federal regulations which in reality provide the means for accurate purchase and inventory control. These two classes of products, however, constitute a relatively small portion of the over-all purchases of an institutional pharmacy. Therefore, the purchase and control of the largest segment of the inventory is left to the administrative staff of the hospital or its duly authorized delegates.

In most general hospitals with an out-patient clinic operation, a pharmacy inventory of $100. to $200. per bed may be considered reasonable. However, many pharmacies, particularly those associated with the large teaching hospitals, include in their inventory parenteral and irrigating fluids, surgical dressings, rubber goods, sutures, surgical instruments, syringes and laboratory supplies. Clearly then, the dollar value of the inventory when expressed in dollars per bed may vary depending upon the variety of the inventory as well as the activity of the institution. In general, the pharmacy inventory should be adapted to the individual hospital's needs taking into consideration its distance from a source of supply, storage facilities, and rapidity of inventory turn-over.

In view of the fact that, throughout this discussion, three words "purchase," inventory" and "control" will be in constant use, it is felt that these terms should be defined.

The word *purchase,* as defined in the dictionary, has numerous meanings, the most appropriate being—"to obtain by paying money or its equivalent; to buy for a price."

The word *inventory* is defined as— "an itemized list of goods with their estimated worth; specifically an annual account of stock taken in any business."

The word *control* is defined as follows—"to exercise, directing, guiding, or restraining of power over."

Purchasing Agent vs. Pharmacist

The hospital literature is replete with articles dealing with the question, "Should pharmaceuticals and related products be purchased by the purchasing agent or the pharmacist?"

One school believes that all institutional purchasing should be centralized under the aegis of the purchasing agent. According to this system the pharmacist, like all other department heads, requests, on a special form, the item to be purchased. The selection of the brand and vendor is thereby left to the discretion of the purchasing agent, unless the pharmacist has prepared a list of specifications which may or may not restrict the selection to the product of a particular manufacturer. This system has certain control and economic merits and can function within the hospital. It must, however, depend upon the close cooperation between the pharmacist and purchasing agent. Each must be aware of the definite contribution which he can make to such a specialized purchase.

The other school believes that pharmaceuticals and related items constitute specialties which require the technical skills of a formally trained individual for their proper selection and purchase.[1]

A leading advocate of this school was Dr. Malcolm T. MacEachern who in his text[2] stated:

> ". . . the purchase of drugs and pharmaceuticals is a specialty which can be carried out to the best advantage by a pharmacist trained in managing a hospital pharmacy. . . . This is the only department in the hospital in which it is usually *not* advisable to have purchasing done by a general purchasing agent."

One of the principles enunciated in the American Society of Hospital Pharmacists' *Minimum Standard for Pharmacies in Hospitals*[3] is that ". . . the pharmacist in charge shall be responsible for specifications both as to quality and source for purchase of all drugs, chemicals, antibiotics, biologicals and pharmaceutical preparations used in the treatment of patients . . ."

This same document under the section on *Elaboration of Responsibilities* goes on to state that

> . . . . "The pharmacist should furnish specifications for the purchase of all drugs, chemicals and pharmaceutical preparations even though a purchasing agent may do the actual procurement through a centralized department.

Since the pharmacist has the responsibility for the compounding, dispensing and manufacture of the drugs used in the hospital he should also have the authority to specify the drugs to be purchased. In large institutions with centralized purchasing, the pharmacist and the purchasing agent should work hand-in-hand, each recognizing the importance of the function of the other. In such a system it is essential that the pharmacist state the specifications for drugs to be purchased and to have authority to reject any article below standard or not complying with specifications so that the purchasing agent may be guided and assisted in his function. The pharmacist will also, in certain instances, wish to consult with the Pharmacy and Therapeutics Committee concerning specifications for drugs."

Francke[4] writing editorially states that "in the application of this principle, the pharmacist is made, in effect, the agent of the medical staff and of the hospital for the specifications of medicinal agents. Justification for this lies in the fact that since the pharmacist has the responsibility for the compounding, dispensing and manufacturing of drugs in the hospital, he should also have the authority for the specifications of drugs to be purchased."

The hospital may follow the intermediate plan whereby the actual function of purchasing is retained by the purchasing department, and yet utilize the benefits of the technical knowledge of the pharmacist by permitting him to develop the necessary specifications for the purchase of the drugs and allied products.

Role of Purchasing Agent in Drug Procurement

The role of the purchasing agent in drug procurement may vary markedly from small to large hospitals. In the small hospital, the purchasing function may be a part-time one and may be handled by the administrator, an administrative assistant or the storekeeper. This, therefore, means that lack of time or pressure from other duties will cause the individual to restrict his activities in this function to a minimum.

In a large hospital, where the purchasing function is of such magnitude that it is a full-time position for one or more individuals, the purchasing agent may assume the following duties in relation to drug purchases:

1. issues purchase orders
2. maintains purchase records
3. follows-up on delayed orders
4. initiates competitive bidding procedures
5. obtains quotations from specified sources

Role of the Pharmacist in Drug Procurement

Pharmaceuticals for hospital use may be purchased in one of the following ways:

1. by direct purchase from the manufacturer
2. by direct purchase from a wholesaler
3. by bid from either manufacturer or wholesaler
4. by purchase from a local retail pharmacy (emergency purchases only)
5. by a contract purchase arrangement with the manufacturer (*e.g.* ampul contract or solutions contract)
6. by a contract purchase through a hospital purchase bureau or corporation.

The hospital pharmacist should acquaint the purchasing agent with the above avenues of drug purchasing. The choice of one over the other may be made by the pharmacist or left to the discretion of the purchasing agent.

With regard to bid purchasing, a word of caution needs to be interjected. If the bids for drugs are released to a select group of reputable manufacturers, then the lowest bidder should receive the purchase order and the hospital may be assured of receiving first-quality merchandise. If, on the other hand, the bids are released to all vendors requesting them, the lowest price does not always mean quality merchandise. Therefore, if this type of bid release program is to be employed, it is strongly recommended that some arrangement be made for the analytical and clinical testing of samples of the product. This testing program may be carried out by a local laboratory or by the hospital.

In addition to the above, the hospital pharmacist should, in collaboration with the purchasing agent, assume the following duties:

1. maintain a list of the names, addresses and telephone numbers of drug manufacturers, wholesalers, and their local representatives
2. prepare detailed specifications for drugs, chemicals and biologicals
3. prepare Request for Purchase Forms
4. prepare Receiving Memo if drugs are received directly by the pharmacy
5. prepare Return Goods Memo, whenever applicable.

With regard to the development of drug specifications, the hospital pharmacist should make liberal use of the latest editions of the *United States Pharmacopeia*, the *National Formulary* and their supplements.

6

These compendia are officially referred to as the "U.S.P." and the "N.F."

Purchasing Procedure

The plan of purchasing procedures herein described assumes that there exists in the hospital a qualified pharmacist and a hospital purchasing agent who have been instructed to cooperate in the purchasing of pharmaceuticals and allied products. The plan further assumes that specifications have been drawn and that all supplies ordered will be received and stored either in the pharmacy or in a storeroom exclusively controlled by the pharmacist.

The pharmacist, or a person authorized by him, should complete a **Purchase Request Form** (Fig. 29) for the product desired. Drugs coming from the same vendor may be grouped upon a single form. This form provides the purchasing department with data concerning the description, specification, packaging, price, quantity needed as well as information concerning the inventory balance and anticipated monthly use. In addition, this form also is the source document for information which is of importance to the accounting office, namely the cost center to be charged and the discount which may or may not be earned upon payment for the merchandise. The original of this form should be forwarded to the administrative officer responsible for the department. Upon his approval, the form is then forwarded to the purchasing agent. The copy is retained by the pharmacist as a record of the fact that the merchandise is in the process of being procured.

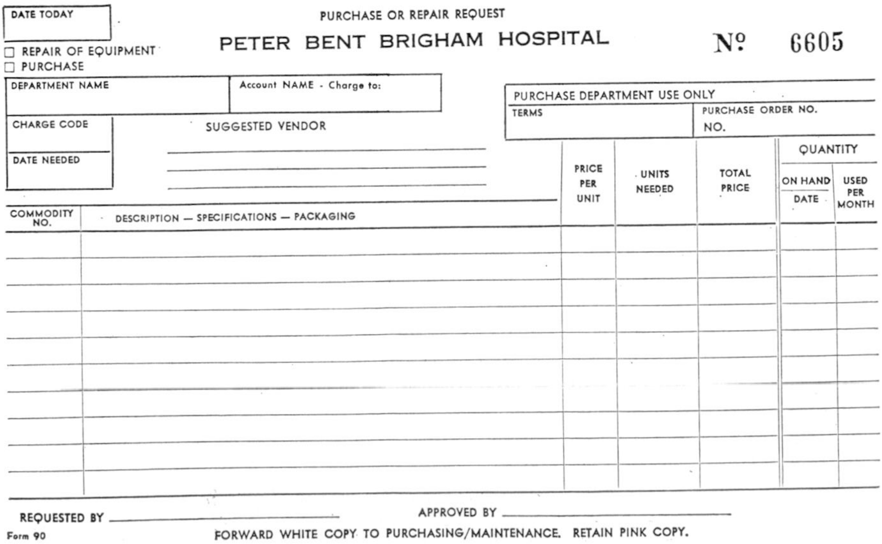
DATE TODAY

PURCHASE OR REPAIR REQUEST

PETER BENT BRIGHAM HOSPITAL

№ 6605

☐ REPAIR OF EQUIPMENT
☐ PURCHASE

DEPARTMENT NAME

Account NAME - Charge to:

PURCHASE DEPARTMENT USE ONLY

TERMS

PURCHASE ORDER NO.
NO.

CHARGE CODE

SUGGESTED VENDOR

DATE NEEDED

COMMODITY NO.	DESCRIPTION — SPECIFICATIONS — PACKAGING	PRICE PER UNIT	UNITS NEEDED	TOTAL PRICE	QUANTITY ON HAND / DATE	QUANTITY USED PER MONTH

REQUESTED BY ____________ APPROVED BY ____________

Form 90

FORWARD WHITE COPY TO PURCHASING/MAINTENANCE. RETAIN PINK COPY.

FIG. 29. Purchase Request Form.

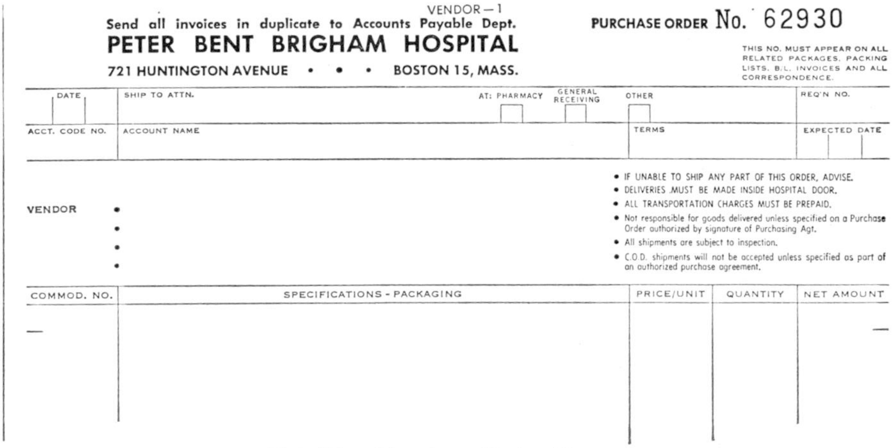
VENDOR—1

Send all invoices in duplicate to Accounts Payable Dept.

PETER BENT BRIGHAM HOSPITAL

721 HUNTINGTON AVENUE • • • BOSTON 15, MASS.

PURCHASE ORDER No. 62930

THIS NO. MUST APPEAR ON ALL RELATED PACKAGES, PACKING LISTS, B/L, INVOICES AND ALL CORRESPONDENCE.

DATE	SHIP TO ATTN.	AT: PHARMACY	GENERAL RECEIVING	OTHER	REQ'N NO.
ACCT. CODE NO.	ACCOUNT NAME			TERMS	EXPECTED DATE

VENDOR

- IF UNABLE TO SHIP ANY PART OF THIS ORDER, ADVISE.
- DELIVERIES MUST BE MADE INSIDE HOSPITAL DOOR.
- ALL TRANSPORTATION CHARGES MUST BE PREPAID.
- Not responsible for goods delivered unless specified on a Purchase Order authorized by signature of Purchasing Agt.
- All shipments are subject to inspection.
- C.O.D. shipments will not be accepted unless specified as part of an authorized purchase agreement.

COMMOD. NO.	SPECIFICATIONS - PACKAGING	PRICE/UNIT	QUANTITY	NET AMOUNT

FIG. 30. Purchase Order Form.

Upon the receipt of the approved Purchase Request, the purchasing agent should then prepare the official **Purchase Order** (Fig. 30). This form utilizes the data from the source document, the Purchase Request. The purchase order may take the form of any number of different types—it may consist of a two-page or a many page snap-out form. The majority of institutions prefer the multi copy snap-out form since it provides a copy for the vendor, accounts payable department of the hospital, purchasing number file, initiating department, two receiving reports and a history copy.

The vendor's copy is either mailed or given to the vendor's representative.

The accounts payable copy is forwarded to the accounting office where it is held until the invoice is received from the vendor and the completed receiving reports from the initiating department. Then and only then may the invoice be processed for payment.

The third copy is retained by the purchasing agent for his "number file." This will serve as a source of information to him whenever a question is raised relative to the issuance of the order.

The fourth copy is returned to the initiating department, in this case, the pharmacy. This copy should be matched with the Request for Purchase to check for accuracy.

Copies 5 and 6 serve as receiving reports and are sent to the receiving department. If the order is received in full, only copy five is required to be completed and forwarded to the accounting office. Should merchandise be back ordered, the second receiving report (copy 6) is utilized.

Copy 7 is known as the history copy and is retained by the purchasing agent for use in ascertaining rates of use, etc.

Some hospitals prefer to use a separate purchase order form and a separate Receiving Notice. The disadvantage in the use of this system is that the individual receiving the merchandise must record by hand the name of each item. This may cause error and, if rushed by the load of work, a delay in receiving the completed memo in the accounting office, thereby causing a loss of the discount for prompt payment.

This form also provides for copies for the accounting department, purchasing agent, initiating department, and storeroom files.

Whenever merchandise that has been received by the hospital is to be returned to the vendor for any cause, a Returned Goods Memorandum must be prepared for it is by this means that the hospital can be assured of receiving credit for the merchandise. This form is of the snap-out type and provides for copies for the accounting department, purchasing agent, storeroom, initiating department and the vendor.

Once the merchandise is received, it is the duty of the pharmacist to record upon a **Purchase Record** (Fig. 31) the transaction for each item purchased. By so doing, he will have available a source of reference for determining rate of use, cost of drug, source, etc. Some pharmacists feel that this card should be maintained by the purchasing agent and made available to them whenever necessary. Whichever way the situation is to be handled is irrelevant so long as the card is prepared and kept up to date. The final decision as to whose responsibility it is rests with the desires of the administrator.

On occasion, merchandise may be ordered from the pharmacy at a time when it is out of stock. This may happen quite frequently in pharmacy departments handling surgical and laboratory supplies as well as drugs. When this happens, an **Out-of-Stock Form** (see Chapter 15, Fig. 65) should be prepared in duplicate and one copy sent to the initiating pavilion or laboratory. The other copy is retained in the pharmacy. This form serves a dual purpose in that it speeds the delivery of merchandise to the floor upon its arrival and it prevents the pavilion or laboratory from reordering and creating a false sense of heavy demand which could result in over ordering by the pharmacy.

No.	VENDOR	No.	VENDOR	No.	VENDOR	No.	VENDOR
1		4		7		10	
2		5		8		11	
3		6		9		12	

Mo.	Yr.	Ven.	Ordered Quantity	Dept.	Price Per	Total Cost	RATE OF USE			
							From	To	Months	

FIG. 31.   A sample of a Purchase Record Form.

Controls on Purchases

Many administrators attempt to exercise a power of control over the volume of purchases by the pharmacist by placing a dollar limitation on the purchase order. This method is archaic and is easily circumvented by the issuance of multiple small orders which in the long run is more costly for the hospital.

A more modern and reliable means is the *computation* of *inventory turnover*. Inventory turnover is computed by dividing the cost of goods sold during the fiscal period by the average of opening and closing inventories. This gives the number of times the inventory has been "turned" during the fiscal period.[5]

A low turnover indicates:

1. duplication of stock
2. large purchases of slow-moving items
3. dead inventory.

A high turnover of inventory may be due to small volume purchasing which is indicative of a failure to take advantage of maximum quantity discounts.

A turnover of four times a year is considered satisfactory for most institutions. However, those in short supply of cash reserves may wish to increase their turnover rate to six times a year. This is a policy decision and should be arrived at by discussion with the administrator.

Hospital pharmacists might well try to control purchase volume and inventory by the use of the EOQ (Economic Order Quantity) and RQL (Reorder Quantity Level).

The RQL is stated to be the inventory level that must be reached before additional stock can be ordered. Ideally, the remaining inventory should be almost depleted before the arrival of the new shipment. Obviously, zero stock level must be avoided because it can cause serious problems. This can usually be avoided by building into the system safety factors for various vendor lead times. Sapp[7] makes utilization of the following table:

SAFETY FACTORS FOR VARIOUS VENDOR LEAD TIMES

Vendor Lead Time (VLT)	Safety Factor
0 to 2 weeks	1.0
2 to 5 weeks	1.5
5 to 8 weeks	2.0
8 to 11 weeks	2.5
11 to 15 weeks	3.0

To determine the RQ, divide the **average usage** rate per month in units of issue (AU) by thirteen weeks; then multiply this figure by the average **vendor lead time** (VLT) plus the safety factor.

In the application of the above formula, Sapp[7] stresses the following points:

(1) Unanticipated large increases in usage.
(2) Shelf life of the items involved.
(3) Unusual delays in delivery caused by strikes or storms.
(4) Necessity for rechecking the RQL periodically to allow for a change in usage rate.

The determination of how much to order is the EOQ factor. In determining the EOQ factor it is important to ascertain the *cost* of *ordering* and the *cost* of *carrying inventory*.

The following must be considered in arriving at the *cost* of *ordering*:[7]

(1) All labor in purchasing except the purchasing manager.
(2) The labor cost in supporting areas such as the stockroom, receiving and material control.
(3) The cost applicable to payment of invoices generated by the purchasing section should apply to ordering cost.
(4) Cost of general operating supplies such as pencils, paper, forms etc.
(5) Freight and telephone costs.

After all of the above are applied to total cost, divide the resulting figure by the total number of purchase orders to obtain the *ordering costs* in *dollars per order*. Ordering cost per order can vary from $5.00 to $8.00.

To determine carrying charges consideration must be given to the following:[7]

(1) Interest on the dollar value of the inventory.
(2) Space charge (rent) for the storage area.
(3) Labor costs for storage operations.
(4) Cost of supplies for storage operations.
(5) Insurance.
(6) Taxes (if applicable).
(7) Obsolescence.
(8) Deterioration.
(9) Pilferage.

Dividing the value of the inventory by the total of the above costs results in the *inventory holding* or *carrying cost*. In general, carrying charges may range from 18 to 30 per cent.

Thus the formula for determining Economic Order Quantity is the following:

$$EOQ = \sqrt{\frac{2 \times 12 \times \text{monthly usage} \times \text{cost of ordering}}{\text{Unit cost} \times \text{Holding Cost}}}$$

On the basis of the above equation, purchasing agents have developed monographs to simplify figuring the EOQ.

Quality of Drugs

As has been stated above, the pharmacist should draw freely upon the specifications detailed in the *United States Pharmacopeia,* the *National Formulary* and their supplements.

Both the U.S.P. and the N.F. are designated as official compendia by the terms of the Federal Food and Drug Law and the Federal Food, Drug, and Cosmetic Act.

The *Pharmacopeia* and the *National Formulary* render "a distinct service to pharmacists and pharmaceutical manufacturers by providing specifications for the procurement of drugs used in dispensing, prescription compounding, and manufacturing, and supplying formulas and working directions for the preparation of dosage forms."[6]

During recent years, there has been a move towards the acceptance and use of the initials A.R.B. (Any Reliable Brand). Certainly, if there exists a situation where the prescriber believes in the use of these initials, well and good; however, these symbols should never be used by a hospital pharmacist or a hospital purchasing agent as a specification for quality merchandise. What one individual considers to be "reliable" may often times be far from the truth. If any symbols are to be used as a means of specification then those of U.S.P. and N.F. are the safest and most reliable.

Oftentimes a hospital pharmacist may desire assistance in the selection of a product for use by the hospital. If the hospital has an active Pharmacy and Therapeutics Committee, this committee may serve as an advisor to the pharmacist. Because of the background and experience of the membership, it behooves the hospital pharmacist to give a great deal of weight to their suggestions.

Certain very large hospitals in this country feel that it is more economical to purchase drugs from manufacturers who might not be listed in the "Class A group." The consensus being that since these small firms do not have to support expensive research and large sales staffs, the savings can be passed along to the purchaser. This premise can be dangerous and should not be followed unless the hospital is in a position to establish a small control laboratory for the purpose of analyzing products purchased from these firms. Oftentimes the cost of operating such a laboratory will far exceed the cost of purchasing under tight specifications from a reliable manufacturer.

Some pharmacists utilize a *Qualified Suppliers List* which is based upon their personal knowledge and experience with the manufacturer and his products.[9]

Other pharmacists make use of a *Suppliers Application Form* to obtain information about prospective suppliers. The information requested includes the company's annual sales, a list of other accounts, the number of employees, type of operation, description of quality control procedures and the company's location and facilities. The use of this form is stated to discourage marginal suppliers and serves as a screening technique for the hospital pharmacist.[8]

Discounts

There are three ways in which merchandise may be purchased at a discount or savings: (1) volume contract, (2) "deals," and (3) discounts.

Volume contracts are usually offered by a majority of the manufacturers and include contracts to cover total purchases of parenteral solutions, ampoules, tablets or even gallon goods. Under this system, the institution approximates its annual consumption of the particular class of product and signs an agreement with the company to purchase this amount. At the end of the contract period, usually a year, if the goal has been reached, the manufacturer will issue a rebate check based on a percentage of the value of the total purchase. A hidden benefit of this type of purchase is the fact that the contract price is usually protected from an increase yet any reduction in price is passed on to the hospital.

"Deals" represent that type of transaction that involves the purchase of a specified volume and receiving certain merchandise at no additional cost (*e.g.* "Three free with the purchase of a dozen"). There is nothing wrong with this type of purchase if the "free goods" remain in the pharmacy inventory. In order that the inventory not be understated, the entry into the hospital inventory accounts should indicate that fifteen units were received for the price paid.

"Deals" which are created by the representative and the pharmacist without the full sanction of the manufacturer should be either avoided or carefully scrutinized by the Administrator or Comptroller since these offer a great temptation for dishonesty.

Discounts may accrue to the institution for the prompt payment of its drug bills. Because of the large volume of drug consumption, these discounts amount to a sizeable sum of money at the end of a year.

Other types of discounts are also available from the manufacturers, *e.g.* discounts to government institutions or to educational institutions. Obviously, the hospital pharmacist should immediately investigate the discount policy of every new firm with which he deals.

Central Storage vs. Pharmacy Storage

The dichotomous storage arrangements of supplies is prevalent in many hospitals, although it is common knowledge that central storage is ideal.

The proponents of centralized storage facilities are quick to demonstrate the reduction in labor and record keeping, as well as the tight control afforded by centralization.

In contrast, it should be pointed out that the responsibility for the storage of drugs should be placed with competent individuals who have been educated, trained and licensed to handle pharmaceuticals. These individuals are the pharmacists.

In order that the pharmacist may properly supervise the storage of drugs, they should be stored in an area directly under his control. This allows him the freedom of stock arrangement, instituting of inventory controls, the adjustment of inventory based upon his knowledge of the prescribing trends of the staff and the preparation of inventory cost reports to management.

Therefore, all merchandise ordered by or for the pharmacy should be shipped directly to the pharmacy receiving area. Should the merchandise be received by the hospital post office or central storeroom, it should immediately be forwarded to the pharmacy in the unopened state.

Upon the receipt of the merchandise in the pharmacy receiving area, the department personnel then process it in the routine manner, namely, checking the receiving slip with the copy of the purchase order and preparing a receiving memorandum.

Storeroom Arrangement

There is no definite rule specifying how a pharmacy storeroom should be arranged. Each individual may so arrange the area to meet both his and the institution's needs.

In general hospitals handling a variety of supplies, the storeroom is divided into the following areas:

1. Alcohol and Liquors
2. Capsules and Tablets
3. Chemicals
4. Gallon Goods
5. Narcotic Vault
6. Ointments
7. Biologicals and other cold room inventory
8. Laboratory Supplies
9. Surgical Instruments
10. Rubber Goods
11. Sutures
12. Medical and Surgical Supplies

Alphabetical arrangement is followed, where possible, within the section. Each shelf, drawer, or bin within the section is numbered to facilitate location of the item during the taking of a physical inventory as well as to locate the item for new personnel.

"Shelf-Stripping" and "Floor Marking"

"Shelf-stripping" consists of applying a strip of tape to the front run of the shelf and marking upon it pertinent information relative to the product being stored. The usual information placed on the tape consists of the name and strength of the product, unit size, maximum level and minimal level, the re-order point being the minimal level.

Where adequate funds are available plastic or metallic strips may be applied to the shelving which will permit the insertion of a card bearing the essential data.

Another means of accomplishing the same goal is to attach the data card to the wooden shelf by means of a thumbtack or stapler.

"Floor-marking" consists of preparing a stencil with the necessary information and painting it on the storeroom floor. This is best done on concrete or wooden floors. In areas where the floor is tiled or marking the floor is not desirable, a good quality tape with adherability may be employed.

By so marking and identifying the storage areas, one provides a definite space for the storage of a particular product, induces orderliness and provides another means of checking inventory to prevent shortages.

Marking of Merchandise

Management consultants all agree that money invested in drug inventories should have a turnover of four to five times a year. A turnover of less than four indicates overstocking and a turnover of more than five may indicate understocking.

One means of sound inventory control is to date and price each item when it is received into inventory. This may be accomplished by the utilization of a marking machine to print small adhesive-backed tags that contain the following information: date received, cost price, and the selling price.

The date is placed on the first line and consists of the month and year. This is usually numerically indicated as "6/65."

The second line represents the cost price of the particular unit. This figure is usually coded in order to preserve confidential price quotations. This figure is of great value in institutions where supplies are sent to areas at cost for it enables the dispensing pharmacist to immediately price the charge slips. In addition, the availability of this figure is of great value in taking and pricing a physical inventory.

The third line represents the retail price to the patient. By placing this figure on the tag, it is possible to save a great deal of time by having the dispensing pharmacist price the charge ticket without having to refer to a charge or rate book.

Control of Dated or Perishable Inventory

Dated inventory such as biologicals or antibiotics requires special control in order to insure potency at the time of dispensing and to be sure that the pharmacy is not carrying in inventory worthless stock.

This can be accomplished by the use of a form such as the **Record of Dated Pharmaceuticals** (Fig. 32).

Each dated product is entered on this sheet which provides the name of the product, the date of purchase, the manufacturer, the control number and the expiration date. By placing a check mark in the box of the appropriate month, the pharmacist can tell at a glance which product is expiring and should be replaced or returned for credit.

Some pharmacists prepare a separate sheet for each dated product. This modified sheet eliminates the need of re-writing the name of the product each time it is purchased. The remaining information and format remains the same.

Taking of a Physical Inventory

The taking of a total physical inventory in the pharmacy is usually required by the auditing firm employed to audit the hospital's fiscal operation. Since the pharmacy inventory usually is the largest in dollar value, it receives a great deal of attention.

HOSPITAL PHARMACY
RECORD OF DATED PHARMACEUTICALS

PRODUCT	DATE OF PURCHASE	MFG.	CONTROL NUMBER	1	2	3	4	5	6	7	8	9	10	11	12	MISC.
										1965						

Fig. 32

On the other hand, some auditing firms will require only a spot check type of inventory on 10 or 20 per cent of the high-cost, fast-moving items.

The actual taking of a physical inventory cannot be undertaken without a great deal of planning and attention to detail. Anything less than one's maximum effort will lead to a faulty inventory and thus to a repeat performance.

Approximately two months before the taking of an inventory, the pharmacist should review his stock and remove from it all merchandise which has not moved since the last inventory. In addition, any merchandise should be removed which has been purchased during the year but has not moved appreciably during the preceding three months. These items should be returned for credit whenever possible; if such a move is not feasible, they should be written off the inventory via an adjustment in the books of account in the business office.

Once this has been accomplished, the inventory should be recorded on the inventory sheets. This recording should consist of only the name of the item, its strength, or other identification. The sheets upon which the recording is to take place should be in duplicate, and should have proper spaces to show the date, location, recorder and caller. (See Fig. 33.)

The actual taking of the inventory may start at the close of a business day or at a time when there is no movement of merchandise. At this time the pharmacy staff and its helpers may arrange themselves

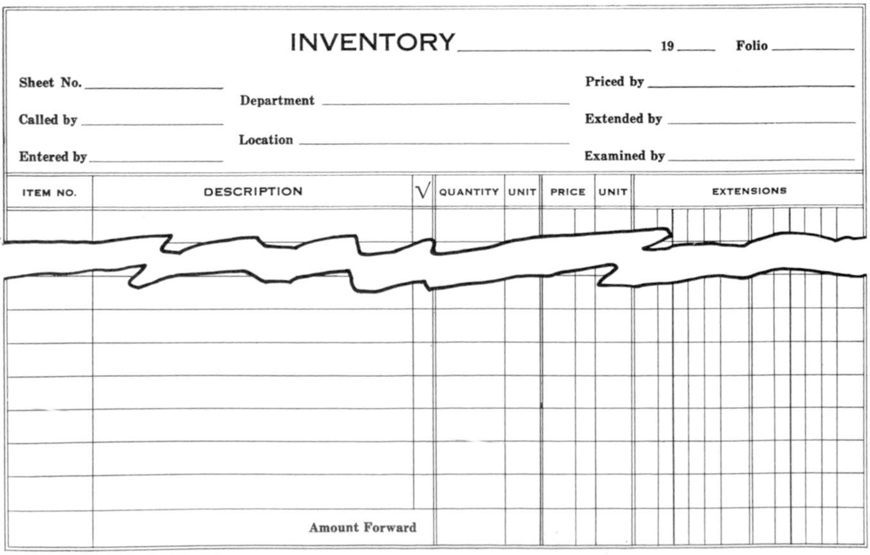

INVENTORY ____________ 19____ Folio ________

Sheet No. ________ Department ________ Priced by ________

Called by ________ Location ________ Extended by ________

Entered by ________ Examined by ________

ITEM NO.	DESCRIPTION	√	QUANTITY	UNIT	PRICE	UNIT	EXTENSIONS
	Amount Forward						

FIG. 33. Sample form for the recording of the inventory.

into teams of two—one to record and the other to call out the name of the item, price, and count. As each sheet is completed, it is handed to the auditor supervising the inventory. It is the prerogative of the supervising auditor as to how many entries he wishes to check out. The usual procedure is to check all large dollar volume items and to random check the less valuable entries.

At the close of the inventory, the sheets may be turned over to the comptroller for extension, or this operation may be delegated to the pharmacist.

Any merchandise ordered prior to the date of inventory and received on the day of inventory or shortly thereafter need not be counted. The invoices pertaining to these purchases should be clearly marked with the fact that they were received "post inventory." The accounting office will make the appropriate adjustment in the final inventory figure to account for this merchandise.

The Perpetual Inventory

The maintaining of a perpetual inventory is, of course, an ideal situation if the record-keeping can be kept up to date. In many small hospital pharmacies, the pharmacist, at the end of each day, summarizes all drug charge slips and makes the proper posting in the perpetual inventory file. The process of tabulation may be accomplished by either the pegboard method or the use of punched cards.

The pegboard method merely requires a pegboard and requisition forms with holes evenly spaced and punched along the top. The forms are then aligned on the board so that the first sheet is entirely visible and subsequent sheets covering all but the section showing the quantities ordered. The forms are then summarized across into one master requisition form which is used for posting the inventory records.

The larger and more complex operations require mechanized equipment such as that provided by the International Business Machine Corporation or the Remington Rand Corporation. The basic operations performed on this specialized equipment are key punching, verifying, sorting, collating, interpreting, calculating, tabulating and reproducing. These systems may utilize a punched card whereby the data are punched in the various fields in the body of the card.

By using this type of system it is possible to have purchase orders, receiving reports and disbursement requisitions forwarded to the tabulating department daily, where transaction cards are punched. These cards are then fed into calculators and tabulators which issue a comprehensive stock status report. This report may be produced on a daily, weekly or monthly basis.

The latest and most sophisticated system for electronic data processing is the computer.

With one of these systems, a hospital can readily obtain a record of all inventory items, and their balances in quantity and dollar value is maintained. Using item numbers already in use, the inventory record can show the following:

1. item number	6. disbursements
2. description	7. vendor number
3. unit size	8. price
4. quantity on hand	9. general ledger number
5. receipts	

The installation of either of these mechanized systems is highly technical as well as costly and therefore the institutional officers, comptroller and pharmacist should avail themselves of the counsel and advice of the various reputable manufacturers or consulting services before embarking upon such a program.

Materials Management

To this point, purchasing and inventory control have been discussed from the viewpoint of the department of pharmacy—that is, complete control over the drugs by the pharmacist from purchase to disposition. In the operation of a modern hospital, it is still possible to provide the control feature even though part of the responsibility may rest in another person—the Director of Materials Management. In some hospitals, the Department of Materials Management has operational responsibility over purchasing, receiving, inventories, print shop, central sterile supply, laundry, distribution, messenger service, traffic and disposal activities.

Simply defined, materials management encompasses all materials and their movement from point of origin to point of use, and then to their final breakdown back into the environment.[9]

In those hospitals utilizing the materials management concept, it is not uncommon to find that the hospital pharmacist plays an important role in developing the program associated with the acquisition, storage, distribution and disposition of biologicals, radioisotopes, drugs and chemicals.

SELECTED REFERENCES

SCHMID, F. W. and KAHN, S.: Pharmacist-Purchasing Agent: A Case Study, Hospitals, *34*:60, July 1, 1960.

AMICARELLA, H.: Pharmacist Makes a Good Purchasing Agent, Modern Hosp., *94*:6:128, 1960.

CARLIN, H. S. and FLACK, H. L.:   Pharmacists' Increased Responsibilities for Purchasing Under the Formulary System, Hosp. Management, 88:1:48, 1959.

SMITH, J. E. and STARR, EILEEN: Electronic Data Processing Applications in Hospital Pharmacy, 1:2:26, 1966.

D'AMBOLA, JOSEPH V.: A Drug Inventory and Purchase System, Hospital Pharmacy, 1:6:11, 1966.

BLAKE, MARTIN I.: Role of the Compendia in Controlling Factors Affecting Bioavailability of Drug Products, J.A.Ph.A., NS11:11:603, November, 1967.

HEARD, JACK S.: Your Role as Purchaser is Important, Hospital Pharmacy, 6:4:12, April, 1971.

DOYLE, JOHN: EOQ Plus ABC Equals Better Purchasing, Health Institution Purchasing, 2:3:19, October, 1971.

WINTERS, B. H. and HERNANDEZ, L.: A Computerized Drug Inventory Control System, Am. J. Hosp. Pharm., 29:9:780, September, 1972.

BIBLIOGRAPHY

1. HASSAN, WILLIAM E., JR.:   Purchase and Inventory Control of Pharmaceuticals, Hospital Progress, October, 1958.

2. MACEACHERN, MALCOLM, T.:   *Hospital Organization and Management,* 3rd Ed. Chicago, Physicians' Record Co., 1957.

3. Minimum Standard for Pharmacies in Hospitals, Am. J. Hosp. Pharm., 15: 11:992, 1958.

4. FRANCKE, D. E.:   Editorial, Am. J. Hosp. Pharm., 13:2:107, 1956.

5. BOWLES, G. C., JR.:   Consulting with Bowles, Am. J. Hosp. Pharm., 15: 9:818, 1958.

6. *The National Formulary,* 12th Ed., Easton, Mack Printing Co., 1965.

7. SAPP, DONALD E.: How We Use EOQ and RLQ for Better Inventory Control, Health Institution Purchasing, 2:3:24, October, 1971.

8. DRAKE, CHARLES E. and KABAT, HUGH F.: A Quality Assurance Program for Pharmaceutical Purchases, J.A.Ph.A., NS11:11:612, November, 1971.

9. MILLER, JAMES G.: Materials Management: Some Guidelines, Hospital Care, 3:3:17, November 1972.

Chapter

10

Detailman-Pharmacist Relationship

EACH year the pharmaceutical industry budgets millions of dollars for the purpose of promoting their products. A sizeable portion of this allocation is devoted to providing the profession with well-trained detailmen or medical service representatives. One of the duties of these people is to carry on a large-scale educational program relative to the use of the latest therapeutic agents. This is usually achieved in hospitals through the media of drug exhibits and "detailing" of the chief of the pharmacy service and physicians.[1]

In a recent survey, it was shown that 92 per cent of the physicians interviewed stated that they saw "some" or "all" detailmen.[2] Of interest to the hospital pharmacist is the further statistic that in answer to the question—Has the Detailman's Contribution Increased or Lessened in the Past Five Years?—30 physicians answered "increased," 29 answered "lessened" and 28 answered "same."[2]

By the same token, there must be rapport between the pharmacist and the detailman. That this does not always exist is supported by such derogatory opinions as—"nothing but order takers"; "detailmen have generally poor attitude"; and "not told what is being detailed."[3]

Although it behooves the manufacturer to exercise extreme care in the selection of his field representative, it is imperative that the hospital pharmacist develop appropriate rapport with the detailman in order that the hospital and medical staff might benefit from his specialized knowledge.

Hospital displays are desirable since they offer a convenient means of contacting a large number of staff physicians in a minimal amount of time. Furthermore, there is, by this approach, a saving of the physician's valuable time when compared to an office visit by the same medical representative.

Many hospital administrators frown upon drug exhibits on the grounds that they promote an aura of commercialism in an otherwise highly professional atmosphere. To avoid the "taunt of commercialism," it behooves the hospital pharmacist to develop basic policies for the conduct of detailmen within the hospital and guiding principles for scheduling drug exhibits.

Appointments

In order to carry on a successful professional relations program and to service hospital inventory requirements, it is necessary for the manufacturer's representatives to make periodic visits to the pharmacy. Faced with a heavy work-load, a shortage of staff, or an unforeseen event, the pharmacist is prone to dismiss him with an "I'll see you the next time around." In other instances, the visit of the detailman is taken too lightly and the time devoted to the interview is rapidly utilized with needless "chit-chat."

After consideration of the above, it should be clear that the direct loser is the hospital pharmacist and the indirect loss is shared by the entire hospital staff. The hospital pharmacist must avail himself of the opportunity to draw upon the specialized knowledge of the detailman.

There are many ways in which this can be accomplished. Those most commonly employed are to arrange the detailman's visit on an "appointment only" basis, the use of a product information sheet, and the development of a controlled method of allowing demonstration and sales promotional displays within the hospital.

While it is relatively easy for the pharmacist to schedule appointments, it may place an undue hardship upon the detailman unless the scheduling is given some forethought.

One method of scheduling appointments is to divide the list of detailmen into three categories: (1) Those on a monthly basis, (2) Those on a bi-weekly basis, and (3) Those to be interviewed whenever they are in the territory.

For each representative in categories 1 and 2, a definite time should be assigned which coincides with the hours he expects to be in the particular section of the community in which the hospital is located. Once the schedule is established, it behooves each party to be prompt, and when necessary to cancel the appointment in advance.

Representatives in the third category must realize that they are being accorded a special privilege. They, therefore, have special obligations which are relatively simple. These entail the courtesy of notifying the pharmacist in advance of the approximate date and hour of the intended visit, and, conversely, the pharmacist should inform the representative of his ability to keep the appointment. Either of the above can be easily accomplished by postcard or telephone.

Proper Utilization of Appointment Time

Having established the routine for visitation, the pharmacist should use the time to best advantage. The nature of the division of time and the topics to be discussed rests with the pharmacist. As a guide, the allocated time may be divided into two units: (1) to discuss inventory needs, and (2) new products. It is in connection with the latter that the greatest amount of time can be saved. This can be accomplished through the use of a *Product Information Sheet* (Fig. 34). The required information can be recorded by the pharmacist while he is being "detailed" by the representative. Since the data on the sheet are con-

PRODUCT INFORMATION SHEET

Name _____   Mfg. _____

Generic Name _____

Chemical Name _____

Synonyms _____   _____   _____

Composition (if a combination)   Therapeutic Uses

_____   _____   _____

_____   _____   _____

_____   _____   _____

_____   _____   _____

_____   _____

Contraindications and Cautions   Toxicology and Antidote

_____   _____

_____   _____

_____   _____

Dosage and Administration   Forms Available   Similar Products

_____   _____   _____

_____   _____   _____

_____   _____   _____

Package Sizes and Prices   Literature   ____Yes ____No

_____   _____   Samples   ____Yes ____No

_____   _____   Date:_____

This Space Reserved for Pharmacy and Therapeutics Committee.

FIG. 34

cise, it serves as a valuable quick reference for pharmacists and medical staff. It may also serve the worthy purpose of providing the members of the Pharmacy and Therapeutics Committee with an "abstract" of a new product.

Promotional Displays

The sponsoring of sales promotional displays within the hospital by pharmaceutical and medical supply representatives can be an interesting and worthwhile venture if properly controlled and supervised. One way to regulate these exhibits is to prepare a set of guiding principles governing displays; develop an application form which requests permission to conduct an exhibit; and finally place the total responsibility for the notification of the clinical and nursing staff of the exhibit as well as the supervision of the display upon the hospital pharmacist.

The rules for conducting the exhibit may vary with each institution, therefore, the following guiding principles are suggested as a model:

1. Demonstration and sales promotional displays by pharmaceutical and hospital supply representatives may be arranged by completing and having approved the "Request for Display Form" available from the pharmacy.
2. Displays or exhibits, for which application is made in the pharmacy, must be of a professional and ethical nature and must be related to hospital function.
3. All displays, not to exceed one per week, are presented in the staff room. Special group meetings, including film presentations, require arrangement through the executive offices.
4. Sales representatives and exhibitors are not permitted entrance to the various hospital departments without administrative approval: this includes the clinics, nursing stations, pavilions and operating suite.
5. Exhibitors must remain by their displays, and shall not solicit orders or approach persons who do not wish to view the displays.
6. Distribution of advertising in the form of samples and brochures must be confined to the display area, and only during the time reserved for the display or exhibit. Distribution of prescription legend items is allowed to physicians only.
7. Notices of any kind are not to be posted throughout the hospital by an exhibitor.
8. Displays and exhibits of each supplier are limited to two annually, and each to one-half day from 9:00 a.m. to 1:00 p.m.

9. Pharmaceutical products to be displayed are limited to those officially included in the latest revisions and supplements of the hospital formulary or those products accepted by the therapeutics committee for clinical trial in the hospital.
10. Representatives should have available a supply of reprints of clinical studies by qualified investigators on each product displayed.

The Request for Display forms (Fig. 35) should always be used because they serve a number of valuable control purposes. From the completed form, the pharmacist may determine exactly what is to be displayed and who is going to conduct the exhibit. In addition, reference to the copy of the Request for Display form will enable the pharmacist to determine whether or not the display of any particular product coincided with its increased use; the frequency of displays by any particular firm; and the frequency which an individual therapeutic category was featured.

REQUEST FOR DISPLAY

I, (We) do hereby agree to abide by the rules and regulations covering displays in the hospital, and request the following date to feature the items listed below in a display.

Date of Application:_____

Company:_____

Representative(s) Covering Display:_____

_____

_____

Display Date Requested:

    1st Choice_____   2nd Choice_____

Do You Need Display Equipment?   _____Yes   _____No

Products to be Displayed:

_____   _____   _____

_____   _____   _____

Display Approved By_____ Date:_____
Please prepare in duplicate. Return *both* copies to the Pharmacy. The approved copy will be returned to you and is your authorization to conduct the display.

FIG. 35

Once the display is scheduled, the pharmacist should notify all clinical and nursing personnel of the date, hour and products to be exhibited. This notification can be accomplished in any number of ways.

1. General memo to clinical and nursing staffs.
2. Posting of a list of displays for the month or season in the Nursing Office and Staff Room.
3. Publication of the display dates in the Pharmacy Bulletin.
4. Specific letter to the Chief-of-Staff and to the Director of Nursing.

On occasion, the question arises as to whether or not the hospital should charge the manufacturer for the right to conduct displays on the hospital premises. The argument advanced is that a certain amount of administrative time is utilized in the scheduling and announcing of displays; guard services are utilized to deter unauthorized personnel or visitors from entering the display area; parking facilities are utilized; and hospital equipment such as tables or small trucks are used by the representative.

There is no single answer to the question. Certainly the above reasons are valid and if it is the policy of the hospital to rent space for various functions, then a rental for a pharmaceutical display is warranted. On the other hand, the donation of the above services and the space for a display provides a return to the hospital in the form of a well-informed staff on the latest developments in pharmacology and therapeutics.[1]

Control of Drug Samples

HOSPITAL mail rooms are deluged with drug samples. Often these samples are addressed to doctors no longer on the staff, and unfortunately the samples are often carelessly handled by the mail room personnel or the physician himself. It should be clear that any unsolicited drug sample entrusted to the general mail has a good chance of being discarded by the physician in such a manner that it unintentionally creates a hazard.

The hazard can be of many different types. (1) By disposing of the drug material into a wastebasket, it becomes readily available to cleaning personnel who may salvage it for the purpose of self-medication or for the illegitimate drug traffic. (2) Improper disposition of the baskets may mean that they could fall into the hands of children with disastrous results and (3) if incinerated by housekeeping personnel an explosion hazard is incurred, particularly if many vials or sealed containers of various drugs have been discarded.

Definition

The words "drug sample" would appear to be clearly self-explanatory, however, in order that there be no misunderstanding, the following definition is presented.

A drug sample may be considered as any quantity of any form of a chemical, drug or drug product which is made available by the manufacturer to an individual legally qualified to receive it. It makes no difference whether the drug is made available in an original trade package, or in a clearly identifiable sample package.

Use of Samples in the Hospital

Any discussion governing the use of drug samples must, of necessity, be divided into two parts—their use by the hospital and secondly, the use of samples by the manufacturer or his representative.

The use of drug samples in the hospital may be as varied as the imagination of the pharmacist in charge. One type of program that falls into this category and is worthy of mention is the pharmacist and the student nurse association "adopt" a hospital located in some remote part of the world and undertake to accumulate and ship the samples to its medical staff for distribution to their indigent patients.

In some hospitals, sample drugs are used in the care of the intern and resident staff as well as the students enrolled in the various nursing, dietary or technician training programs.

One pharmacist has gone on record[4] as recommending the availability of drug samples as a means of inducing widespread clinical use. Another[5] has described a method whereby drug samples are utilized in the care of the indigent ill irrespective of whether they were ambulatory clinic patients or admitted to the hospital.

Insofar as the manufacturer is concerned, drug samples are used as a means of introducing the physician to a new product and to induce him to try it clinically.

Use of Samples in Competitive Buying

Some manufacturer's representatives have used drug samples as a means of offsetting the company's higher price for a particular product, especially when competitive prices are lower. Whether or not this is ethical conduct on the part of the medical service representative and the hospital pharmacist is a difficult point to debate. Certainly those pharmacists who do not permit such transactions are to be commended and those who are prone to permit this practice under the guise that they are doing their job—namely, obtaining the best drugs available for the lowest net cost—should be cautioned to make every aspect of the negotiation open to the scrutiny of those in authority lest their individual integrity become the subject of question.

Control of Samples

The best place to control sample distribution in the hospital is at the source of the sample's entry into the institution—the detailman, drug displays and in the mail receiving room.

All detailmen or medical service representatives whether on private calls to physicians in the hospital or conducting displays should be fully informed of the hospital's policy governing the distribution of drug samples. Although a conscientious medical service representative will acquaint himself with the rules, it behooves the hospital pharmacist to call them to the attention of the representatives prior to each display request.

In brief, a good drug sample control policy would dictate that no samples may be left in the clinics, on the pavilions or nursing stations, nor may large quantities be left with physicians for the purpose of being dispensed by him for clinical trial.

Any physician desirous of using sample drugs for clinical trial should arrange to have the material deposited in the pharmacy from whence his prescriptions for the material will be honored. In this case the hospital may or may not collect a small handling fee from the patient.

Furthermore, the policy should also prohibit the distribution of drug products to hospital personnel even though the particular product to be distributed may have an over-the-counter status.

Some manufacturer's have adopted an excellent policy in requiring the physician to write a prescription for the material requested, whereas others do not distribute samples during a display but will mail samples of the requested products directly to the physician.

Mass mailings to physicians in hospitals create problems in drug control, as these samples are or may be carelessly discarded and thereby fall into the wrong hands, or they are easily pilfered while awaiting distribution.

One way of mastering this problem is to have all mass mailings of drugs delivered directly to the pharmacy. Here, under the control of pharmacists, the samples may be sorted and properly stored or, if necessary, adequately destroyed or discarded. Any physician desiring the sample material may obtain a reasonable supply from the pharmacy.

Cataloguing of Drug Samples

Once the packages of drug samples are delivered to the pharmacy, they should be sorted, exterior mailing cartons removed, catalogued and properly stored in a sample section. The pharmacist is reminded that sample drugs, like their purchased counterpart, should not have their control number identification removed as it may be the only means of identifying a particular batch of drug being recalled due to untoward side effects or reactions or possible error in preparation.

The cataloguing procedure should be reasonably detailed and accurate if it is to serve its purpose. The recording may be done on cards for storage in a card file or on punched paper suitable for storage in a binder. Irrespective of the choice, the following data should be recorded for each drug sample received:

(a) Trade Name	(f) Control Number
(b) Generic Name	(g) Expiration Date (if any)
(c) Manufacturer	(h) Date Received
(d) Strength	(i) Quantity Received
(e) *Pharmaceutical Form*	(j) Location: Shelf #_: Drawer #_

Once catalogued and stored, any pharmacist removing a portion or the entire supply of sample must then record on the back of the page or card the following information concerning its disposition:

(a) Date	(c) To Whom
(b) Amount Dispensed	(d) Signature of dispensing pharma-cist.

If the sample material is given to a physician his name is placed in the space after "(c) To whom;" if a patient on a physician's prescription, then the prescription serial number is entered; if to a house patient, his name and hospital number should be entered.

Effect of Samples on Fiscal Operations

Drug samples that are not obtained in the process of competitive buying are not usually considered a part of the pharmacy inventory.

However, if a relatively large volume of sample material is solicited and dispensed from the pharmacy, two obvious results may be immediately noted: (a) there will usually be a reduction in pharmacy income and (b) the volume of purchases will decline. The long range effect will invariably manifest itself by a reduction in the "turn-over rate" of the inventory.

On the other hand, if the drug samples are being dispensed to indigent patients, there should be a corresponding decrease in the the allowances associated with the patient's inability to pay the hospital's bills for drugs.

Both aspects of the effect of the use of large amounts of drug samples on income, inventory and allowances have been briefly presented in order that the pharmacist may be forewarned of these possible repercussions.

Controlled Substances Act of 1970

The Controlled Substances Act of 1970 amends the Federal Food, Drug and Cosmetic Act by placing additional controls over *stimulant and depressant* drugs through increased record keeping and inspection requirements providing control over intrastate traffic in these drugs, and making possession of them illegal except under certain specified conditions. (See Chapter 16.)

SELECTED REFERENCES

TEPLITSKY, B.:   Drug Exhibits in Hospitals, Am. Profess. Pharmacist, *23*:6: 550, 1957.

SR. M. JUNILLA: Delineated Policy for Pharmaceutical Representatives, Bull. Am. Soc. Hosp. Pharm., *13*:1:63, 1956.

MORAVEC, D. F.:   Drug Samples, Hosp. Management, *86*:5:102, 1958.

ZUGICH, J. J.:   Code for Detailing in Hospitals, Am. Profess. Pharmacist, *23*: 11:980, 1957.

PARKER, P. F.:   Detailing in the Hospital, J. Am. Pharm. Assoc. Pract. Pharm. Ed., *18*:4:217, 1957.

JEFFREY, L. P.:   Simple Methods of Facilitating Communications Between Medical Service Representatives and Physicians, Am. J. Hosp. Pharm., *15*:7:584, 1958.

BURKHOLDER, D.:   The Role of the Pharmaceutical Detailman in a Large Teaching Hospital, Am. J. Hosp. Pharm., *20*:6:274, 1963.

MARIEL, SR.:   Handling Drug Samples, Hosp. Progress, *38*:74, 1957.

JEFFREY, L. P.:   The Pharmacy Should Control Drug Samples, Modern Hosp., *90*:2:90, 1958.

Anon.:   What Happens to Drug Samples After They Reach Hospitals? Am. Prof. Pharm., *27*:1:60, 1961.

ENO, D. M. and SPERANDIO, G. J.:   Drug Samples in Hospital Pharmacy: A Study of Distribution and Control, Am. J. Hosp. Pharm., *17*:11:679, 1960.

OWENS, C. V.:   An Answer to Physician Sampling—Scriptstarter, J. Am. Pharm. Assoc. NS3, *10*:524, 1963.

NAIMARK, G. M.:   A New Approach to the Sampling of Drugs, J. Amer. Pharm. Assoc. NS3, *10*:521, 1963.

BIBLIOGRAPHY

1. HASSAN, WILLIAM E., JR.:   Pharmaceutical Detailman—Liability or Asset? Hospital Management, *88*:1:40, 1959.
2. ————:   The Physician and the Detailman, Medical Marketing & Media, *4*:4:8, April, 1969.
3. LECCA, PEDRO J., GOLD, STUART, and SMITH, MICKEY C.:   Pharmacists' Response to a Program to Improve Pharmacist-Manufacturer Relations, J.A.Ph.A., NS*11*:11:592, November, 1971.
4. MORAVEC, D. F.:   Drug Samples, Hosp. Management, *86*:102, November, 1958.
5. JEFFREY, L. P.:   A Method for the Control of Drug Samples, Bull. Am. Soc. Hosp. Pharm., *14*:415, July-August, 1957.

Chapter

11

The Pharmacy Procedural Manual

JOURNALS and texts concerned with the broad subject of management are replete with articles and chapters on the importance of written policies as a managerial control tool. The hospital, in general, and the pharmacy, in particular, should have written policies for a number of reasons:

a. They serve as a guide for the training of new employees.
b. They prevent error resulting from the verbal transmission of the policy from one employee to another.
c. They insure the fact that the same policy will apply in all like situations.
d. They serve as a control tool in ensuring a defined procedure for performing a task, thereby eliminating waste of materials through error or carelessness.
e. In the hands of the supervisor, they serve as a means of evaluating job performance.
f. In a legal suit, they may serve as an important element in the hospital's defense of an action in tort arising out of a pharmacy error.

The management of the department of pharmacy in the hospital utilizes the same concepts which are commonly utilized in industry; namely, the pharmacist-in-chief as the manager or supervisor must coordinate people, supplies and equipment in such a manner as to produce efficiently an end-product which in the case of a hospital pharmacy is efficient and economical drug service.

Because of the number of people who may become involved, as well as the myriad of processes which must be utilized and controlled, the manager should, for the sake of uniformity and control, record the policy and technics in a manual.

Unfortunately, too many hospital pharmacists do not develop a policy manual for a number of reasons, the most common of which may be simple procrastination or lack of appreciation of its value. In other instances, it may be due to a false sense of security resulting from the belief that if no one else knows how to do a particular job, the individual who does know how is an indispensable being. And finally, the plain truth in many instances is the fact that many pharmacists do not even know what a procedural manual is nor how to commence work for its development.

Definition

A procedural manual may be defined as a series of administrative and professional policies which may serve as a guide to the hospital pharmacist in the development and execution of effective and proficient pharmaceutical services in the hospital.

Scope

Of necessity, the scope of the pharmacy procedural manual must be as broad as that of the department which it is to serve.

Berenice[1] in describing operational manuals in hospital pharmacy provides an example of the comprehensiveness of a good manual:

> "The first operational manual of any pharmacy department must contain the recorded development of the operation of the department from its very beginning, its objectives, philosophy, motivation, policies, regulations, departmental procedures, staffing pattern, job specifications, organizational plan and chart, floor plans, plot plans, description of the department, listing of physical facilities and library holdings, its intradepartmental, and interdepartmental relationships, description of its Formulary System, its Pharmacy and Therapeutics Committee and its activities, guidance manual for Internship and/or Residency Program in Hospital Pharmacy when such a program is offered. At the outset, one should give a short history of the institution and also state the purpose of the manual itself."

Contents and Format

The organization of the wealth of administrative and professional policy material requires a great deal of thought and planning, for to do otherwise will result in a chaotic presentation which may complicate rather than elucidate matters.

Latiolais[2] has suggested that the procedural manual be divided into four general sections: Organization; Facilities; Personnel; Services and Activities, with this section being subdivided into an Administrative and a Professional division.

This concept is adequate and is recommended to those who may wish to organize and develop a procedural manual for their hospital pharmacy. One must, however, bear in mind that no two manuals or hospitals will have the exact same policy and, therefore, in some instances even this general classification will not suffice. For the purpose of this chapter, the four sections suggested above will be developed in order that the student may have some insight into the subject.

The following is a presentation of a format which may be readily adapted to a specific operation by any pharmacist.

The main sections are identified by a numeral from 1 to 4. Therefore, each subject under each main section is identified by the section number plus a second number to identify the subject. For example, the first topic under Organization would be identified by the numerals 1-1; the second by 1-2, etc.

In addition, the student is provided with a reasonably comprehensive check list under each main heading which will serve as a guide, as well as a reminder as to the type of subject material which might well fall within the scope of a particular section.

1. *ORGANIZATION*

    1–1. Organization of the hospital
    1-2. Organization of the pharmacy
    1-3. Services offered by the department
    1-4. Intra and Interdepartmental Relationships
    1-5. The Pharmacy and Therapeutic Committee
    1-6. The Antibiotics Committee

2. *EQUIPMENT and PHYSICAL PLANT*

    2-1. General policies relating to the use, maintenance and repair of equipment
        2-1-1. The distilled water still
        2-1-2. Ointment Mill
        2-1-3. High speed mixer
        2-1-4. Variable speed mixer
        2-1-5. Homogenizer
            etc.
    2-2. Policy and procedure governing the loan of pharmacy equipment.
    2-3. Obtaining maintenance department services for the pharmacy.
    2-4. Obtaining engineering department services for the pharmacy.
    2-5. Policy governing the use of Central Sterile Supply Department autoclaves and sterilizers.
    2-6. Policy governing the use of laboratory equipment in control procedures.

3. *PERSONNEL POLICIES*

    3-1. Job descriptions
    3-2. Fringe benefits—General Policy
        3-2-1. Sick leave
        3-2-2. Vacation
        3-2-3. Holidays
        3-2-4. Jury duty
        3-2-5. Attending institutes, seminars or conventions
            etc.

4. *SERVICES* and *ACTIVITIES*

4-1. *ADMINISTRATIVE*

    4-1- 1. Hours of operation
    4-1- 2. Purchasing procedure
    4-1- 3. Pricing policy
    4-1- 4. Refund policy
    4-1- 5. Handling of cash receipts
    4-1- 6. Requisitioning of charge floor stock
    4-1- 7. Requisitioning of non-charge floor stock
    4-1- 8. Requisitioning of special patient charge drugs
    4-1- 9. Requisitioning of ancillary surgical and medical supplies
    4-1-10. Alcohol records and controls
    4-1-11. Controlled substances records and controls
    4-1-12. Inventory taking and its records
    4-1-13. Compounding records
    4-1-14. The monthly and annual report
            etc.

4-2. *PROFESSIONAL*

    4-2- 1. Narcotic regulations
    4-2- 2. Use of research drugs
    4-2- 3. Automatic stop orders
    4-2- 4. The Formulary System
    4-2- 5. Policy governing drugs brought to the hospital by patients
    4-2- 6. Labels and labelling
    4-2- 7. Use of the metric system
    4-2- 8. Prepackaging of bulk drugs
    4-2- 9. Dispensing policies
    4-2-10. On-call service
    4-2-11. Bulk compounding
            (Formula, procedure, etc. for each product.)
    4-2-12. Sterile compounding
            (Formula, procedure, etc. for each product.)
    4-2-13. The residency training program in the hospital pharmacy
    4-2-14. Poison Control Center
    4-2-15. Information Services
            4-2-15-1. Pharmacy Library
            4-2-15-2. Pharmacy Bulletin
            4-2-15-3. Lecture Service
            4-2-15-4. Drug Displays
    4-2-16. The addition of drugs to intravenous solutions by nurses

Sample Bulletins for a Manual

The style of writing the procedural manual need not be restricted; it may be in outline form or in text style. The language used should be simple and direct. Verbosity should be avoided for the sake of clarity, brevity and safety.

Division 1–16
Bulletin -5-

Requisitions for Pharmacy Supplies

In order to account accurately for the distribution of Pharmacy supplies issued to the various hospital departments the proper requisition must be completed.

Ward Stock Medications must be requisitioned on Form No. 16.

Laboratory and Medical and Surgical Supplies must be requisitioned on Form No. 16A.

Prescription drugs for personal use must be requisitioned on Form 29-12-59.

All of the above requisition forms must be legibly and completely filled out including the proper code number to which the charge is to be made.

Division 1–16
Bulletin -6-

Hospital Prescriptions

Hospital policy requires that a prescription be written for any drug, prescribed for clinic patients, discharge patients, or employees regardless of its nature, which is to be issued from the Hospital Pharmacy.

As the Hospital Pharmacy is not a licensed retail drug outlet, and in order that the Hospital may meet fully the requirements of the State Board of Registration in Pharmacy, all such prescriptions must be written on Hospital prescription blanks (white for discharge patients, yellow for clinic patients and employees).

Division 1–16
Bulletin -7-

Automatic Stop Order for Dangerous Drugs

All orders for CONTROLLED SUBSTANCES must be re-written every 24 hours. All P. R. N. (pro re nata) and standing orders for all medications except narcotics, sedatives, and hypnotics shall expire at 10:00 a.m. on the seventh day unless renewed.

Division 1–16
Bulletin -8-

Separation of Internal Use Preparations from Those for External Use

The licensure rules and regulations for hospitals in Massachusetts specifically state that "poisons and medications for external use shall be kept in a separate compartment."

Accordingly, all drug supplies shall be arranged in such manner as to comply with the above regulation.

If you have any question as to what products should be classed in the category "poisons and medications for external use," please call the Pharmacist-in-Chief, Ext. xxx or the Associate Director, Ext. xxx.

Division 1–16
Bulletin -10-

Pharmacy Hours

The Pharmacy is open during the following hours for use by both clinic and house patients.

    Monday–Saturday - - - - - - - 8:00 A.M.–9:00 P.M.
    Sunday and Holidays - - - - - - 9:00 A.M.–9:00 P.M.

House patients requiring special medications after these hours may have them dispensed by the Nursing Supervisor from the Emergency Drug Cabinet.

The Nursing Supervisor may not mix or compound medications. Should this be necessary, the Nursing Supervisor shall call in the "on call" pharmacist.

A list of the "on call" pharmacists is maintained by the switchboard operator.

Division 1–16
Bulletin -11-

Intravenous Solutions, the Addition of Drugs by Nurses

1. The addition of drugs for intravenous administration to intravenous solutions is often most conveniently and expeditiously performed by the Nursing Service and may thereby facilitate patient care.
2. In all circumstances this may be performed only under specific written order in the appropriate order book by the doctor responsible for the patient's care.
3. This addition may be performed only by graduate nurses and senior class nursing students under supervision of a graduate nurse.
4. No medication may be given by the Nursing Service directly intravenously, *i.e.* without further dilution by an appropriate and specified volume of intravenous fluid.
5. Also excluded specifically are phenolsulfonphthalein (PSP), sulfobromophthalein sodium (Bromsulphalein, BSP), similar testing drugs and solutions commonly used without dilution, and experimental drugs and solutions not yet accepted for routine use by the Pharmacy and Therapeutics Committee.
6. The following medications and solutions in preparations specifically for intravenous use may be added under the rules of this bulletin.
   a. Antibiotics
   b. Electrolyte solutions, *e.g.,* sodium bicarbonate, potassium chloride, sodium lactate, sodium iodide, sodium chloride and all other intravenous electrolyte solutions
   c. Vasopressors, *e.g.,* Phenylephrine (Neo-Synephrine), l-arterenol (Levophed) and other such agents
   d. Vitamins
   e. Aminophylline
   f. Barbiturates
   g. Diphenylhydantoin (Dilantin)
   h. Hormonal preparations for intravenous use, *e.g.,* hydrocortisone
7. The following drugs may be administered by a graduate nurse provided that the initial dose has been administered by a physician, the dosage and its dilution are specifically written in the Doctor's Order Book and the medication order is re-written on a *daily basis.*
   a. 5-fluouracil
   b. **Heparin**

Medications, Preparation and Administration by Nurses

Purpose: To prepare and administer medications as ordered by the physician safely, accurately and efficiently.

Responsibilities of the Nurse

1. The nurse must know the nature of the drug, the desired effect, the average dose, the mathematical preparation of the dose, the toxic symptoms, the method of preparation and administration and the antidote before administering any medication.
2. The nurse must clearly understand all medication orders before carrying them out.
3. The nurse must administer and chart only those medications which she herself has prepared.
4. Medications poured but not administered must be discarded and may not be returned to the drug bottle.
5. See Bulletin 1–16–2 for reporting adverse drug reactions
   1–16–3 for reporting drug intoxication
   1–16–4 for emergency drugs
   1–16–5 and 1–16–6 for ordering from Pharmacy
   1–16–7 for automatic stop orders
   1–16–8 for the storage of internal and external preparations

Regulations Concerning Narcotics

1. See Bulletin 1–16–1 for federal and hospital regulations.
2. All narcotics must be counted at each change of shift by two nurses, one from each tour of duty. Both nurses must sign that the count was made and was correct. Errors in the count must be reported to the supervisor.
3. All narcotics obtained from the Pharmacy are to be counted and signed for by a professional nurse. Any discrepancy is to be reported to the pharmacist at once.

Medications at Bedside

1. Nitroglycerine tablets may be left at the bedside if so ordered by the doctor. No more than ten tablets should be left with the patient. At 7 A.M. and 7 P.M., the tablets are to be counted, the number used by the patient recorded and additional tablets added to the bedside supply to maintain the supply of ten.
2. Medication brought to the hospital with the patient is not kept at the bedside. It is shown to the physician, then sent home with a responsible family member or friend. If this is not possible, the medication is labelled with the patient's name, locked in the medication cabinet and, with the permission of the physician, sent home with the patient at the time of his discharge.
3. No medication other than nitroglycerine is maintained or left at the bedside of any patient.

Administration of Medications

1. *Policies*
   a) Medication cards are made out by the nurse in charge, noting the patient's name, full name of the drug, dose, route of administra-

tion, times ordered or frequency of administration. Each card is initialled by the nurse who makes it out. All 'stat' and single dose orders are written on red cards; all other medications on white cards.

b) The medicine card is checked against the Kardex and/or Doctor's Order Book for drug, route, patient's name, date and time.

c) The drug label is checked with the medication card at least three times: before removing the bottle from the shelf, before pouring, when returning to the shelf.

d) At the bedside, before the medication is administered, the patient is identified by checking the medication card against the name on the wrist band, with the name on the bed card and by asking the patient to state his name if he is able to do so.

e) The nurse remains at the bedside until the patient has taken the medication; medication is never left at the bedside.

f) The medication is charted immediately after administration.

g) Any untoward situation (patient refuses medication, is absent from the pavilion etc.) is reported to the Head Nurse and noted on the Kardex.

2. *Intravenous Medication*

No medication may be given intravenously by nurses at this hospital.

3. *Liquid Medications*

a) Spirits and tinctures must be kept tightly capped since the strength of the drug increases as the solvent evaporates.

b) Acids are to be given through a straw to avoid discoloration of the teeth.

c) Iodine preparations are to be given in milk or well diluted with fruit juice or water.

4. *Rectal Medications*

a) Rectal medications may be administered by retention enema or by suppository.

b) It is explained to the patient that the medication is to be given rectally and to be retained. The patient is assisted to turn on his left side.

c) If medication is given by suppository, the nurse puts on a glove or finger cot, lubricates the tapered end of the suppository and inserts it well beyond the sphincter.

d) If medication is given by retention enema, the least amount of solution which will dissolve the drug and provide safe dilution is used and the solution is allowed to run in slowly.

e) The patient remains quietly on the left side for a few minutes to aid in retention.

5. *Parenteral Medications*

a) Policies—Graduate Nurses

Nurses may give parenteral medications (subcutaneous, intramuscular, intradermal) if they have had adequate instruction and supervision in the method used and have adequate knowledge of the drug.

Nurses may not administer tetanus anti-toxin.

Special restrictions may be imposed on non-formulary drugs. The nurse must check with her immediate superior (head nurse or supervisor) before administering these drugs.

7

No more than 5 ml. of medication may be injected intramuscularly into one site at any one time.

b) Policies—Student Nurses

Student nurses may not administer narcotics without first obtaining the permission of the head nurse. The student must be prepared to give the following information: patient's full name, medication and dose ordered, frequency with which medication may be given, time medication was last given, pulse and respiration of the patient.

Student nurses may never administer medication intravenously or into the I.V. tubing.

Student nurses may add medication to intravenous solutions only under the direct supervision of an instructor.

c) Administration of Parenteral Medications

Medication is prepared in the syringe. With a transfer forceps, a sponge moistened with benzalkonium chloride (Zephiran) 1:750 is removed from the container and placed in a medicine cup. The cup and syringe with needle protected by a needle guard are carried to the bedside.

Disposable needles are bent after use to prevent re-use and discarded *only* in the container provided for needles.

Injection sites and methods:

Subcutaneous—injected at a 45° angle into the lateral aspect of the upper arm.

Intramuscular—injected at a 90° angle. The injection is given in the upper portion of the upper outer quadrant of the buttocks, two inches below the crest of the ileum. The deltoid or the lateral aspect of the thigh may also be used. Sites of injection should be rotated.

Intradermal—injected as nearly parallel as possible in the skin of the anterior forearm. Only the tip of the needle should be inserted in the skin and a wheal should appear as soon as the medication is injected.

Special Manuals

Hospital pharmacies within large teaching hospitals generally require, in addition to the standard procedural manual, a special manual to cover specific aspects of the operation. These may be for use in such areas as the control laboratory, sterile technics laboratory, manufacturing laboratory, hyperalimentation unit and unit dose section.

In preparing the sections of the special manuals, it is essential that specific detail be provided in order that the special manual be useful. Note the following examples:

Cleaning and Preparation of Rubber Closures Process G[4]
(W.F.I. Treated)
"1. Thoroughly rinse washer with distilled water. Use large home-laundry type agitator washer for 43 mm. black disc

closures. Use small Southern Cross stainless steel agitator washer for 20 mm. closures.

2. Place closures in washer and sufficient *hot* 0.5 per cent sodium pyrophosphate solution in distilled water to the fill mark on the washer or to adequately cover the closures. Suspend disc closures in washer in nylon mesh bag.
3. Agitate for 20 minutes for new closure and 30 minutes for reused closures. Keep cover on washer.
4. Rinse thoroughly with repeated quantities of distilled water until closures are free from detergent. The conductivity of the final rinse water should be not more than that of the distilled water. Remove closures from rinse water by lifting out of the water (do not pump out water first).
5. Immerse the closures in W.F.I. and autoclave at 121°C. for 20 minutes.
   Containers to be used: for 43 mm. black discs—use stainless steel bucket with glassine paper under aluminum foil cover, double thick.
   for 20 mm. closures—use Pyrex wide mouth screw cap jars, cover with nylon cloth, screw cap in place over nylon after autoclaving.
6. Pour off the water and rinse with W.F.I. Lift out of the W.F.I., rinse and transfer to another container. Add sufficient W.F.I. to cover the closures and again autoclave at 121°C. for 20 minutes.
7. If supernatant liquid is clear (if not, repeat step 6 until clear), pour off the liquid and allow closures to drain before use. Keep covered with original sterile covering until used."

Cleaning and Preparation of Filters for Reuse Process E[4]
(Ertel Filters)
"1. After use, dismantle the assembly and discard filter pads.
2. Thoroughly scrub the assembly components until clean.
3. Remove the porous stone disc and boil for 15 minutes in 0.5 per cent sodium pyrophosphate solution. Rinse thoroughly with distilled water. Soak in fresh distilled water for at least 30 minutes.
4. Immerse the stone disc in 10 per cent hydrochloric acid for one hour. Rinse thoroughly with distilled water. Leach in fresh distilled water for at least one hour, changing the water three or more times during the leaching period.
5. Assemble filter, including new asbestos pads.
6. Pass at least 2000 ml. of W.F.I. through the assembly by filtration.
7. Loosen bolts, cover outlets with glassine paper, wrap unit in kraft paper and autoclave for 45 minutes at 121°C. Write, with indelible ink on the paper wrapping, the asbestos pad number, date of sterilization, and product for which to be used (if applicable).
8. Do not use without resterilization, if stored for more than two weeks.
9. Tighten bolts before use. Discard the first portion of filtrate (approx. 200 ml.), that is passed through the filter."

Sampling Plans For Sterility Testing and Quantitative Assay[4]
"The same product units are to be used for sterility test, pyrogen test (when required), and for quantitative assay or other tests.

Plan AA

1. Used for products sterilized by autoclaving. Ten product units are selected.
2. Select one product unit from each "corner" of the top and bottom shelves or layers and two product units from the center of the load.
3. If there is but one layer of product units, take duplicate units from each "corner" and from the center of the load.
4. Affix tag to nine units with manufacturing lot number of product.
5. Affix tag to tenth unit with manufacturing lot number and formula of product.

Plan BB

1. Used for products filled aseptically, without terminal sterilization. Ten product units are selected.
2. Select the first two product units filled, one unit each after approximately 10, 20, 40, 60, and 90 per cent of the filling procedure, and the last two product units filled.
3. Affix tag to nine units with manufacturing lot number of product. Number consecutively in the order in which selected.
4. Affix tag to tenth unit with lot number and formula of product."

After all is said and done with regard to this topic of procedural manuals, the student as well as the seasoned hospital pharmacist will benefit greatly from the wisdom afforded by the following excerpt from an editorial.[3]

"Procedural manuals can be a great asset in the proper management of the Pharmacy Department and the coordination of its activities with other departments and the professional and administrative staffs. Hospital pharmacists will find them valuable tools, tools however, which can never replace the professional judgment of the pharmacist."

SELECTED REFERENCES

ROURKE, SR. MARY VERA: Mercy Hospital Pharmacy Policies, Am. J. Hosp. Pharm., *16*:6:274, 1959.

BOWLES, GROVER C.:   Written Policies and Procedures Improve Hospital Pharmacy Management, Modern Hosp., *96*:5:117, 1961.

MARIE, SR. RUTH: Job Description and Procedure Manuals in Hospital Pharmacy, Hosp. Pharm., *16*:28, 1963.

BEAR, SR. ALICE: How to Prepare a Procedural Manual, Hosp. Topics, *42*:8: 85, 1964.

BIBLIOGRAPHY

1. BERENICE, SR. MARY: Operational Manuals in Hospital Pharmacy, Am. J. Hosp. Pharm., *16*:6:269, 1959.
2. LATIOLAIS, CLIFTON J.:   Pharmacy Procedure Manual, Hospitals, J.A.H.A., *33*:13:77, 1959.
3. FRANCKE, DON E.:   An Editorial Procedural Manuals as Administrative Tools, Am. J. Hosp. Pharm., *16*:6:267, 1959.
4. AVIS, KENNETH E., CARLIN, HERBERT S., FLACK, HERBERT L.: Procedure Manual for Parenteral and Other Sterile Preparations (1960), Sterile Technics Laboratory, Jefferson Medical College, Philadelphia, Pa.

Chapter

12

Drug Distribution—Floor Stock System

EACH pavilion in the hospital, regardless of its size or specialty care, has a supply of drugs stored in the medicine cabinet even though the nursing unit is serviced by a unit dose system. These medications may be classified under two separate headings, each of which serves a specific purpose. Drugs on the nursing station may be divided into *"charge floor stock drugs"* and *"non-charge floor stock drugs."* It is the responsibility of the hospital pharmacist, working in cooperation with the nursing service, to develop ways and means whereby adequate supplies of each are always on hand and, in the appropriate situation, that proper charges are made to the patient's account.

This chapter will deal with the means whereby floor stock drugs are selected, and leave the methods whereby they are requisitioned by nursing service, distributed by pharmacy personnel and methods of issuing charges to patients, where the situation so warrants, to a later chapter on dispensing and distribution systems in the hospital pharmacy.

Definitions

Charge floor stock drugs may be defined as those medications that are stocked on the nursing station at all times and are charged to the patient's account after they have been administered to him.

Non-charge floor stock drugs represent that group of medications that are placed at the nursing station for the use of all patients on the pavilion and for which there may be no direct charge to the patient's account. In fact, the cost of this group of drugs is usually calculated in the per diem cost of the hospital room.

Today, there are four systems in general use for dispensing drugs for in-patients. They may be classified as follows: (i) Individual Prescription Order System, (ii) Complete Floor Stock System and (iii) Combinations of (i) and (ii) and the unit dose method. (To be discussed in Chapter 13.)

Individual Prescription Order System

As has been previously stated, this system is generally used by the small and/or private hospital because of the reduced manpower requirements and the desirability for individualized service. Inherent in this system is the possible delay in obtaining the required medication and the increase in cost to the patient. At the same time, there are very definite advantages: (i) all medication orders are directly reviewed by the pharmacist; (ii) provides for the interaction of pharmacist, doctor, nurse and patient and (iii) provides closer control of inventory.

The "Complete" Floor Stock System

Under this system, the nursing station pharmacy carries both "charge" and "non-charge" patient medications. Rarely used or particularly expensive drugs are omitted from floor stock but are dispensed upon the receipt of a prescription or medication order for the individual patient.

Although this system is used most often in governmental and other hospitals in which charges are not made to the patient or when the all inclusive rate is used for charging, it does have applicability to the general hospital.

Obviously, there are both advantages and disadvantages to the complete floor stock system. Advantages include: (i) ready availability of the required drugs; (ii) elimination of drug returns; (iii) reduction in number of drug order transcriptions for the pharmacy and (iv) reduction in the number of pharmacy personnel required. The disadvantages of such a system are: (i) medication errors may increase because the review of medication orders is eliminated; (ii) increased drug inventory on the pavilions; (iii) greater opportunity for pilferage; (iv) increased hazards associated with drug deterioration; (v) lack of proper storage facilities on the ward may require capital outlay to provide them and (vi) greater inroads are made upon the nurses' time.

To be borne in mind by the student is the fact that in some hospitals the complete floor stock system is successfully operated as a decentralized pharmacy under the direct supervision of a pharmacist.

Obviously, when this occurs, many of the disadvantages associated with such a system disappear. In addition, the use of the decentralized pharmacy concept provides for a "home base" for the clinically oriented pharmacist.

Combinations of Individual Drug Order and Floor Stock Systems

Falling into this category, are those hospitals which use the individual prescription or medication order system as their primary means of dispensing, but also utilize a limited floor stock. This combination system is probably the most commonly used in hospitals today and is modified to include the use of unit dose medications.

Selection of Charge Floor Stock Drugs

The final decision as to which drugs shall be placed on the pavilions should rest with the Pharmacy and Therapeutics Committee, because this representative group of clinicians possesses a unique and intimate knowledge of the medicinal requirements of the patients within the institution.

This does not mean that the decision as to which drug shall or shall not be admitted to floor stock status should be arbitrarily arrived at. Representatives of nursing service, pharmacy and administration should be consulted for guidance and advice.

Once a floor stock list has been determined, it becomes the responsibility of the hospital pharmacist to make the drugs available, enforce the decision of the Pharmacy and Therapeutics Committee by not permitting deviations, and periodically to re-submit the list to the Pharmacy and Therapeutics Committee for re-evaluation in the light of later experience and therapeutic trends.

In arriving at a list of charge floor stock drugs, the Pharmacy and Therapeutics Committee will be concerned, in all probability, with having available for immediate use drugs of proven efficacy and which the average clinician considers necessary to administer to the patient as soon as a diagnosis is made or, at least, for the immediate symptomatic treatment.

Aside from the storage problem on the pavilion, there should be no valid reason why the decision of the Committee in this respect should not be honored, since each of these agents is chargeable to the patient's account. The only really important criteria to be considered here are the patient's clinical needs. The patient's financial status or ability to pay should have no bearing on his clinical need.

The following represents a typical list of injectable charge floor stock drugs in common use in a large teaching hospital:

Anti-allergenics
Diphenhydramine HCl 10 mg./ml.
Hydrocortisone Sodium Succinate 100 mg.

Antibiotics
   Penicillin G Potassium 20 million units
   Procaine Penicillin 300,000 units/ml.
   Chloramphenicol Sodium Succinate 1 Gm./10 ml.
   Streptomycin Sulfate 1 Gm./2 ml.

Anticoagulant
   Heparin 10,000 units/ml.

Anti-epileptic
   Sodium Diphenylhydantoin 50 mg./ml.

Antihypertensive
   Reserpine HCl 0.5 mg./2 ml.

Antinauseants
   Trimethobenzamide HCl 100 mg./ml.
   Prochloperazine 10 mg./2 ml.

Cardiovascular Agents
   a. Depressant
         Procaine Amide 100 mg./ml.
   b. Antifibrillator
         Quinidine HCl 0.18 Gm./1.5 ml.
   c. Vasoconstrictors
         Phenylephrine HCl 10 mg./ml.
         L-Arterenol 0.2%
         Metaraminol Bitartrate 10 mg./ml.

Coagulant
   Protamine Sulfate 50 mg./5 ml.

Diuretics
   Meralluride 2 ml.
   Mercaptomerin 125 mg./2 ml.

Spasmogenics
   Bethanecol Chloride 5 mg./5 ml.
   Neostigmine Methylsulfate 0.5 mg./ml.

Tranquilizers
   Chlordiazepoxide 100 mg./2 ml.
   Trifluoperazine 2 mg./ml.

Miscellaneous
   Potassium Chloride 40 mEq./20 ml.
   Dextrose 50%
   Mannitol Injection 25%

Selection of Non-Charge Floor Stock Drugs

With regard to the non-charge floor stock drugs a different set of criteria are employed. Here, consideration is usually given to the cost of the preparation, the frequency of use, the quantity used, and the effect upon the hospital budget and reimbursement from third party payors.

In many hospitals, this list is exceptionally small and therefore the patient is billed for numerous single doses of drugs. This, of course, produces bad public relations and the pharmacist should do all in his power to correct the situation.

A list of pharmaceutical and related preparations that are considered to be non-charge floor stock drugs in a 315-bed university teaching hospital will be found in Chapter 13. Each hospital should, of course, arrive at its own list based upon the needs of the staff and the type of patient cared for. Too brief a list will necessarily mean frequent small charges for pharmaceuticals. The sum of several such charges for each dose is usually more than would be charged for a like number of doses issued in one package. This has been a prime cause of adverse public relations for the hospital and should be guarded against whenever possible.

Prescribing of Floor Stock Drugs

There are three techniques employed in transmitting drug order information from the nursing stations to the pharmacist. They are:

   (i)   Prescription order is written on a separate blank by the physician (Fig. 36).
   (ii) Carbon or other copy of the chart order (Physician's Order Sheet) is sent to the pharmacist.
   (iii) Chart order is transcribed by hospital personnel assigned to the nursing station.

Some of the smaller hospitals continue to require separate prescriptions for all medications. The student must bear in mind that there is nothing wrong with this in that it establishes the same professional relationship and fosters the same practice existing in the community practice of pharmacy. In the larger hospitals, this system is not favored by the physicians.

A second method consists of using a carbon or other copy of the doctor's written order as a prescription order. In this system the pharmacist receives a copy of the original medication order. No transcribing or copying is required of hospital personnel assigned to the nursing station in order to obtain prescribed medication as initially ordered. It has been demonstrated that this system reduces medication errors because of the review by pharmacists of all drug orders for each patient in the original handwriting of the physician ordering the medication.

		John Doe
		Hosp. #12-34-56
PHYSICIAN'S ORDERS		Location B25
		Dr. Smith

Date Ordered	Date Discontinued	ORDERS
1/1/65		Digitoxin 0.1 mg. one at 7:00 a.m.
		Hexavitamin Capsule one daily
1/2/65		Secobarbital 100 mg. one h.s. prn
1/3/65	1/5/65	Potassium Chloride 1 Gm. one daily in a.m.

FIG. 36. An example of a Physician's Order Sheet found in the patient's medical record. The orders shown here are typed. Under normal circumstances, these are written by the physician in ink.

In one version of this system, physicians are allowed to mix all types of orders for the patient on one sheet. Although this has the advantage of providing the pharmacist with a total picture of what is happening to the patient, it is preferable to educate the physicians to limit the writing of their drug orders to a single medication order sheet (Fig. 36). Once written, it behooves the responsible party to promptly remove the copy portion of the medication order and transmit it to the pharmacy in order to obviate dispensing delays.

The method most widely employed at present is that in which the nurse, nursing unit manager, or ward secretary transcribes or copies via a mechanical copying device the physician's written order on to another document (Figs. 40 and 41), sometimes called a drug requisition slip, and sends it to the pharmacy for reviewing and dispensing. This transcribed or copied order is also used by the pharmacist to create his *patient drug profile* and to initiate the medication charge.

If the medication ordered is a non-charge drug, the nurse makes an entry on her records and at the proper time will remove the drug from the ward stock container and administer it to the patient.

Labeling of Floor Stock Drugs

Of further interest to the non-hospital pharmacist members of the profession is the fact that none of the ward stock drugs are labeled with the directions for use. This is so because of the fact that many

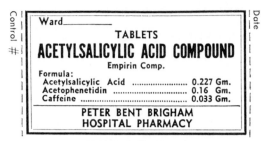

FIG. 37.   An example of a non-charge floor stock medication label.

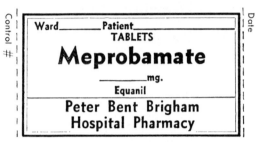

FIG. 38.   An example of a charge floor stock medication label.

patients may be receiving the same drug but under a different therapeutic regimen. If one set of directions was affixed to the container under these circumstances, then it is obvious that confusion and error may result. Therefore, packages containing non-charge as well as generally used charge floor stock medications bear a label which shows the name of the ward and the name and strength of the preparation as well as any other pertinent information (Fig. 37).

In contrast, medications being sent to the floor for the specific use of a single patient bear a similar label with the addition of the patient's name (Fig. 38). Once again, the specific directions for use are eliminated because of the fact that the therapeutic regimen may be altered from day to day by the physician in charge. Therefore, the nurse must make frequent checks of the patient's record in order to keep informed of the latest treatment prescribed.

Nursing Procedure for Administration of a Drug

Although the hospital pharmacist does not become involved with this aspect of patient care, he should become thoroughly familiar with the procedure used in his particular institution.

There are many different procedures for the administration of drugs by nurses employed in the hospitals of this country; therefore, space will permit only the methodology employed by one hospital.[1] For newer techniques, see Chapter 13.

Medications (Preparation and Administration)

Purpose: To prepare and administer medications as ordered by the physician safely, accurately and efficiently.

Responsibilities of the Nurse

1. The nurse is to know the nature of the drug, the desired effect, the average dose, the mathematical preparation of the dose, the toxic symptoms, the method of preparation and administration and the antidote before administering any medication.
2. The nurse must clearly understand all medication orders before carrying them out.
3. The nurse must *administer* and chart only those medications which she herself has prepared.
4. Medications poured but not administered must be discarded and may not be returned to the drug container.

Regulations Concerning Narcotics

1. See Chapter 16 for Federal and hospital regulations.
2. All narcotics must be counted at each change of shift by *two nurses, one from each tour of duty.* Both nurses must sign that the count was made and was correct. Errors in the count must be reported to the supervisor at once.
3. All narcotics obtained from the pharmacy are to be counted and signed for by a professional nurse. Any discrepancy is to be reported to the pharmacist at once.

Medications at Bedside

1. Nitroglycerine tablets may be left at the bedside if so ordered by the doctor. No more than ten tablets should be left with the patient. At 7 A.M. and 7 P.M. the tablets are to be counted, the number used by the patient recorded and additional tablets added to maintain the supply of ten.
2. Medication brought to the hospital with the patient is not kept at the bedside. It is shown to the physician, then sent home with a responsible family member or friend. If this is not possible, the medication is labeled with the patient's name, locked in the medication cabinet and, with the permission of the physician, sent home with the patient at the time of his discharge.
3. No medication other than nitroglycerine is maintained or left at the bedside of any patient.

Administration of Medications

1. Policies
   a. Medication cards are made out by the nurse in charge, noting the patient's name, full name of the drug, dose, route of administration, times ordered for or frequency of administration. Each card is initialled by the nurse who makes it out. All 'stat' and single dose orders are written on red cards; all other medications, on white cards (Fig. 39).

Orders and Sample Medication Cards

Note: Red medication cards are used for narcotic,
single, and stat orders.
Hours from 7 P.M. to 7 A.M. are written in red on
the medication card.

1. Gantrisin 0.5 gm. (PO) Q 4 h

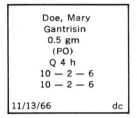

2. Phenobarbital 30 mgm (PO) Tid

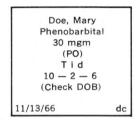

3. Penicillin 100,000 units (I.m) Qid

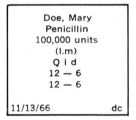

4. Streptomycin 0.5 gm (I.m.) Q 6 h

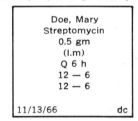

5. Demerol 100 mgm Q 4 h PRN (I.m)

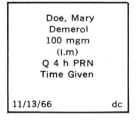

6. Bufferin Q 4 h PRN (PO)

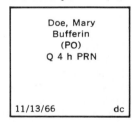

FIG. 39.

b. The medicine card is checked against the Kardex and/or doctor's
order book for drug, dose, route, patient's name, date and time.

c. The drug label is checked with the medication card at least three
times: before removing from the shelf, before pouring, when
returning the container to the shelf.

d. At the bedside, before the medication is administered, the patient
is identified by checking the medication card against the name on
wrist band, with name on bed card and by asking the patient to
state his name if he is able to do so.

e. The nurse remains at the bedside until the patient has taken the medication; medication is never left at the bedside.

f. The medication is charted immediately after administration.

g. Any untoward situation (patient refuses medication, is absent from the pavilion etc.) is reported to the Head Nurse and noted on the Kardex.

2. Intravenous Medication

a. No medication may be given intravenously by nurses.

3. Liquid Medications

a. Spirits and tinctures must be kept tightly capped since the strength of the drug increases as the solvent evaporates.

b. Acids are to be given through a straw to avoid discoloration of the teeth.

c. Iodine preparations are to be given in milk or well diluted with fruit juice or water.

4. Rectal Medications

a. Rectal medication may be administered by retention enema or by suppository.

b. It is explained to the patient that the medication is to be given rectally and retained. The patient is assisted to turn on his left side.

c. If medication is given by suppository, the nurse puts on a glove or finger cot, lubricates the tapered end of the suppository and inserts it well beyond the sphincter.

d. If medication is given by retention enema, the least amount of solution which will dissolve the drug and provide safe dilution is used and the solution allowed to run in slowly.

e. The patient remains quietly on the left side for a few minutes to aid in retention.

5. Parenteral Medications

a. Policies—Graduate Nurses

Nurses may give parenteral medications (subcutaneous, intramuscular, intradermal) if they have had adequate instruction and supervision in the method used and have adequate knowledge of the drug.

Nurses may not administer Tetanus Anti-Toxin.

Special restrictions may be imposed on non-formulary drugs. The nurse must check with her immediate superior (head nurse or supervisor) before administering these drugs.

No more than 5 ml. of medication may be injected intramuscularly into one site at any one time.

b. Policies—Student Nurses

Student nurses may not administer narcotics without first obtaining the permission of the head nurse. The student must be prepared to give the following information: Patient's full name, medication and dose ordered, frequency with which medication may be given, time medication was last given, pulse and respiration of the patient.

Student nurses may never administer medication intravenously or into the intravenous tubing.

Student nurses may add medications to intravenous solutions only under the direct supervision of an instructor.

c. Administration of parenteral medications.

Medication is prepared in the syringe. With a transfer forceps a sponge moistened with benzalkonium chloride (Zephiran) 1:750 is removed from the container and placed in a medicine cup. The cup and the syringe with needle protected by needle guard are carried to the bedside.

Disposable needles are bent to prevent re-use and discarded *only* in the container provided for needles.

Injection sites and methods:

Subcutaneous—injected at 45-degree angle in the lateral aspect of the upper arm.

Intramuscular—injected at a 90-degree angle. The injection is given in the upper portion of the upper outer quadrant of the buttocks, two inches below the crest of the ilium. The deltoid or the lateral aspect of the thigh may also be used. Sites of injection should be rotated.

Intradermal—injected as nearly parallel as possible in the skin of the anterior forearm. Only the tip of the needle should be inserted in the skin and a wheal should appear as soon as the medication is injected.

Inspection of Nursing Drug Cabinets

Once a large supply of drugs is placed in the nursing station, the hospital pharmacist's responsibility is increased. The only way the pharmacist can be sure that the drug supplies on the pavilions are being properly cared for is by personal inspection of the drug cabinets.

Too often, this facet of the pharmacist's responsibility is taken too lightly and may oftentimes be delegated to nursing supervisory personnel who, although well motivated, are not trained to evaluate the state of deterioration of drugs.

In order that the inspection program be successful, it should be carried out by pharmacy and nursing personnel on a regular basis. In addition, there should be developed a regular check list of points to be looked for during each inspection tour.

The following is a ten-point check list which may, with modification, be used for the inspection of the drug cabinets on the nursing station of any hospital.

1. Check lock mechanism for security.
2. Check lighting and refrigeration within the drug cabinet.
3. Check the uniformity of containers.
4. Check the uniformity and completeness of labeling.
5. Check to see that minimal and maximal inventories are being adhered to.
6. Check to see that internal use medications are separated from external use products.
7. Ascertain that all dated pharmaceuticals and related products are still usable.
8. Determine whether non-dated drugs have deteriorated.

9. Check whether research drugs are properly labeled and segregated.
10. Eliminate any samples, non-approved drugs, or non-drug items from the cabinet.

SELECTED REFERENCES

TEPLITSKY, BENJAMIN: Nursing Drug Cabinets—Their Inspection. *Hospital Pharmacy Handbook,* Vol. 2, Chicago, Clissold Publishing Co., p. 8.
McKINLEY, J. D.: Floor Stock Control, Am. Prof. Pharm., *26*:389, 1960.
ARLOW, SAMUEL E.: The Use of Supplementary Labels in Hospital Pharmacy, Am. J. Hosp. Pharm., *18*:10:601, 1961.

BIBLIOGRAPHY

1. Current Practice Manual of the Peter Bent Brigham Hospital, Bulletin 4-1, 1964.

Chapter

13

Dispensing to In-Patients

THE increased demand for the utilization of hospitals coupled with the growing shortage of professional personnel—nurses, pharmacists, dietitians and social workers—has stimulated thought and research in work simplification through the establishment of criteria which define each and every job performed by this category of personnel.

A great deal of nursing time was consumed by frequent trips to the pharmacy to obtain medications and other ancillary supplies. As a direct result thereof, many administrators have requested the hospital pharmacist and nursing administrative staff to scrutinize present procedures and develop new systems for the distribution and dispensing of drugs.

In the interim, many stop-gap measures were taken simply because they appeared to be the most expedient but which, when viewed in the light of experience and reasoning, were in reality a direct violation of the law.

One such approach was the indiscriminate stocking of drugs on the nursing station in bulk quantities, thereby eliminating the pharmacist's control, for here the physician prescribed, the nurse *dispensed,* and the nurse *administered.* Clearly, in a situation such as this the nurse in performing the dispensing act is infringing upon the professional as well as the legal prerogatives of the pharmacist.

Archambault[1] has stated that drug administration is a nursing act which consists of the removal or withdrawal of a single dose from a drug container and its administration to a patient on the order of a physician or dentist. He has further stipulated that dispensing is a pharmacy act and consists of the pharmacist removing two or more doses from a bulk drug container and placing them in another container for subsequent use.

Pharmacists should be alert to such infringements and should not lend their approval to such procedures. Most hospital administrators would support the pharmacists' stand on this if the matter is brought to his attention with adequate particularity.

Another hasty decision, in some areas, was the installation of vending type machines, only to have the attorneys-general of several states rule that they were illegal. Most of the decisions were based on the fact that state laws provide that registered nurses are not authorized under statute to dispense drugs, but may "administer" them after the prescription has been "dispensed" by a licensed person.

A more rational approach to the subject might be the installation of a messenger service between the pharmacy and the nursing stations, installation of mechanical conveyor systems or pneumatic tube systems or to develop emergency boxes, or the placing of charge floor stock drugs on the pavilion after a limited selection of drugs for this use has been made by the Pharmacy and Therapeutics Committee.

In order to alleviate the nursing burden, some hospital administrators contend that hospital pharmacists must assume responsibility for medications from the time of their selection to the time of their administration. Yet, in designing a system which incorporates this concept, consideration must be given to alleviate the burden placed upon the nursing service for the ordering, preparation and administration of medications.[2]

Many examples are recorded in the literature that illustrate the relationship between a drug distribution system and the nursing system.

One study of nursing activities indicated that approximately 15 per cent of a professional nurses' time is spent in the communication aspects of medication procedures.[3] This is not unusual when compared to other studies which show that: a 22-per cent increase in the amount of time nurses were able to spend at the patient's bedside as a result of changing the drug dispensing system[4]; 5.5 hours per day of nursing time were saved as a result of the installation of a unit dose system[5]; 14.4 hours per day of nursing time for four medical wards were freed by the use of a unit-dose system.[6]

Guidelines for Hospital Drug Distribution Systems

Because of the importance of drug distribution systems in the hospital, the American Society of Hospital Pharmacists approved and the American Hospital Association endorsed a *Statement on Hospital Distribution Systems*.[7]

The following guidelines for planning and evaluating hospital drug distribution systems is abstracted from the aforementioned statement:

Traditional methods of distributing drugs in hospitals are now undergoing reevaluation, and considerable thought and activity is being directed toward the development of new and improved drug distribution systems. Some of the newer concepts and ideas in connection with hospital drug distribution systems are centralized or decentralized (single, or unit-dose) dispensing, automated (mechanical and/or electronic) processing of medication orders and inventory control, and automated (mechanical and/or electronic) storage and delivery devices. Several investigators are at work in each of these areas, and the results of their studies may greatly alter current practices and procedures.

Because of the present state of uncertainty regarding the proper scope and optimum design of drug distribution systems for the modern hospital, and as an aid to pharmacists, nurses, physicians, and administrators who are faced with making decisions concerning drug distribution systems during this period of change, the following guidelines for evaluating proposed changes or new ideas or equipment are presented.

Though some of the practices recommended may not be widespread at the present, the adoption of these practices is believed to be a desirable and practical goal. Therefore, it is urged that they be given prime consideration in the design of new drug distribution systems and in modifications of existing ones (particularly where such changes would commit a hospital to a considerable financial investment in a system not including, or not easily altered to include, the recommended practices).

1. Before the initial dose of medication is administered, the pharmacist should review the prescriber's original order or a direct copy.

2. Drugs dispensed should be as ready for administration to the patient as the current status of pharmaceutical technology will permit, and must bear adequate identification including (but not limited to); name or names of drug, strength or potency, route(s) of administration, expiration date, control number, and such other special instructions as may be indicated.

3. Facilities and equipment used to store drugs should be so designed that the drugs are accessible only to medical practitioners authorized to prescribe, to pharmacists authorized to dispense, or to nurses authorized to administer such drugs.

4. Facilities and equipment used to store drugs should be designed to facilitate routine inspection of the drug prior to the time of administration.

5. When utilizing automated (mechanical and/or electronic) devices as pharmaceutical tools, it is mandatory that provision be made to provide suitable pharmaceutical services in the event of failure of the device.

6. Such mechanical or electronic drug storage and dispensing devices, as require or encourage the repackaging of drug dosage forms from the manufacturer's original container, should permit and facilitate the use of a new package, which will assure the stability of each drug and meet U.S.P. stand-

ards for the packaging and storing of drugs, in addition to meeting all other standards of good pharmacy practice.

7. In considering automated (mechanical and/or electronic) devices as pharmaceutical tools, the distinction between the accuracy required in accounting practices versus that required in dispensing practices should be clearly distinguished.

Accordingly, this chapter will be devoted to the various means employed by the hospital pharmacist to dispense and distribute various categories of drugs throughout the hospital.

Dispensing of Charge Non-Floor Stock Drugs

Perusal of a modern hospital formulary will quickly show the large number of therapeutic agents available to the physician. They also indicate that the ordering, dispensing and accounting of these drugs must consume an inordinate amount of time on the part of nursing service and pharmacy personnel. Therefore, it has become necessary to streamline the paperwork involved through the adoption of semi-automated processes and technics. Having previously discussed the method whereby a physician orders a drug for a patient (Chapter 12), this section will deal with the forms of accounting.

One method adopted by the hospital to identify patients is the principle of the charge plate. Here, by the use of a plastic or metal card prepared on the patient's admission to the hospital or clinic, much nursing time is conserved. As a matter of fact, all newly-printed hospital forms usually reserve a 1 $\times$ 3 inch space in the upper right or left hand corner of the form for the information on the identification plate. Accordingly, all charge stations are equipped for using this time saving device which yields an important by-product—legibility of identity.

Many drug order forms may have such information as name of drug, dosage form and route of administration preprinted on it, thereby again conserving time by requiring only a minimal effort to select the drug, the desired form and route of administration.

Items with an extremely heavy demand have specific cards with all the information preprinted. All that is necessary is the patient's identity which is quickly supplied through the use of the charge plate.

Drug order forms may be prepared on duplicate or triplicate snap out forms which provide a copy for the pharmacy, accounting department and a control copy for the pavilion.

Some hospitals have developed a procedure whereby the hospital pharmacy receives a copy of the nurse's drug administration record or the physician's drug order sheet. Pharmacists then prepare periodic charges to the patient's account and re-stock the pavilions with the items consumed.

In large hospitals with extensive computer and automatic data processing systems, drug orders usually begin with a pre-punched card bearing all the necessary information except the identity of the patient. These cards are sent to the pavilion along with a predetermined number of ampuls, vials, capsules, etc. Each time a drug is administered, the nurse imprints the patient's identity upon the card and forwards it to the accounting department. In addition to the billing aspect, these same cards should also be "run through" to provide the pharmacy with a tabulation of items consumed and thereby serve as an order to replenish supplies.

One example of a simple snap-out form utilizing the principles of the charge plate system is shown in Figure 40. This form is prepared in duplicate on the ward by the charge nurse or other responsible individual. The original is then forwarded to the pharmacy and the duplicate retained on the ward as a control copy. In addition to dispensing the requested medication, the pharmacist is also required to complete the form by inserting the cost price, the selling price and the number of units dispensed. This information is deemed to be necessary for internal auditing purposes.

A second example of a snap-out form that may utilize the principle of the charge plate is that shown in Figure 41. This form differs from that shown in Figure 40 in that the original portion entitled *Requisition for Medication* is forwarded to the pharmacy and contains on its face complete information relative to the administration of the drug by the nursing service. The second copy is utilized in the billing procedure whereas the third copy is used in the accounting department for internal audit purposes.

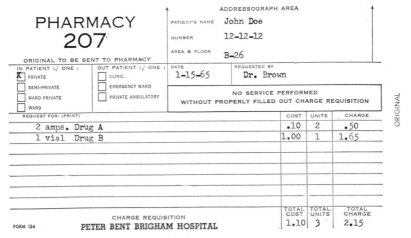

FIG. 40.   Pharmacy charge floor stock requisition form formerly used at the Peter Bent Brigham Hospital.

NEW ENGLAND CENTER HOSPITAL Requisition for **MEDICATION** IN PATIENT USE ☒ HOME USE ONLY ☐ :	Mary Doe 12-12-50 Room 25 Dr. Roe IF OFFICE ACC'T. DR.'S NAME:

ORDERED BY DR.: Dr. Roe		ORDER MADE OUT BY:	JK		FILLED BY:	WH	
DRUG	DOSE	How Often	Route of Admin.	Quant. Issued	COST	CHARGE
1. Drug A	10 mg.	daily	I.M.	1 amp	1.00	1.65
2. Drug B	15 mg.	t.i.d.	oral	20 tab.	.30	.50
3.						
REQUISITION NO.: 12345				**TOTAL**	1.30	2.15

F-515 1/63

SEND THIS COMPLETE SET TO B.D. PHARMACY

FIG. 41.   Combination Requisition for Medication, Charge Slip and Internal Audit Slip developed by the New England Center Hospital

The Envelope System

One hospital has developed a system whereby an envelope is used to dispense drugs to the nursing station and at the same time is also used as a charge ticket.[9] Under this system the pharmacist fills pre-labeled envelopes with the specific drugs and places a predetermined quantity on the nursing unit. When the drug is administered to the patient, the nurse places the patient's name and room number on the envelope and places it in her "out" basket. This is later picked up by the messenger service and is delivered to the pharmacy where it is priced and forwarded to the accounting office.

Allowance or Credit Procedures on Unused Charge Drugs

Much has been written and spoken of the desirability and the moral and legal obligation to extend credit for unused medications consonant with necessary legal and fiscal controls.

Where a credit is to be issued, two things must be done; first, criteria for issuing credit on pharmaceuticals must be established, and second a proper credit form must be developed.

Many state pharmacy laws prohibit accepting pharmaceuticals for credit return unless the container is an unopened original package. To this should be added the caution that such containers should not have been out of the pharmacist's control for an unreasonable period of time. Most hospital pharmacists accept for credit most unopened

JEFFERSON MEDICAL COLLEGE HOSPITAL
Philadelphia, Pa.

CHARGE - CREDIT VOUCHER

Date_____

Name
Room—
Ward
Admission
Number
Sex
Doctor

Complete or Imprint with Address-O-Plate

Explanation of Charge / Credits	√	DEBIT (CHARGE)	CREDIT
		$	

Signature of Person Preparing Voucher

Below this line for Main Office use only.

CODE
1 - Service
2 - Laboratory
3 - Drugs
4 - Operating Rm.
5 - Anesthesia
6 - X-Ray
FORM 14

7 - Physical Therapy.
8 - EKG
9 - Blood or Plasma
10 - Med.-Surg. Sup.
11 - 3 Telephone
11 - 4 Guest Trays

11 - 5 Formula & Bracelet
11 - 6 BMR
11 - 7 Oxygen
11 - 8 Nursery
11 - 9 Trfn Lab Svc
11 - 10 Shock Treat.

11 - 11 Hearing & Speech Center
11 - 12 Guest
B C Blue Cross
B D Bad Debts
B R Board Refunds

D C Discount Credits
T B Transfer of Balance
P P Part Pay

A   D   P   S   W
Circle Appropriate Letters

FIG. 42. The multi-purpose Charge-Credit Voucher developed at the Jefferson Medical College Hospital.

PRINT SERVICE AREA NAME AND CODE NUMBER

ADDRESSOGRAPH AREA
PETER BENT BRIGHAM HOSPITAL
PRINT PATIENT'S FULL NAME & ADMITTING NO.

IN PATIENT (✔ ONE)	OUT PATIENT (✔ ONE)	STREET
☐PRIVATE	☐CLINIC	
☐SEMI-PRIVATE	☐EMERGENCY WARD	CITY STATE
☐WARD PRIVATE	☐PRIVATE AMBULATORY	DATE
☐WARD		

No Credit Allowed Without Writing Procedure and Code Number

CREDIT PATIENT FOR FOLLOWING PROCEDURES:	CODES	UNIT	CREDIT
DISCHARGE DATE			

FORM 284-9-63

VALID ONLY IF AUTHORIZED AND SIGNED BY:
☐ CONTROLLER
☐ ASS'T CONTROLLER
☐ OFFICE MANAGER
☐ OPD SUPERVISER
☐ ADMINISTRATION _____

CREDIT

TOTAL UNIT	TOTAL CREDIT

FIG. 43. The separate or specific type of credit voucher developed by the Peter Bent Brigham Hospital.

ampuls, vials, tubes, and sealed containers of capsules and tablets which are returned from the pavilions. In order to avoid too great a loss to the patient when his therapy is suddenly changed, most hospitals restrict the amount of drug dispensed. A common number of tablets or capsules dispensed to a hospitalized patient is 20.

In some hospitals, a multi-purpose Charge-Credit Slip is utilized for extending credit to the patient's account for returned medications (Fig. 42). On the other hand, some institutions prefer to separate the functions of the two procedures and utilize two separate slips. One specifically for the charge and the other for extending credit. See Figure 43 for this type of form.

Dispensing and Distribution of Non-Charge Floor Stock Drugs

This category of drugs and related products being predetermined and stable is amenable to a variety of unique methods whereby the drugs are conveyed from the pharmacy to the nursing station.

Basic to all the distribution systems is the preparation of a printed list which indicates the name and strength of the product, the size of the unit, and its location on the nursing station. Figure 44 represents one such form which encompasses non-charge floor stock drugs as well as various lotions, germicides, mouthwashes and sterilizing solutions.

Drug Basket Method

One method routinely used by hospitals for stocking non-charge floor stock drugs and related products on the nursing station is the "drug basket method." Under this system, the night nurse checks the medicine closet, utility room and drug refrigerator inventory of supplies against a master list provided by the pharmacy through the nursing service. The nurse places a check mark on the number required for each drug on the requisition for floor stock supplies (Fig. 44). Where there is an empty container, she places it in the drug basket. Once the procedure is completed, the drug basket containing the empty containers and requisition for floor stock supplies, is then sent to the pharmacy.

Immediately upon opening in the morning the pharmacy staff commences to fill each container and dispense the requested ampuls and vials as ordered. Once the basket is completed, it is delivered to the floor via a messenger service or, in the newer institutions, via a dumb-waiter or basket ejector delivery system.

PETER BENT BRIGHAM HOSPITAL

PHARMACY REQUISITION FOR FLOOR STOCK

AREA............CODE............   DATE............

Drugs listed below are to be considered floor stock and supplied Monday
—Wednesday—Friday. All other drugs must be ordered as charge drugs.

MEDICINE CLOSET

Amt.	AMPULS	Price
	Adrenalin 1 ml. 1 : 1000	
	Aminophylline 10 ml. 250 mg.	
	Atropine Sulfate 20 ml. 0.4 mg./ml.	
	Digitoxin 1 ml. 0.2 mg.	
	Digoxin 2 ml. 0.25 mg./ml.	
	Lidocaine HCl 50 ml. 1%	
	Lidocaine HCl 50 ml. 2%	
	Lidocaine HCl 1% with Epinephrine 1 : 1000 50 ml.	
	Phenolsulfonphthalein (P.S.P.) 1 ml. 6 mg./ml.	
	Saline for Injection 30 ml.	
	Scopolamine H. Br 1 ml. 0.65 mg.	
	Sodium Dehydrocholate (Decholin) 5 ml. 1 Gm./5 ml.	
	Sulfobromophthaelin Sod. (B.S.P.) 3 ml. 50 mg./ml.	
	Water for Injection 30 ml.	

Amt.	CAPSULES & TABLETS	Price
	Acetylsalicylic Acid (Aspirin) 0.3 Gm.	
	Acetylsalicylic Acid Buffered	
	Acetylsalicylic Acid Compound	
	Ammonium Chloride E.C. 0.5 Gm.	
	Amobarbital Sodium 0.2 Gm.	
	Atropine Sulfate T.T. 0.65 mg.	
	Bisacodyl (Dulcolax) 5 mg.	
	Bishydroxycoumarin (Dicoumarol) 25 mg.	
	Cascara Sagrada Ext. 0.3 Gm.	
	Chloral Hydrate 0.5 Gm.	
	Digitalis 0.1 Gm.	
	Digitoxin 0.1 mg.	
	Digoxin 0.25 mg.	
	Ferrous Gluconate 300 mg.	
	Ferrous Sulfate 0.3 Gm.	
	Nitroglycerin H.T. 0.3 mg.	
	Nitroglycerin H.T. 0.6 mg.	
	Pentobarbital 50 mg.	
	Phenobarbital 15 mg.	
	Placebos	
	Polyvitamins	
	Potassium Chloride E.C. 1 Gm.	
	Propoxyphene HCl (Darvon) 32 mg.	
	Propoxyphene HCl Darvon Compound—65 mg.	
	Quinidine HCl 0.2 Gm.	
	Secobarbital 50 mg.	
	Sodium Bicarbonate 0.6 Gm.	

Amt.	SOLUTIONS—INTERNAL		Price
	Ammonium Chloride Syr.	8 oz.	
	Belladonna Tr.	2 oz.	
	Benzoin Comp. Tr.	4 oz.	
	Cascara Fldext Aromatic	4 oz.	
	Castor Oil	8 oz.	
	Chloral Hydrate 1 Gm./5 ml.	8 oz.	
	Glyceryl Guaiacolate- (Robitussin)	4 oz.	
	Kaolin-Pectin Mixture	8 oz.	
	Opium Tr. Camphorated	4 oz.	
	Peppermint Spirit	2 oz.	
	Potassium Chloride Elixir	8 oz.	
	Potassium Iodide Sat. Sol.	2 oz.	
	Potassium Triple Ion Elixir	8 oz.	
	Terpin Hydrate Elixir	4 oz.	
	Terpin Hydrate & Codeine Elixir	8 oz.	
	Vanilla Flavor	4 oz.	

Amt.	POWDERS		Price
	Dextrose (D-Glucose)	100 Gm. Units	
	Sodium Bicarbonate	16 oz.	
	Talcum—Individual Units°		
	Thymol Iodide (Aristol)°	2 oz.	
	°Store in Utility Room		

Amt.	MISCELLANEOUS	Price
	Amyl Nitrite	
	Aromatic Ammonia	

REFRIGERATOR

Amt.	SUPPOSITORIES		Price
	Acetylsalicylic Acid	0.6 Gm.	
	Aminophylline	500 mg.	
	Bisacodyl (Dulcolax)	10 mg.	

Amt.	LIQUID		Price
	Hydrogen Peroxide 3 Vol.	16 oz.	
	Magnesia, Milk of	32 oz.	
	Petrolatum, Liquid	32 oz.	

FIG. 44. (*Continued on opposite page*)

UTILITY ROOM

Amt. SOLUTIONS—EXTERNAL Price

	Amt.		Price
	Alcoholic Sponge Lotion	32 oz.	
	Alkaline Aromatic Solution (Mouth Wash)	32 oz.	
	Amphyl—2%	Gal.	
	Back Rub Lotion	Ind.	
	Benzalkonium Chloride 1:750	gal.	
	Benzalkonium Chloride 1:1000	gal.	
	Benzalkonium Chloride 1:20,000	gal.	
	Benzalkonium Chloride Tr.	16 oz.	
	Benzoin Tr.	4 oz.	
	Calamine Lotion	8 oz.	
	Chlorinated Soda—5%	32 oz.	
	Collodion Flexible	4 oz.	
	Creo-Napol 1 : 50	Gal.	
	Denatured Alcohol for Lamps	8 oz.	
	Deodorizing Spray	16 oz.	
	Ether—Not For Anesthesia	8 oz.	
	Ether—Alcohol Mixture	8 oz.	
	Glycerin	8 oz.	
	Hand Lotion	8 oz.	
	Hexachlorophene Deterg.	32 oz.	
	Hexachlorophene Liquid Soap	32 oz.	
	Iodine Aqueous—2%	8 oz.	
	Iodine Tr.—2%	8 oz.	
	Instrument Sterilizing Solution	32 oz.	
	Isopropyl Alcohol—50%	32 oz.	
	Magnesium Sulfate—Glycerin Solution	16 oz.	
	P.C.G. Solution	8 oz.	
	Thermometer Germicide Solution	32 oz.	

Amt.   OINTMENTS & CREAMS   Price

	Amt.		Price
	A & D Oointment	1 oz.	
	Lanolin	1 oz.	
	Lanolin—Stearin Cream	4 oz.	
	Petrolatum	1 oz.	
	Surgical Lubricant—Single use unit		
	Zinc Oxide Ointment	1 oz.	

Amt.   REAGENTS   Price

	Amt.		Price
	Actone	8 oz.	
	Acetic Acid—50%	4 oz.	
	Benzidine Reagent	4 oz.	
	Schiller's Solution	8 oz.	
	Sulfuric Acid—50%	2 oz.	
	Sulfuric Acid—0.5%	2 oz.	
	Toluene	8 oz.	
	Topfer's Reagent	4 oz.	
	Wright's Stain	8 oz.	

THIS SPACE FOR PHARMACY OFFICE USE ONLY

Filled by . . . .

Checked by . . . .

Price Total for sheet . . . . $ . . . .

Previous Total $ . . . .

Current Total $ . . . .

Form 16-Drug

FIG. 44.   Pharmacy requisition for non-charge floor stock supplies.

Mobile Dispensing Unit

A mobile dispensing system, previously described, for the hospital pharmacy[8] utilizes a specially constructed stainless steel truck measuring 60 inches high, 48 inches wide and 25½ inches deep. The main body of the truck is mounted on six 8-inch balloon tires, the center wheels being stationary while the remaining four are swivel-type. The main compartment is provided with two locking sliding doors, a handle for steering and pushing, a heavy duty steel and rubber protective bumper and a 2-inch rim on the top to permit carrying empty containers being returned to the pharmacy.

The interior of the unit consists of four shelves which allow for the transport of all size containers. Figure 45 shows a view of the truck.

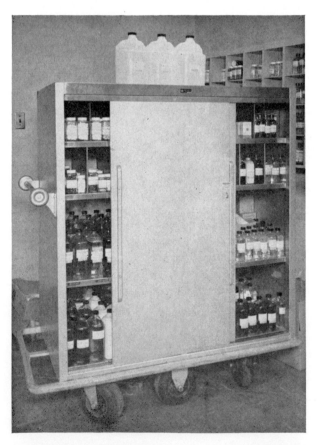

Fig. 45.   A mobile unit for dispensing non-charge floor stock drugs at the Peter Bent Brigham Hospital.

Under this system, two mobile units are put into operation in order to permit one unit to be in use while the other is being serviced. The frequency of delivery and the hours during which the mobile unit will visit the pavilion can be selected in cooperation with the Nursing Service.

By using this system, it will not be necessary for the night nurse to check the pharmacy inventory or have empty containers transported to the pharmacy. Instead, the pharmacist or the pharmacy aide manning the mobile unit will inventory the pavilion drug cabinets and check off the items and quantity of supplies left. The carbon copy of the *Requisition for Floor Stock Supplies* is left on the pavilion as a record of the delivery, and the original is returned to the pharmacy where it will serve three purposes:

1. to re-stock the mobile unit
2. to determine rate of use or consumption
3. to serve as a charge document for the internal allocation of costs.

Although it would appear that this method primarily conserves nursing personnel time, it has a number of advantages which are beneficial to the pharmacy, particularly if the truck is manned by a pharmacist.

For example, the drugs and the nursing station drug cabinets will always be under the supervision of professional personnel. The pharmacist is brought out of the pharmacy and made available for on the spot consultations by clinical and nursing staffs, and through the routine checking of the medicine closet, deteriorated, out-dated and non-approved drugs and drug samples may be quickly removed.

Mechanical Dispensing

Hospital pharmacists during the past ten years have been engaged in various forms of research aimed at the mechanization of dispensing procedures both within the pharmacy and on the nursing station.

One such machine, known as the "Brewer System" (see Fig. 46) is currently available. This machine is arranged to dispense a maximum of 8 packages of 96 different items; however, the pharmacist may decrease the variety of drugs and thereby cause the machine to contain more than 8 packages of any single item.

The packaging of drugs to be dispensed by the machine is basically the same as for a non-machine type of operation, namely, the pharmacist places the capsules, tablets or ampuls into a cardboard box, which is sized to fit the unit, prepares a pre-packaging control sheet and finally, instead of placing the pre-packaged units into bins in the pharmacy dispensing area, loads them into the machine.

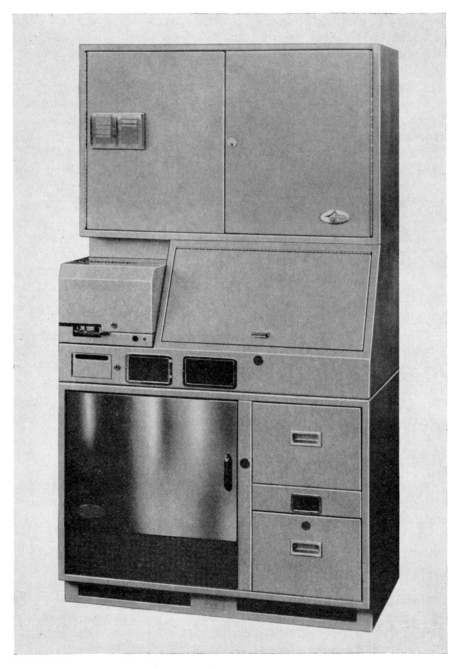

FIG. 46.   (*Legend on opposite page*)

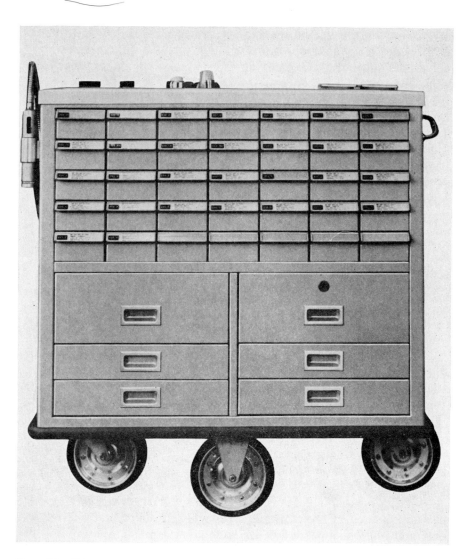

FIG. 47. The Brewer Drug Station and Brewer Drug Cart. (Courtesy of the Brewer Pharmacal Engineering Corporation, Upper Darby, Pennsylvania.)

In order to operate the machine, the nurse must use three plates: one giving the patient's identification, one identifying the desired medication and one identifying the nurse. When all three plates are inserted into position, the machine becomes activated and dispenses the package of medication, prints a label, prints a charge ticket, and records the entire transaction on an internal tape via a charge recorder within the system.

The installation of such a system in the hospital is a significant investment to control drugs on the nursing station although advocates of the system make some interesting claims relative to the elimination of drug losses and of medication errors.

Amongst the claims made for the installation of such a system are: provides maximum drug control, reduces pharmacy inventory, reduces clerical labor for the pharmacy staff, assures control of drug inventory on the nursing station, reduces clerical duties of the nurse, eliminates illegible charge slips, expedites patient charges and facilitates cost accounting.

Legal Problems

Some state attorneys general and boards of registration in pharmacy have ruled that use by hospital nurses of a mechanical device for dispensing drugs is "illegal." The reasoning behind these rulings is that the nurse by selecting and withdrawing drugs from the mechanical dispensing machine is in effect performing a "dispensing act" which is usually reserved for duly-licensed pharmacists or physicians.

Unfortunately, this reasoning is not applicable to the situation in view of the fact that nurses perform this very act each and every time that they withdraw a physician-ordered medication for a patient from the ward floor stock. Floor stock medications exist in nearly every hospital, whether mechanical drug distribution equipment is used or not, and is considered to be one of the accepted methods of drug distribution in hospitals.

Although mechanical devices for the dispensing of drugs have not been adjudicated by the courts to be illegal*, any hospital pharmacist contemplating the installation of such a system should obtain the view of the local board of registration in pharmacy and/or the attorney general of the state.

Unit-Dose Dispensing

Unit-dose medications have been defined[10] as—

> "those medications which are ordered, packaged, handled, administered and charged in multiples of single dose units containing a predetermined amount of drug or supply sufficient for one regular dose, application or use."

*The AMA News, March 22, 1965. A letter on Drug Dispensing by H. M. Trowern, Jr.

The concept of unit-dose dispensing is not a new innovation to pharmacy and medicine. For many years, pharmaceutical manufacturers have prepared and sold prefilled, single dose disposable syringes of medications and single-unit foil or cellophane wrapped capsules and tablets. Because the concept is broad, one might even consider the individual ampul or single dose containing vial as the precursor to unit dose dispensing.

Although unit dose dispensing is a pharmacy responsibility, it cannot be instituted in the hospital without the cooperation of the nursing, administrative and medical staffs. Thus, it is recommended that a planning committee be created and charged with the responsibility of developing the approach to the utilization of a unit dose system in the hospital. Despite the motivation of the committee membership, experience dictates that the hospital pharmacist should take the time to thoroughly educate them in the concepts of unit dose dispensing. This may be accomplished via literature reprints, film strips and visitations to institutions who have implemented a unit dose system. Throughout this educational and developmental period, liaison must be maintained with the medical, nursing and administrative staffs by the hospital pharmacist.

The following are some advantages attributed to a unit dose system:

(1) Patients receive improved pharmaceutical service 24 hours a day and are charged for only those doses which are administered to them.
(2) All doses of medication required at the nursing station are prepared by the pharmacy thus allowing the nurse more time for direct patient care.
(3) Allows the pharmacists to interpret or check a copy of the physician's original order thus reducing medication errors.
(4) Eliminates excessive duplication of orders and paper work at the nursing station and pharmacy.
(5) Eliminates credits.
(6) Transfers intravenous preparation and drug reconstitution procedures to the pharmacy.
(7) Promotes more efficient utilization of professional and non-professional personnel.
(8) Reduces revenue losses.
(9) Conserves space in nursing units by eliminating bulky floor stock.
(10) Eliminates pilferage and drug waste.
(11) Extends pharmacy coverage and control throughout the hospital from the time the physician writes the order to the time the patient receives the unit-dose.
(12) Communication of medication orders and delivery systems are improved.

8

(13) The pharmacists can get out of the pharmacy and onto the wards where they can perform their intended function as drug consultants and help provide the team effort that is needed for better patient care.

The unit-dose dispensing concept may be introduced into the hospital in either of two ways—the choice depending upon the individual hospital and its pharmacist. The first method is the **centralized unit-dose drug distribution system,** often abbreviated as CUDD, and the **decentralized unit-dose drug distribution system,** often abbreviated as DUDD. Some pharmacists have developed a plan whereby they use a combination of the two methods.

The initiation of a unit-dose dispensing system in the hospital is not an easy task and requires a great deal of planning both within the pharmacy and with the nursing service. The hospital pharmacist should enter into such a program a step at a time. He should commence by distributing as many injectables as possible in individual disposable syringes; he may commence the distribution of tablets and capsules in strip-packages; certain lotions, creams and ointments are already available on the drug market in single dose aluminum foil or plastic containers and thus lend themselves to the concept of unit-dose dispensing.

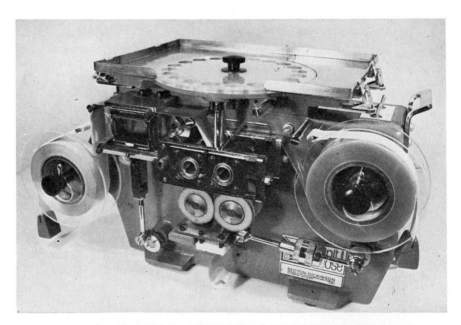

Fig. 48. Una-Strip Packer, Model SA Oral Solid Packaging Machine. (Courtesy of Becton, Dickinson and Co., Rutherford, New Jersey)

The adaption of a unit-dose dispensing system in the hospital can save personnel time both in the pharmacy and on the nursing service; provide contamination free positive identification of the medication up to the time of administration; eliminate labeling errors; permit far more accurate medication charges; and prevent the loss of partially used medications.

Personnel time can be saved in the pharmacy because under the unit dose system it no longer becomes necessary for the pharmacy to repackage and label the product in smaller dispensing units. Since this step is eliminated, so, too, is the cumbersome procedure for the

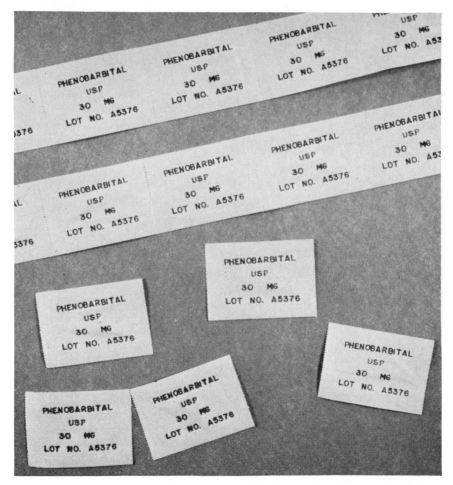

FIG. 49. Samples of packages produced by the Una-Strip Packer (Model SA or Mark 11). Other side of packages not shown can be made of transparent or opaque materials. (Courtesy of Becton, Dickinson and Co., Rutherford New Jersey.)

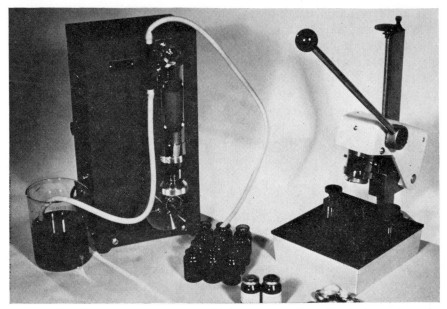

Fig. 50.   Brewer Pipetter, manual bench capper, aluminum three-piece closures and amber glass vials. (Courtesy of Becton, Dickinson and Co., Rutherford, New Jersey.)

preparation of adequate records for the purpose of recalling all available containers of a specific product should the occasion arise.

Unit-dose dispensing of medications can be accomplished in many ways. One means is through the use of strip-packaging and vial and syringe filling equipment in the hospital. (See Chapter 20 Pre-Packaging in the Hospital). Figure 48 shows a solid oral packaging machine for convenient, economical, and reliable institutional use. Packages resulting from the use of the Una-Strip®* Packer are shown in Figure 49. The other side of the package not shown can be made of transparent or opaque materials. Vials of 15, 30 and 60 ml may be filled by the use of a Brewer Pipetter along wth a manual bench capper as shown in Figure 50 or by the use of a hand capper as shown in Figure 51. An example of one product in a 30-ml. vial with the cap properly applied is shown in Figure 52. Injectable drugs may also be prepared for the unit dose system within the hospital. Disposable glass syringes in 0.5, 1, 2.5, 5 and 10-ml. sizes are commercially available (Fig. 53) and can be filled in the hospital using the syringe filling stand and transfer needle as shown in Figure 54. Once filled, the syringes are placed in a plastic tray and labeled as shown in Figure 55. Before commencing such a program, the student should

* Una-strip® Becton, Dickinson and Co.

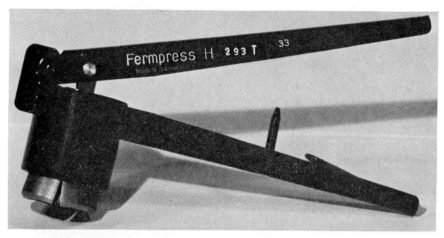

FIG. 51. Fermpress hand capper. Applies unit dose three-piece aluminum closures to 15-, 30- and 60-ml. glass vials. (Courtesy of Becton, Dickinson and Co., Rutherford, New Jersey.)

become familiar with the American Society of Hospital Pharmacists' *Guidelines for Single Unit Packages of Drugs.* See Chapter 20, page 322.

A second method may be to purchase the packaging service from an outside contractor or by the joint purchase and sharing of equipment with a neighboring hospital.

The third method is to purchase all drugs in unit dose packages. For example, Philips Roxane Laboratories distribute unit of use galenicals, magmas and suspensions whereas Wyeth Laboratories, via the "Wyeth System," makes available a combination of single packaged and labeled tablets and capsules and pre-filled, single unit disposable sterile cartridge-needle units (Tubex®) † and a specially designed medication dispensing cabinet. Other manufacturers produce solid orals in unit dose packages and produce injectables in ready-to-use plastic syringes.

It should be noted at this point that the Wyeth medication dispensing cabinet differs completely from the dispensing machine type of unit which is a component of the Brewer System. Where the Brewer unit requires various "control plates" to cause it to operate, the Wyeth unit requires none. Where the Brewer unit can imprint labels and drug charge information, the Wyeth unit does not. These differences are stated here merely for the purpose of impressing upon the student that one is not similar to the other in either design or concept. Each performs a special type of function or service.

† Tubex® Wyeth Laboratories.

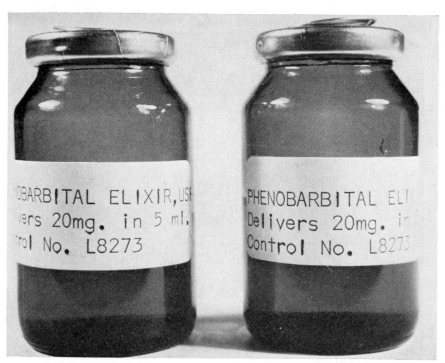

FIG. 52. An example of a 30-ml. vial with closure properly applied and labeled. (Courtesy of Becton, Dickinson and Co., Rutherford, New Jersey.)

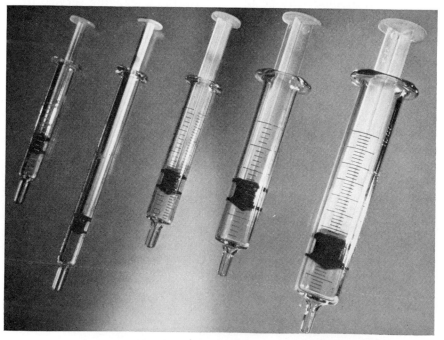

FIG. 53. B-D Glaspak disposable glass syringes in 0.5, 1, 2.5 and 10 ml. sizes. The 2.5-ml. size is available in tray packs of 10 with special black ceramic scale. (Courtesy of Becton, Dickinson and Co., Rutherford, New Jersey.)

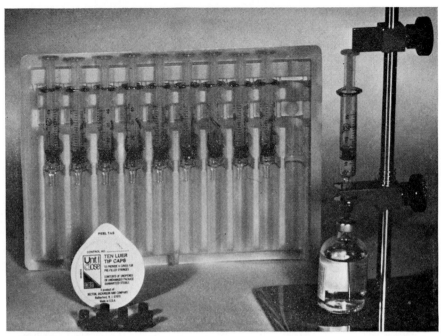

FIG. 54. Tray of ten Glaspak syringes, Luer tip cap and a view of a syringe filling stand and transfer needle. (Courtesy of Becton, Dickinson and Co., Rutherford, New Jersey.)

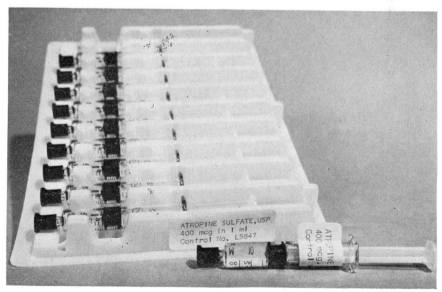

FIG. 55. Tray pack of B-D Glaspak 2.5-ml. syringes filled and with B-D Luer tip caps. A possible labeling method is shown. (Courtesy of Becton, Dickinson and Co., Rutherford, New Jersey.)

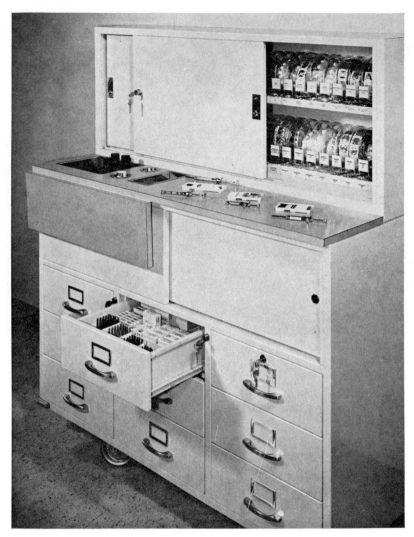

FIG. 56.   Wyeth mobile drug station. (Courtesy of Wyeth Laboratories,
Philadelphia, Pennsylvania.)

One interesting feature of the Wyeth system is its adaptability to
utilize three different packagings of oral unit doses—a soft-pack strip
pack consisting of a roll of single dose medications which can be dispensed from a re-usable reel-type of dispenser, the Redipak® strip
pack, the same cellophane roll of single dose medications described
above except that here the outer casing is a disposable cardboard box,
and finally, the commonly used strip pack.

The medication dispensing cabinet is available in two styles; a large stationary unit for use at the nursing station or a smaller mobile unit (see Fig. 56) which may be used as a complete medication cart.

By introducing a full-line single unit package of drugs, the hospital pharmacist has the advantage of what has been described as a "pre-system" phase-in from which accrue the following:[11]

    (i)   "acquaint nurses with the various new containers from which they will be administering medication;

    (ii) assist in planning for and stocking of various inventory levels;

    (iii) provide the many benefits of single unit packaging itself even though a unit dose system is not operational."

Unit-Dose Dispensing Procedure

The characteristic features of centralized unit-dose dispensing are that all in-patient drugs are dispensed in unit-doses and all the drugs are stored in a central area pharmacy and dispensed at the time the dose is due to be given to the patient. To operate the system effectively, electronic data processing equipment is not required, however delivery systems such as medication carts and dumbwaiters are needed to get the unit-doses to the patients; also suction tube systems (called pneumatic tubes) or other means are required to send a copy of the physician's original medication order to the pharmacy for direct interpretation and filling.

The *decentralized* unit-dose system, unlike the centralized system, operates through small satellite pharmacies located on each floor of the hospital. The main pharmacy in this system becomes a procurement, storage, manufacturing and packaging center serving all the satellites. The delivery system is accomplished by the use of medication carts. This type of system can be used for a hospital with separate buildings or old delivery systems.

Although each hospital introduces variations, the following is a step-by-step outline of the procedure entailed in a decentralized unit-dose system:

    (i)   Upon admission to the hospital, the patient is entered into the system. Diagnosis, allergies and other pertinent data is entered on to the Patient Profile card.

    (ii) Direct copies of medication orders are sent to the pharmacist.

    (iii) The medications ordered are entered on to the Patient Profile card.

    (iv) Pharmacist checks medication order for allergies, drug-interactions, drug-laboratory test effects and rationale of therapy.

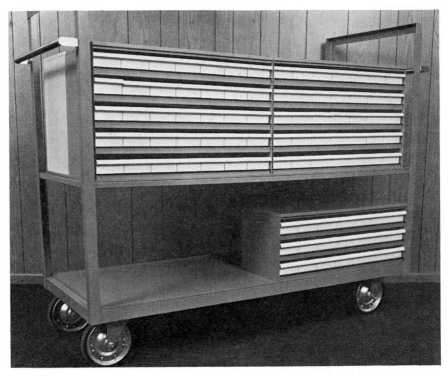

Fig. 57. B-D Transfer Cart shown with transfer units in place. Transfer units are sold separately and do not come with the transfer cart. (Courtesy of Becton, Dickinson and Co., Rutherford, New Jersey.)

(v)   Dosage scheduled is coordinated with the nursing station.

(vi) Pharmacy technician picks medication orders, placing drugs in bins of a transfer cart per dosage schedule (Fig. 57).

(vii) Medication cart is filled for particular dosage schedule delivery (Figs. 58 and 59).

(viii) Pharmacist checks cart prior to release.

(ix) The nurse administers the medication and makes appropriate entry on her medication record.

(x)   Upon return to the pharmacy, the cart is rechecked.

(xi) Throughout the entire sequence, the pharmacist is available for consultation by the doctors and nurses. In addition he is maintaining a surveillance for discontinued orders.

New Concepts in Dispensing

Of late, much has been written about placing a pharmacist on the nursing station to assume all responsibility concerning the ordering, stocking and preparation of drugs for administration as well as to be readily available for consultation by the clinical and nursing staffs.

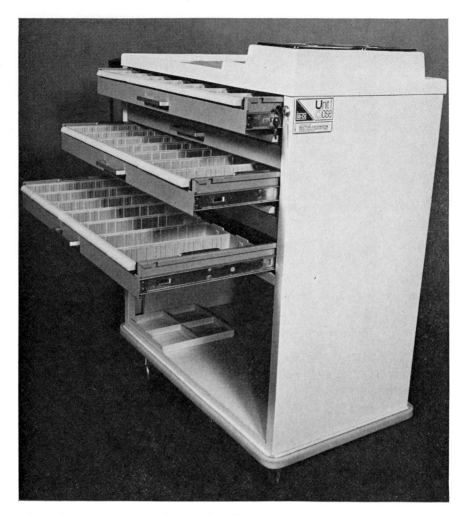

Fig. 58. B-D Nursing Cart with sliding drawers. This model has capacity for 35 patients. Models with 24, 28 and 42 patient capacity are also available. (Courtesy of Becton, Dickinson and Co., Rutherford, New Jersey.)

If funds and a sufficient number of pharmacists were available, all would agree that this would be a desirable step forward in ensuring drug safety through a marked reduction in medication errors.

This would be possible because the pharmacist is sufficiently trained and legally licensed to deal with all aspects of drug selection and handling with the exception of administering it to the patient. On the pavilion, the pharmacist may help the physician in the selection of the most therapeutically beneficial drug, assist the nurse by interpreting the physician's order as well as the preparation of each

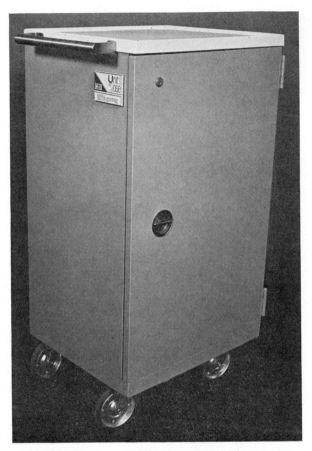

Fig. 59.   B-D Nursing Cart with door. (Courtesy of Becton, Dickinson and
Co., Rutherford, New Jersey.)

dose for administration, and the ordering, storage, charging and
control of all drugs and related products on the nursing station.

Because the funds and personnel are not presently available, some
pharmacists[12,13] have experimented with a centralized unit-dose system. Under this method, the department of pharmacy prepares a
single dose of medication ready for administration to the patient
and delivers it to the pavilion a few minutes before it is to be administered by the nurse.

Both of these studies indicated that nursing time could be saved,
that the incidence of error was in all probability reduced and that
the system gained "nurse acceptance" in a relatively short time.

Researchers at the University of Arkansas Medical Center have
been involved in an extremely interesting study whereby they are

attempting to develop a centralized unit-dose system for general hospital use.[14,17]

As described, the methodology requires that a carbon copy of the physician's order be forwarded to an IBM Keypunch operator who interprets the order via a code system onto the cards which are then processed through a sorter, reproducer and card-type converter.

Another of these sophisticated electronic data systems permits the physician to write his order and insert the written sheet into a machine, which then transmit a view of the order on to a videoscope in the pharmacy. Here it is checked for accuracy by the pharmacist and if correct, he may activate the dispensing portion of the machine by pressing a button which automatically activates a computer and an entire series of events takes place. The drug is dispensed, the nurse is alerted to administer the medication, a charge is entered upon the patient's account and upon the administration of the drug by the nurse, another press of a button enters the fact upon the patient's hospital record. The computer can also notify the doctor if the drug is not in inventory, is not prescribed according to the dose or route of administration recommended in the hospital formulary and will alert the nurse if she has failed to administer the drug within a predetermined period of time.

It should be clear that the use of electronic data processing equipment in conjunction with the dispensing of unit-dose medications can provide a broad spectrum of useful statistical data governing drugs and their use. Obviously then, such equipment must already be in use in the hospital in order to make the undertaking of a comprehensive automated dispensing program a feasible venture.

One method which does not make use of mechanical or electronic dispensing devices for the distribution of patient-charge drugs is employed at the Massachusetts General Hospital in Boston and is entitled MOSAICS—an abbreviation for **Medication Order Supply and Individual Charge System.**[18] This system places all of the drugs in current use at the hospital in the nurses' drug cabinet.

The Mosaic system is stated to reflect a simple but basic change, namely, that in the past the patient was admitted first and the drug was then requisitioned. Under the Mosaics plan, the drug is already on the floor awaiting the patient. The modus operandi is relatively simple in that a pharmacist visits the patient floor on a regular schedule, re-stocks the unit and makes a charge to the patient or patients consuming the drugs. The information necessary for the charging procedure comes from the Doctor's Order Sheet, Nursing Kardex or Medication Charting Sheets.

The architects of the Mosaics system have demonstrated that by placing the pharmacist on the patient pavilion it was possible for him to serve as a drug advisor and consultant to the medical and nursing staffs. In addition, he was in a better position to perform the pharmaceutical functions of checking upon the storage, administration, expiration date, contamination and degredation of drugs and biologicals.

Self-Medication Program

The large number of effective therapeutic agents which are now available has created a serious problem in the proper treatment of patients. Because of the specificity of pharmacological response of many of these drugs, it is often necessary to employ several in order to obtain the desired clinical response. Frequently, this has led to confusion, improper administration of the drug on the part of the patient and poor therapeutic results.

In an informal survey conducted by the Nursing Service and the Department of Pharmacy of a metropolitan teaching hospital, it was learned that approximately 50 per cent of the ambulatory patients receiving medications were not aware of the reasons for taking the drugs and that nearly 40 per cent exhibited errors in the way they were taking their medications. Upon closer scrutiny of this figure, it was clearly demonstrated that an extremely high percentage of the errors were made when the signa of the precription indicated "As directed" and the patient received more than one prescription.

Since the above observations were being similarly made in other hospitals throughout the country, many physicians, pharmacists and nurses have become interested in the development of a program for the education of patients relative to the *what, why* and *when* of the drugs which have been prescribed for their use.

One way whereby such a program may be initiated is to place patients, who are capable of cooperating, on a self-medication program while they are in the hospital. After the initial stage of alarm caused by proposing such a radical departure from standard hospital procedure has given way to sound reasoning, many will agree that this concept is really no different from that of progressive patient care or that of the ill patient at home who, of necessity, must resort to self administration of prescribed medications.

There are many advantages that would accrue from a satisfactorily developed program, the most important being the education of the patient whereby medication would be taken as intended by the physician when the patient was discharged from the hospital and secondly, while an in-patient, much nursing time could be conserved and devoted to other forms of patient care.

In response to a question as to whether or not physicians may order a medication to be left at the patient's bedside to be taken at the patients discretion, Kenneth B. Babcock, M.D., former Director of the **Joint Commission on Accreditation of Hospitals** replied[19]—

> "The answer is an emphatic 'No.' No medication should ever be left at the patient's bedside to be taken at his or her discretion. Every dose of any medication should be administered by a qualified person and recorded on the chart. This is important not only from the standpoint of the welfare of the patient, but also from a legal aspect."

Based on this opinion, the hospital pharmacist is advised to proceed with caution in the recommendation of such a program for use in the hospital. However, if such a program is, for one reason or another approved for use in a particular hospital, the hospital pharmacist should make every effort to assist in the design of a procedure that would ensure maximal safety for the patient yet protect the hospital and its staff from medicolegal implication.

Since Dr. Babcock's 1964 statement, there have been a number of hospitals and hospital pharmacists who have experimented with self-medication programs.[20,21,22] Some of the projects have been conducted at a physical rehabilitation hospital,[23,24] in an extended care facility,[25] on a geriatric ward of a large New York City hospital and on a cardiology unit of a medical center.[26]

A review of the literature reveals that most investigators conducting these studies believe them to be successful. Thus, the new Joint Commission on Accreditation of Hospitals standards allow for self-medication programs.[27]

SELECTED REFERENCES

TESTER, W.: A Study of Patient Care Involving a Unit-Dose System, Final Report 1967, U.S.P.H.S. Grant No. HM-00328-01, College of Pharmacy and University Hospitals of the University of Iowa, Iowa City, Iowa, Jan. 1, 1967.

————: Hospital Medication Systems Study Guide, American College of Hospital Administrators, Chicago, Illinois, 1969.

KLEINMANN, KURT: Tailoring Pharmacy Systems to Today's Technology, Hospitals, J.A.H.A., *42*:23:59, Dec. 1, 1968.

PARKER, PAUL F.: Unit-Dose Systems Reduce Error, Increase Efficiency, Hospitals, J.A.H.A., *42*:23:65, Dec. 1, 1968.

HELLER, WILLIAM M.: Data Processing in Drug Distribution Systems, Hospitals, J.A.H.A., *42*:23:73, Dec. 1, 1968.

232   **Dispensing to In-Patients**

BOGASH, ROBERT C.: Tomorrow's Drug Distribution System is Already Here, Hospitals, J.A.H.A., *42*:23:79, Dec. 1, 1968.
HASSAN, WM. E.: Quo Vadis Drug Packaging? Hospital Pharmacy, *4*:7:9, July, 1969.
SIMON, G. L., SILVERMAN, H. M., VETTER, T. G. and VOLPERT, B.: A Semi-automated Approach to Unit Dose Dispensing, Am. J. Hosp. Pharm., *29*: 6:491, June, 1972.
MUELLER, WILLIAM J.: Establishing Unit Dose Medication Distribution, Hospital Pharmacy, *7*:12:402, December, 1972.
ZILZ, DAVID A.: Budget and Financial Implication in Implementing and Maintaining Unit Dose Drug Distribution Systems, Hospital Pharmacy, *7*:12: 405, December, 1972.
GARRISON, THOMAS J.: Designing a Unit Dose Medication System, Hospital Pharmacy, *7*:12:413, December, 1972.

BIBLIOGRAPHY

1. ARCHAMBAULT, GEORGE F. L.: The Law of Hospital Pharmacy, Am. J. Hosp. Pharm., *15*:7:593, 1958.
2. CONNORS, EDWARD J.: The Hospital Administrator's Responsibility for Drug Distribution, Hospitals, J.A.H.A., *42*:23:46, Dec. 1, 1968.
3. HSIEH, R.: Evaluation of Formal Communication Systems in a Hospital, Health Serv. Res., *1*:222, Winter, 1966.
4. ———: Hospital Medication Errors, J.A.M.A., *195*:31, Jan. 17, 1966.
5. FREUND, R. G.: How the Centralized Unit-Dose Concept Works in a Community Hospital, J.A.H.A., *40*:152, Sept. 16, 1966.
6. TESTER, W.: A Study of Patient Care Involving a Unit-Dose System, College of Pharmacy, University Hospital, University of Iowa, Iowa City, Iowa, 1967.
7. Statement on Hospital Drug Distribution Systems, Am. J. Hosp. Pharm., *21*:11:535, 1964.
8. HASSAN, WILLIAM E., JR.: Mobile Dispensing for the Hospital Pharmacy, Am. J. Hosp. Pharm., *17*:8:490, 1960.
9. BJERKE, P. and MISSMAN, L. C.: An Envelope System for Floor Medications, Hospitals, J.A.H.A., *34*:63, Aug. 1, 1960.
10. Unit Dose Medication Dispensing, Wyeth Laboratories, Philadelphia, Pa.
11. ———: A Brief Review of the Physical, Mechanical, and Packaging Requirements in Unit-Dose Distribution Systems—Part II, Philips Roxane Laboratories, Columbus, Ohio, 1971.
12. SCHWARTAU, N. and STURDAVANT, M.: A System of Packaging and Dispensing Drugs in Single Doses, Am. J. Hosp. Pharm., *18*:9:542, 1961.
13. McCONNELL, W., BARKER, K. and GARRITY, L.: Centralized Unit-Dose Dispensing, Am. J. Hosp. Pharm., *18*:9:531, 1961.
14. BARKER, KENNETH N. and HELLER, WILLIAM M.: The Development of a Centralized Unit-Dose Dispensing System, Part I, Description of the U.A.M.C. Experimental System, Am. J. Hosp. Pharm., *20*:11:568, 1963.
15. ———: Ibid., *20*:12, 612, 1963.
16. ———: Part III, An Editing Center for Physicians' Medication Orders, Am. J. Hosp. Pharm., *21*:2:66, 1964.
17. HELLER, WILLIAM M., SHELDON, ELEANOR C. and BARKER, KENNETH N.: The Development of a Centralized Unit-Dose Dispensing System for U.A.M.C. Part IV, The Roles and Responsibilities of the Pharmacist and

Nurse Under the Experimental System, Am. J. Hosp. Pharm., 21:8:230, 1964.
18. TUCCI, RALPH G. and WEBB, JOHN W.: Mosaics, Medication Order Supply and Individual Charge System, Am. J. Hosp. Pharm., 21:8:307, 1964.
19. BABCOCK, KENNETH B.: Accreditation Problems, Hospitals, J.A.H.A., 38: 41, July 16, 1964.
20. GORDON, H. L., KELLER, C. J. and LENTINI, V.: Self-Medication Programs in Public Hospitals I. A Survey of Practices in Veterans Administration Hospitals, Hosp. Comm. Psych., 17:355, Dec. 1966.
21. POPE, H. L.: Self-Medication Programs in Public Hospitals II. A Prelude to Discharge, Hosp. Comm. Psych., 17:357, Dec. 1966.
22. HENDERSON, J. H.: Self-Medication in a Psychiatric Hospital, Lancet, 1: 1055, May 13, 1967.
23. REIBEL, E. M.: Study to Determine the Feasibility of a Self-Medication Program for Patients at a Rehabilitation Center, Nurs. Res., 18:65, Jan.-Feb., 1969.
24. JOHNSON, E. W., ROBERTS, C. J. and GODWIN, H. N.: Self-Medication for a Rehabilitation Ward, Arch. Phys. Med. Rehab., 51:300, May 1970.
25. LIBOW, L. S. and MEHLE, B.: Self-Administration of Medications in Hospital or Extended Care Facilities, J. Amer. Geriat. Soc., 18:81, Jan. 1970.
26. BUCHANAN, E. C., BROOKS, M. R. and GREENWOOD, R. B.: A Self-Medication Program for Cardiology Patients, Am. J. Hosp. Pharm., 29:11:928, Nov. 1972.
27. TOUSIGNAUT, D. R.: New JCAH Standards and Modern Hospital Practice, Am. J. Hosp. Pharm., 28:178, Mar. 1971.

Chapter

14

Dispensing to Ambulatory Patients

IT has been shown that about 64 per cent of the hospitals in this country provide out-patient prescription service and that more than 32 million prescriptions were dispensed from out-patient pharmacies in the year 1957.[1]

In contrast, in 1970, 762,862,000 prescriptions were dispensed from hospital pharmacies in the United States. Of this number, 613,863,000 were for in-patients and 148,997,000 for ambulatory patients.[2]

The growth of out-patient clinics may be attributed to the following:

(a) The need of the hospital to supplement its in-patient teaching program.

(b) The demand by the community, lay as well as professional, for comprehensive diagnostic and treatment centers.

(c) The new philosophy of hospitals—to take a more active role in the community health programs.

(d) The need of the hospital and physician to exercise greater control over patients receiving investigational use drugs.

(e) The lack of a sufficient number of physicians in some areas, thereby causing the population to travel to the medical center for comprehensive care.

(f) The fact that the emergency service of a hospital is always available, whereas a physician, in some rural areas, may not always be available.

Because of this volume and the prospect of growing larger within the next twenty years, many community pharmacists have been quick to cite the economic hardship this trend may create in the community. Although this is an important factor to be considered, it would appear that the crux of the problem is the lack of understanding by the community practitioner of the purpose and scope of a complete or comprehensive ambulatory service.

With the aim of alleviating this situation, the American Pharmaceutical Association and the American Society of Hospital Pharmacists established a Commission to study out-patient hospital pharmacy service and related hospital-community-pharmacy problems.

The Commission and Its Report

The two groups recognized that the goal of such a commission would not be realized without the cooperative effort of the medical and hospital associations. Thus an invitation to participate was extended to the American Medical Association and to the American Hospital Association.

The Commission, on October 22, 1964, modified its original name of Commission on Out-Patient Dispensing to read, **Commission on Pharmaceutical Services to Ambulant Patients by Hospitals and Related Facilities.**

One of the objectives adopted by the Commission was—"To obtain accurate data and reliable information regarding pharmaceutical services to out-patients by hospitals and other facilities."

Upon the completion of its studies, the Commission published a report entitled *The Challenge to Pharmacy in Times of Change.* This scholarly publication should be read by every student and practitioner of pharmacy.

Because of the depth of the study and the limited nature of this textbook, it is necessary to concentrate only on the following portion of the Commission's summary[3]—

> 2. **Hospital out-patient pharmaceutical service:** As a general rule, hospitals do not solicit private out-patient prescription patronage. The hospital out-patient department is in a very favorable position to attract private patients because of the convenience factor, but the location of the pharmacy in the hospital, a limited stock of health supplies, and the limitations of the formulary system, are often deterrents to maximum out-patient services. The hospital pharmacist is burdened with the care of hospital patients and has little time to develop a personal consumer loyalty with private patients. The community pharmacist, on the other hand, can develop a personal relationship through a high level of professional and individualized service that will permit him to compete favorably with the convenience advantage that a hospital or a medical center-based pharmacy service offers the patient. The patient has the same right to select his pharmacist as he does his physician or other health practitioner, and none of the parties involved should adopt procedures that circumvent this right.

Location of Out-Patient Dispensing Area

There is no set rule as to the best area to locate an out-patient dispensing pharmacy. This is evidenced by the fact that in today's practice three equally suitable provisions are made for this area:

(*a*) A separate out-patient pharmacy is available.

(*b*) A combined in-patient and out-patient unit with service provided from the same "window."

(*c*) A combined in-patient and out-patient unit with service provided from separate "windows."

A separate out-patient pharmacy is usually established whenever the out-patient department and the pharmacy are geographically widely separated. Although this arrangement has the advantage of being a separate and distinct unit with a specialized function, it possesses the disadvantages of requiring a separate staff as well as consuming a great deal of time, on the part of other pharmacy department personnel, in transporting supplies and drugs to the area.

The above disadvantages are obviously eliminated whenever both in-patient and out-patient facilities are combined. An additional advantage to this arrangement is that the director of the pharmacy service is able to exert a greater degree of control and supervision.

Types of Prescriptions Received

Depending upon the location and kind of hospital, the prescriptions received in the out-patient department pharmacy will generally include those of private patients (where permitted by the state board of registration in pharmacy), indigent patients, non-indigent patients, employees, and patients being discharged from the hospital. It is a known fact that in any large metropolitan teaching hospital, the largest volume of prescriptions comes from the indigent or partially indigent group of patients. It is also established that every patient who visits the clinics does not have his prescription filled in the hospital. Indeed, hospitals with 500 or more beds fill approximately 1 prescription per 3 out-patient visits, whereas the 100 to 199-bed hospitals average about 1¼ prescriptions for each visit.[4]

Because many of these indigent patients are supported by some type of welfare program, their prescriptions require special identification, and the billing for such must be in accord with the requirements of the particular agency. In some states, a special pricing system for the drugs dispensed is in effect. See Chapter 19 for an example and discussion of one such system.

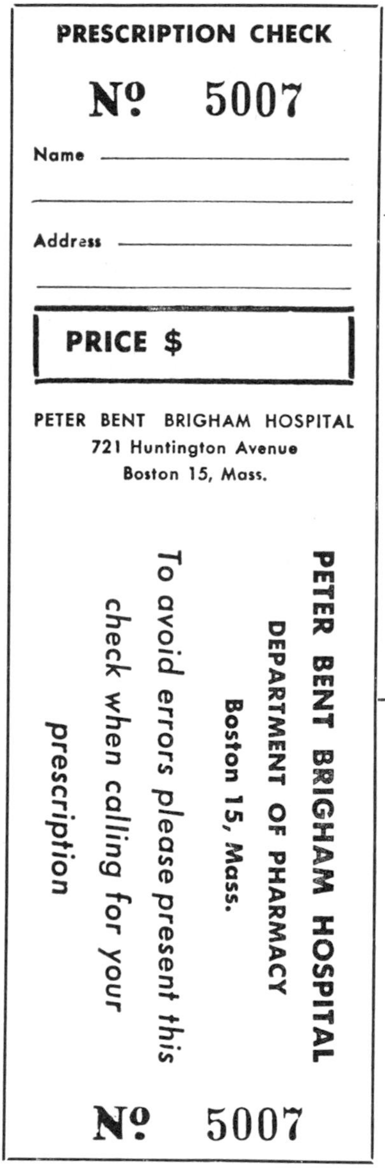

PRESCRIPTION CHECK

No 5007

Name ______________________

____

Address ______________________

____

PRICE $

PETER BENT BRIGHAM HOSPITAL
721 Huntington Avenue
Boston 15, Mass.

PETER BENT BRIGHAM HOSPITAL
DEPARTMENT OF PHARMACY
Boston 15, Mass.

To avoid errors please present this check when calling for your prescription

No 5007

FIG. 60. Prescription Call Check used in the out-patient dispensing pharmacy as a means of matching the correct patient and prescription.

The Dispensing Routine

The dispensing pattern involved in providing clinic patients as well as those patients being discharged with "take home drugs" is identical with that carried on by a community pharmacy.

In both instances, a prescription is written by the physician and the patient takes it to the pharmacy where it is compounded by a pharmacist. If there is to be a waiting period, the pharmacist will make use of a prescription call check which numerically identifies the patient, and the finished prescriptions (Fig. 60). Once in the hands of the pharmacist, the prescription and label are numbered by a numbering machine; the directions and other pertinent information are placed on the label; ancillary labels are affixed; the proper medication is then placed in the container; a check for accuracy is then conducted; and finally the prepared prescription is wrapped and dispensed.

For internal audit purposes, hospital prescriptions are separated into out-patient and in-patient discharges and therefore may utilize two different colored blanks.

Figure 61 represents one type of hospital prescription.

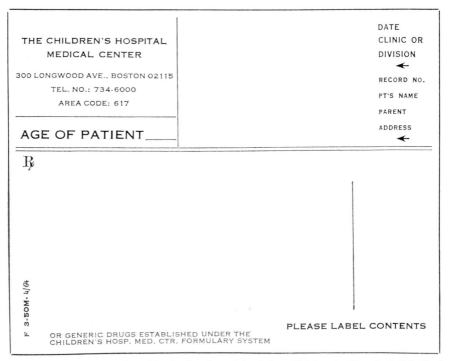

FIG. 61. A prescription blank developed by The Children's Hospital Medical Center in Boston. Note the emphasis on the patient's age.

A rather ingenious combination of prescription call check, prescription and label in a single form is that of the Philadelphia General Hospital. This form (Fig. 62) has many advantages in that it combines three forms into one; it saves the pharmacist's time in handing

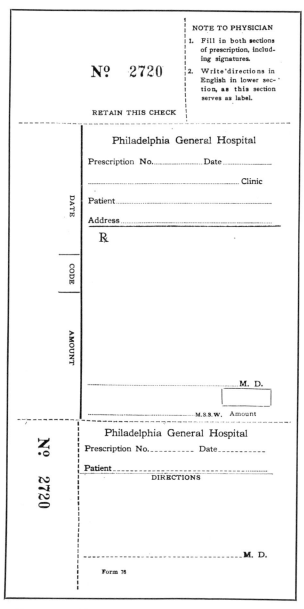

FIG. 62.   A combination prescription call check, prescription and label, all in one form.

out a call check and typing a label; and finally, it is probably more economical. It would seem that its only disadvantages are that the prescription on file does not carry the directions for use and that the directions for use written by the physician on the label portion of the form, more often than not, will be illegible to the patient.

Many other types of prescription forms are in current use in the hospitals of the nation. Some consist of multiple pages attached to a prepunched card ready for use in a computer system; others consist of a prescription blank the back of which is affixed with coded magnetic tape thereby rendering the prescription suitable for use in automatic billing and electronic data-retrieval systems.

Prescriptions Involving Research Projects

The department of pharmacy in a teaching hospital is often called upon either to assist in or to conduct a special research program designed to ascertain the prescribing habits of the staff physicians, the correlation between diagnosis and drug prescribed, as well as cost studies which involve the cost of drugs to both hospital and patient.

Such studies usually involve designing a special prescription blank, an example of which is shown in Figure 63. This two part carbonized prescription form is designed to provide, in addition to the usual information obtained on a prescription, special data required for the particular study. The days of therapy and cost information are provided by the pharmacist compounding the prescription, and the information concerning the diagnosis is obtained by research personnel from the medical record.

The prescription number, patient number, date, age, sex, drug prescribed, quantity prescribed, directions for use, physician's code, days of therapy, cost data and diagnosis are then transferred to a punched tape. The tape is then processed and fed into a computer for a final analysis of the information thus gathered.

I.R.S. Rulings on Out-Patient Dispensing

Revenue received by a non-profit hospital pharmacy for filling prescriptions for in-patients or out-patients is not considered "unrelated business taxable income" and is not subject to federal income tax, the Internal Revenue Service has ruled.

But, if a hospital pharmacy is open to the general public and prescriptions are filled for patients walking in from the street or if sales of non-prescription items are made under the same conditions, this revenue is subject to taxation. One of the rulings permits prescription sales without taxation by a hospital which fills occasional prescriptions written by staff physicians who practice in consultation rooms provided by the hospital. IRS has ruled that these were merely "casual" sales, made as a courtesy to staff physicians.

In ruling that out-patients may have prescriptions filled in hospital pharmacies without subjecting the income received by the institution to federal taxations, IRS also included refills for former patients or prescriptions originally written when the patients were receiving hospital treatment. It also extended the non-taxable income rule to treatment received in home care and extended care facilities operated by or supervised by a hospital.[4]

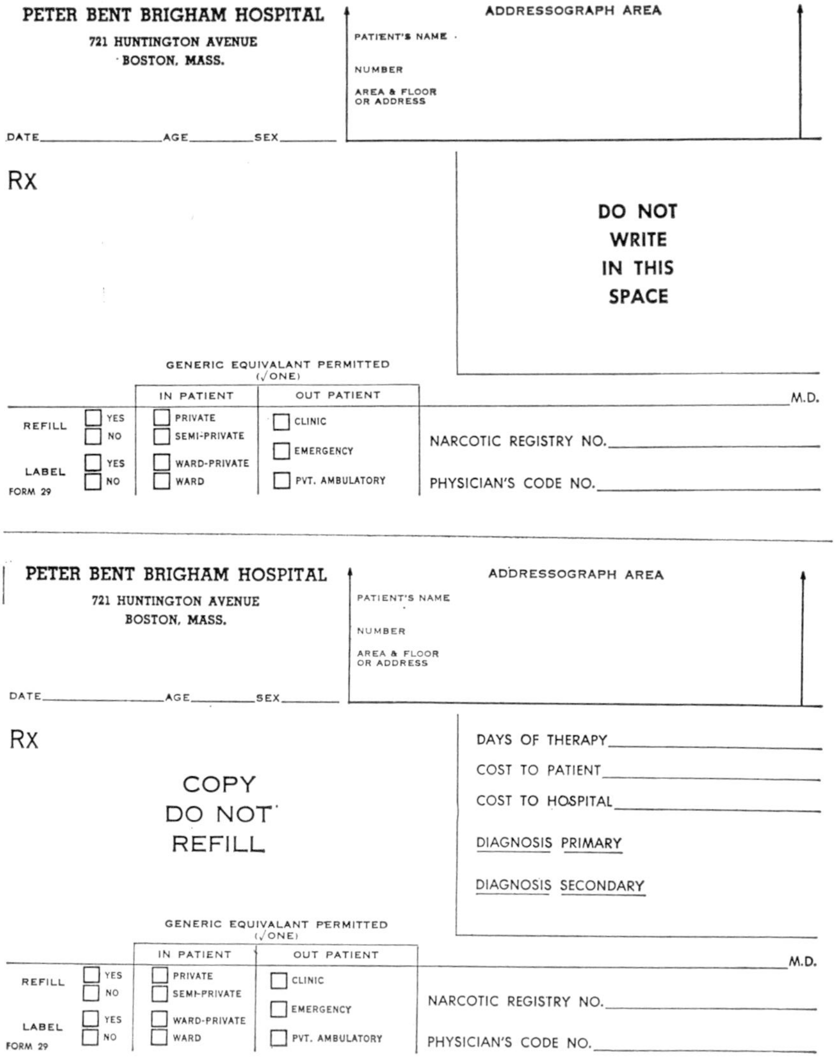
PETER BENT BRIGHAM HOSPITAL
721 HUNTINGTON AVENUE
BOSTON, MASS.

ADDRESSOGRAPH AREA
PATIENT'S NAME
NUMBER
AREA & FLOOR OR ADDRESS

DATE______ AGE______ SEX______

RX

DO NOT WRITE IN THIS SPACE

GENERIC EQUIVALANT PERMITTED (√ONE)

		IN PATIENT	OUT PATIENT	
REFILL	☐ YES ☐ NO	☐ PRIVATE ☐ SEMI-PRIVATE	☐ CLINIC ☐ EMERGENCY	M.D. NARCOTIC REGISTRY NO.______
LABEL	☐ YES ☐ NO	☐ WARD-PRIVATE ☐ WARD	☐ PVT. AMBULATORY	PHYSICIAN'S CODE NO.______

FORM 29

PETER BENT BRIGHAM HOSPITAL
721 HUNTINGTON AVENUE
BOSTON, MASS.

ADDRESSOGRAPH AREA
PATIENT'S NAME
NUMBER
AREA & FLOOR OR ADDRESS

DATE______ AGE______ SEX______

RX

COPY DO NOT REFILL

DAYS OF THERAPY______
COST TO PATIENT______
COST TO HOSPITAL______
DIAGNOSIS PRIMARY
DIAGNOSIS SECONDARY

GENERIC EQUIVALANT PERMITTED (√ONE)

		IN PATIENT	OUT PATIENT	
REFILL	☐ YES ☐ NO	☐ PRIVATE ☐ SEMI-PRIVATE	☐ CLINIC ☐ EMERGENCY	M.D. NARCOTIC REGISTRY NO.______
LABEL	☐ YES ☐ NO	☐ WARD-PRIVATE ☐ WARD	☐ PVT. AMBULATORY	PHYSICIAN'S CODE NO.______

FORM 29

FIG. 63. Two-part prescription blank used in a prescription data survey.

Revenue Rule 68-374 provides as follows:

"Section 513 of the Code defines the term 'unrelated trade or business' as any trade or business the conduct of which is not substantially related (aside from the need of such organization for income or funds or the use it makes of the profit derived) to the exercise or performance by such organization of its exempt functions.

To the extent relevant here, section 513 (a)(2) of the Code further states that the term 'unrelated trade or business' does not include any trade or business which is carried on by an organization described in section 501(c)(3) primarily for the convenience of its patients."

Section 512 of the Code defines the term 'unrelated business taxable income' as the income as computed in this section derived by organizations from any unrelated trade or business regularly carried on.

Section 1.513-1(c)(1) of the Income Tax Regulations states that "in determining whether trade or business from which a particular amount of gross income derives is 'regularly carried on' within the meaning of section 512, regard must be had to the frequency and continuity with which the activities productive of the income are conducted and the manner in which they are pursued."

Section 1.513-1(c)(2)(ii) of the regulations states that "in determining whether or not intermittently conducted activities are regularly carried on, the manner of conduct of the activities must be compared with the manner in which commercial activities are normally pursued by non-exempt organizations. In general, exempt organization businesses which are engaged in discontinuously or periodically will not be considered regularly carried on if they are conducted without the competitive and promotional efforts typical of commercial endeavors."

Section 1.513-1(c)(2)(ii) of the regulations further states that "where an organization sells certain types of goods or services to a particular class of persons in pursuance of its exempt functions 'primarily for the convenience' of such persons within the meaning of section 513(a)(2), casual sales in the course of such activity which do not qualify as related to the exempt function involved or as described in section 513(a)(2) will not be treated as regular. On the other hand, where the non-qualifying sales are not merely casual, but are systematically and consistently promoted and carried on by the organization they meet the section 512 requirement of regularity."

SELECTED REFERENCES

Moravec, D. F.:   Hospital Out-patient Dispensing, Hosp. Management, *89*: 3:80, 1960.

Anon.:   R$_x$ Men Help Finance Pharmacy That Will Compete With Them, Am. Druggist, *141*:22, 1960.

Sowinski, R. P.: Current Trends in Out-patient Pharmacy Service, Am. Prof. Pharmacist, 26:1:56, 1960.

Martin, Eric W.: *Dispensing of Medication*, 7th Ed., Easton, Mack Publishing Co., 1971.

McKelvey, Cornelius P. and Lamy, Peter P.: Patient Care Information in an Ambulatory Health Care Environment. Am. J. Hosp. Pharm. 29:5:401, May 1972.

Mehl, Bernard and Kissner, Edward A.: Ambulatory Pharmaceutical Services in a Changing Urban Community. Am. J. Hosp. Pharm., 29:5:407, May 1972.

Johnson, Richard E., Myers, John E. and Egan, Douglas M.: A Resource Planning Model for Outpatient Pharmacy Operations, Am. J. Hosp. Pharm., 29:5:411, May 1972.

Klienman, Kurt: Outpatient Pharmacy—New Design Encourages Comprehensive Pharmaceutical Service, Am. J. Hosp. Pharm., 29:5:419, May 1972.

BIBLIOGRAPHY

1. Francke, Don E., Latiolais, Clifton J., Francke, Gloria N., and Ho, Norman, F. H.: *Mirror to Hospital Pharmacy*, Washington, D.C., Am. Soc. Hosp. Pharm., p. 117.

2. ———: American Druggist, Aug. 9, 1971, p. 58.

3. Brodie, Donald C.: *The Challenge to Pharmacy in Times of Change*, A.Ph.A. and A.S.H.P., Washington, D.C., 1966.

4. Francke, Don E., Latiolais, Clifton J., Francke, Gloria N., and Ho, Norman, F. C.: *Mirror to Hospital Pharmacy*, Washington, D.C., p. 120.

5. Internal Revenue Bulletin No. 1968-29, July 15, 1968.

Chapter

15

Dispensing Ancillary Supplies

A recent trend in hospital pharmacy is the assumption of responsibility for the purchase, stocking and distribution of the various ancillary medical, surgical and laboratory supplies. The range of inventory for this type of goods is extremely broad and may consist of costly surgical instruments, catheters, sutures, needles, syringes, sphygmomanometers, and laboratory ware.

Whether or not this is a desirable trend depends upon the individual pharmacist and the hospital administration. Certainly the assignment of this added special type of responsibility to the pharmacist is a clear indication of the administration's respect for his multiple talents. In addition, a few years of experience in handling these supplies will better qualify him to assume responsibility for the central sterile supply room or for the purchasing division if the occasion should ever arise.

Certainly, in the very small hospital such an assignment is highly desirable for it may mean the difference between hiring a pharmacist or not hiring one on the basis of insufficient pharmaceutical duties.

Qualifications of the Pharmacist

There should be no doubt about the fact that the pharmacist is certainly capable of undertaking such a task for he, in all probability, will have had greater training than the lay person who might be assigned the task. In addition, he will have a greater understanding relative to the use to which these items are to be put to and therefore may be able also to act in an advisory capacity relative to the selection of one item over another. Furthermore, because of his experience in the handling and accounting of pharmaceuticals, the hospital will be assured of proper control.

Purchasing

Because of the nature of ancillary supplies, they are usually purchased from sources other than a pharmaceutical house or drug wholesaler. Therefore, the pharmacist must acquaint himself with the various agencies, distributors and general wholesaler. Due to the extremely keen competition in this area, the pharmacist is cautioned to take the time to ascertain the integrity and reliability of the vendor, as well as his ability and desire to be cooperative and render special services when called upon in an emergency situation.

Since many distributors have the agency for the same product, it is wise to purchase as many items via the bid process with the right to bid being open to all, but the specifications and other service demands associated with the shipping, billing, etc. being set at a level that only the most reliable vendors can meet.

The purchasing of the supplies should not be mixed with the purchasing of pharmaceuticals and separate records and inventories should be maintained. Depending upon the scope of the ancillary supply inventory, some items may be extremely slow in turn-over; therefore unless a separate physical inventory is maintained and recorded, it is possible to warp the true operation of the drug portion of the pharmacy by reducing the number of times of turn-over of the true pharmacy inventory.

Once the responsibility of handling these items is assigned to the pharmacist, it is suggested that the procedure for the purchase of drugs discussed in Chapter 9 be followed.

Distribution

Ancillary supplies are of such a nature that the laboratories, pavilions and special service areas can predict their rate of use and consequently order them from the pharmacy on a weekly or bi-weekly basis.

The day on which these orders are placed is arbitrary, but it is recommended that a specific day be selected in addition to a time deadline. This is necessary if the supplies are to be ready for pick-up and distribution by the hospital messenger service.

There are two methods whereby the pavilions, laboratories and special service areas may be informed as to exactly what is carried in inventory. They are via a pre-printed requisition form which lists all the supplies or by issuing a catalogue.

If the total number of items stocked is not too great, then a pre-printed requisition form is ideal and the most practical.

On the other hand, the best way to inform those who must requisition the supplies for their area is by means of a published catalogue listing the materials alphabetically under a major heading. The catalogue should be cross-indexed to facilitate its use and should show the unit size of the package to be dispensed. This will save a

PETER BENT BRIGHAM HOSPITAL
REQUISITION TO PHARMACY FOR WARD AND LABORATORY SUPPLIES ONLY

For use in .... Ward A .... Date 1/4/65 ....

Requisitions for Ward and Laboratory Supplies must be in the Pharmacy by 10:30 A.M. daily. Supplies may be picked up any time between 3:30 P.M. and 5:00 P.M. There will be only one order daily. No requisitions will be filled on Sundays and holidays. Please watch your stock supplies, and see that you are well supplied.

WANTED		DESCRIPTION OF ITEM	√	COST
Amount	Size			
1	100	Sugar Testing Tablets		
12	1"	Adhesive Tape		
12	---	Oral Thermometers		
1	2oz.	Benzidine Test Reagent		

Requested by .... Jane Doe, Head Nurse ....

Approved by .... Mary Doe, Supervisor ....   Received by .... Helen Doe, Ward Clerk ....

Form 16A - Drugs

FIG. 64. A requisition to the pharmacy for ward and laboratory supplies. This form is prepared on the ward or in the laboratory and sent to the pharmacy. The pharmacist checks off each item dispensed, prices it, and forwards the completed requisition form to the pharmacy accounting section.

Form 191   ### PETER BENT BRIGHAM HOSPITAL

PHARMACY

DATE   1-5-65

DEPT.   Operating Room

NAME ON ORIGINAL REQ.   Jane Doe

We are temporarily out of the following:

Quantity	ITEMS
1 doz.	Sutures # 123
	☐ Charged ☒ Not charged

When these items are available, your order will be completed.

PLEASE DO NOT REORDER

FIG. 65. Out of Stock Notice.

great deal of time for the dispensing personnel as well as for the pricing clerk.

In hospitals where a catalogue has been published, a special requisition form must also be put into use. This form must, of necessity, be quite simple and yet capable of being used for any type of supply. A sample of such a form is shown in Figure 64.

When preparing this requisition, the department head usually prepares it in duplicate in order that he may retain a copy of the original order as a receiving slip to make sure that all supplies ordered have been received.

Because some items will at one time or another be out of inventory, it is advisable to use an OUT OF STOCK NOTICE to so inform the requisitioning department. A sample of this form is shown in Figure 65. This form is initiated in duplicate by the pharmacist filling the requisition. The original is retained in the pharmacy and the duplicate is sent to the requisitioning department. When the supplies are again in inventory, it is a simple matter to forward the item to the laboratory or ward without their issuing a new request.

Economic Order Quantity Model

If the pharmacist assumes the managerial responsibility for the dispensing of ancillary supplies, then he must utilize modern techniques to maintain control over the investment in inventory. One such method is the utilization of the economic order quantity model (see Chapter 9).

A number of economic order quantity models have been devised to assist one in the control of inventory locked dollars. Basically, these mathematical models determine the optimum inventory level by calculating the optimum order quantity and re-order points. In addition, such additional information as *procurement cost, average holding cost per unit, average investment per unit,* and *optimum turn-over rate,* should be considered.

A model for this purpose has been presented and described in Chapter 9 *Purchasing and Inventory Control.* The same model has application for the control of any type of inventory be it drugs or ancillary supplies.

SELECTED REFERENCES

AHA Health Careers Series—1, Hospital Purchasing Agent Code No. 162-158, American Hospital Association, Chicago, Illinois.
The VOICE of the Pharmacist, *15*:2, December 16, 1971.

Chapter

16

Dispensing of Controlled Substances

THE Federal Harrison Narcotic Act was originally passed in 1914 and was designed to protect the health of the American people and to serve as a source of tax revenue to the Government. Regulation No. 5 of the Harrison Narcotic Act and subsequent treasury department decisions concerned themselves with the practical application of this law.

In 1965, the Federal Food, Drug and Cosmetic Act was amended by the passage of the Drug Abuse Control Amendments of 1965. Thus, the combination of the Federal Harrison Narcotic Act and the Drug Abuse Control Amendments of 1965 formed the basis for the control of the majority of special drugs within the hospital environment. In 1970, the Congress enacted the Comprehensive Drug Abuse Prevention and Control Act, which in effect, combined the Federal Harrison Narcotic Act and Drug Abuse Control Amendments of 1965 and imposed stricter controls over a large number of stimulant and depressant drugs. Thus, the new law required the profession of pharmacy to devise new ways to control a large segment of the medications dispensed.

Comprehensive Drug Abuse Prevention and Control Act of 1970

The above act, also known as Public Law 91-513, and as the Controlled Substances Act, has as its purpose "to amend the Public Health Service Act and other laws to provide increased research into, and prevention of, drug abuse and drug dependence; to provide for treatment and rehabilitation of drug abusers and drug dependent persons; and to strengthen existing law enforcement authority in the field of drug abuse."[1]

The Act is divided into four "titles" dealing with the following subjects:

Title I   —Rehabilitation Programs Relating to Drug Abuse
Title II   —Control and Enforcement

Title III —Importation and Exportation; Amendments and Repeal of Revenue Laws

Title IV —Report on Advisory Councils

Title I, Rehabilitation Programs Relating to Drug Abuse amends Part D of the Community Mental Health Centers Act to include under its provisions persons with drug abuse and drug dependence problems. In addition, it provides for increased budgetary allocations for drug abuse education programs; funding for special projects for narcotic addicts and drug dependent persons; broader treatment authority in public health service hospitals; and research under the Public Health Service Act in drug use, abuse and addiction.

Title II, dealing with control and enforcement is also known as the Controlled Substances Act. In passing this Act, the Congress made the following findings and declarations:

1. Drugs included under this title have a legitimate and useful medical purpose and are necessary to maintain the health and general welfare of the American people.
2. Illegal importation, manufacture, distribution, possession and improper use of controlled substances have a detrimental effect on the health and welfare of the American people.
3. The manufacture, local distribution, and possession of controlled substances have a direct effect upon interstate commerce.
4. Local distribution and possession of controlled substances contribute to the interstate traffic in such substances.
5. It is not a practical matter to attempt to differentiate between controlled substances manufactured and distributed interstate and controlled substances manufactured and distributed intrastate.
6. Federal control of both types of traffic is essential.
7. The United States must establish effective control over domestic and international traffic in controlled substances to be in compliance with the Single Convention on Narcotic Drugs of 1961 to which it was a party.

In order to understand the contents of Title II completely, it is necessary first to be familiar with the definitions contained within the text:

> *Addict:* any individual who habitually uses any narcotic drug so as to endanger the public morals, health, safety or welfare, or who is so far addicted to the use of narcotic drugs as to have lost the power of self-control with reference to his addiction.
>
> *Administer:* the direct application of a controlled substance to the body of a patient or research subject by a practitioner or his agent or by the patient or research subject at the direction and in the presence of the practitioner.

9

Agent: an authorized person who acts on behalf of or at the direction of a manufacturer, distributor or dispenser; exceptions being common contract carriers and warehouse men.

Control: the addition of a drug or other substance, or immediate precursor, to a schedule under Part B of this title, whether by transfer from another schedule or otherwise.

Controlled Substances: a drug or other substance, or immediate precursor, included in Schedule I, II, III, IV or V of Part B of this title. The term does not include distilled spirits, wine, malt beverages or tobacco, as those terms are defined or used in subtitle E of the Internal Revenue Code of 1954.

Counterfeit Substance: a controlled substance whose container or label has, without authorization, the identification of a producer other than the actual producer.

Deliver or Delivery: the actual, constructive, or attempted transfer of a controlled substance, whether or not there exists an agency relationship.

Depressant or Stimulant Substance:

(A) a drug which contains any quantity of (1) barbituric acid or any of the salts of barbituric acid; or (2) any derivative of barbituric acid which has been designated by the Secretary as habit-forming under section 502 (d) of the Federal Food, Drug, and Cosmetic Act [21 U.S.C. 352(d)]; or

(B) a drug which contains any quantity of (1) amphetamine or any of its optical isomers; (2) any salt of amphetamine or any salt of an optical isomer of amphetamine; or (3) any substance which the Attorney General, after investigation, has found to be, and by regulation designated as, habit-forming because of its stimulant effect on the central nervous system; or

(C) lysergic acid diethylamide; or

(D) any drug which contains any quantity of a substance which the Attorney General, after investigation, has found to have, and by regulation designated as having, a potential for abuse because of its depressant or stimulant effect on the central nervous system or its hallucinogenic effect.

Dispense: to deliver a controlled substance to an ultimate user or research subject by, or pursuant to the legal order of a practitioner, including the prescribing and administering of a controlled substance and the packaging, labeling, or compounding necessary to prepare the substance for such delivery.

Dispenser: a practitioner who so delivers a controlled substance to an ultimate user or research subject.

Distribute: to deliver (other than by administering or dispensing) a controlled substance.

Distributor: a person who so delivers a controlled substance.

Drug: the same as that provided by section 201 (g) (1) of the Federal Food, Drug, and Cosmetic Act.

Immediate Precursor: a substance which

(A) the Attorney General has found to be and by regulation designated as being the principal compound used, or produced primarily for use, in the manufacture of a controlled substance;

(B) which is an immediate chemical intermediary used or likely to be used in the manufacture of such controlled substances; and

(C) the control of which is necessary to prevent, curtail, or limit the manufacture of such controlled substances.

Manufacture: the production, preparation, propagation, compounding, or processing of a drug or other substance, either directly or by extraction from substances of natural origin, or independently by means of chemical synthesis or by a combination of extraction and chemical synthesis, and includes any packaging or repackaging of such substance or labeling or relabeling of its container; except that such term does not include the preparation, compounding, packaging, or labeling of a drug or other substance in conformity with applicable state or local law by a practitioner as an incident to his administration or dispensing of such drug or substance in the course of his professional practice. The term "manufacturer" means a person who manufactures a drug or other substance.

Manufacturer: a person who manufactures a drug or other substance.

"Marihuana": all parts of the plant *Cannabis sativa L.,* whether growing or not; the seeds thereof; the resin extracted from any part of such plant; and every compound, manufacture, salt, derivative, mixture, or preparation of such plant, its seeds or resin. Such term does not include the mature stalks of such plant, any other compound, manufacture, salt, derivative, mixture, or preparation of such mature stalks (except the resin extracted therefrom), fiber, oil, or cake, or the sterilized seed of such plant which is incapable of germination.

Narcotic Drug: means any of the following, whether produced directly or indirectly by extraction from substances of vegetable origin, or independently by means of chemical synthesis, or by a combination of extraction and chemical synthesis.

(A) opium, coca leaves and opiates.

(B) a compound, manufacture, salt, derivative, or preparation of opium, coca leaves or opiates.

(C) a substance (any compound, manufacture, salt, derivative, or preparation thereof) which is chemically identical with any substance referred to in (A) or (B) above. Excluded are decocainized coca leaves or extracts of coca leaves which do not contain cocaine or ecgonine.

Opiate: any drug or other substance possessing an addiction-forming or addiction-sustaining liability similar to morphine or being converted into a drug having such capabilities.

Opium Poppy: the plant (excluding the seeds) of the species *Papaver somniferum L.*

Practitioner: a physician, dentist, veterinarian, scientific investigator, pharmacy, hospital, or other person licensed, registered, or otherwise permitted, by the United States or the jurisdiction in which he practices or does research, to distribute, dispense, conduct research with respect to, administer, or use in teaching or chemical analysis, a controlled substance in the course of professional practice or research.

Production: includes the manufacture, planting, cultivation, growing or harvesting of a controlled substance.

Ultimate User: a person who has lawfully obtained and who possesses, a controlled substance for his own use or for the use of a member of his household or for an animal owned by him or a member of his household.

Authority to Control

Part B of Title II authorizes the Attorney General to apply the provisions of this title to the controlled substances listed within Section 202 of this title and (a) add to such a schedule or transfer between such schedules any drug or other substance if he finds that such material has a potential for abuse, and (b) remove any drug or other substance from the schedules if he finds that the drug or other substance does not meet the requirements for inclusion in any schedule. In making these decisions, the Attorney General is required to give consideration to the following factors:

1. The drug's or other substances' actual or relative potential for abuse.
2. Scientific evidence of its pharmacological effect, if known.
3. The state of current scientific knowledge regarding the drug or other substance.
4. Its history and current pattern of abuse.
6. What, if any, risk there is to the public health.
7. Its psychic or physiological dependence liability.
8. Whether the substance is an immediate precursor of a substance already controlled under this title.

The Attorney General may disregard the requirements of this title and control any drug or substance if control of such is required by United States obligations under international treaties, conventions or protocols. He may also, without regard to the findings required by this title, place an immediate precursor in the same schedule in which the controlled substance of which it is an immediate precursor is placed or in any other schedule with a higher numerical designation. Excepted is the drug dextromethorphan although the exclusionary wording allows for its control at some future time if such becomes necessary.

Schedules of Controlled Substances

The key section of Public Law 91-513 is Section 202(a) for within it is created the five schedules of controlled substances, known as Schedules I, II, III, IV and V. The listings within each schedule must be updated and republished one year after the date of enactment and annually thereafter.

Except where control is required by a United States obligation, a drug or other substance may not be placed in any schedule unless the findings required for each schedule are made with respect to such drug or other substance. The findings required for each of the schedules are as follows:

(1) SCHEDULE I
   (A) The drug or other substance has a high potential for abuse.
   (B) The drug or other substance has no currently accepted medical use in treatment in the United States.
   (C) There is a lack of accepted safety for use of the drug or other substance under medical supervision.
(2) SCHEDULE II
   (A) The drug or other substance has a high potential for abuse.
   (B) The drug or other substance has recurrently accepted medical use in treatment in the United States or a currently accepted medical use with severe restrictions.
   (C) Abuse of the drug or other substances may lead to severe psychological or physical dependence.
(3) SCHEDULE III
   (A) The drug or other substance has a potential for abuse less than the drugs or other substances in schedules I and II.
   (B) The drug or other substance has a currently accepted medical use in treatment in the United States.
   (C) Abuse of the drug or other substance may lead to moderate or low physical dependence or high psychological dependence.
(4) SCHEDULE IV
   (A) The drug or other substance has a low potential for abuse relative to the drugs or other substances in schedule III.
   (B) The drug or other substance has a currently accepted medical use in treatment in the United States.
   (C) Abuse of the drug or other substance may lead to limited physical dependence or psychological dependence relative to the drugs or other substances in schedule III.
(5) SCHEDULE V
   (A) The drug or other substance has a low potential for abuse relative to the drugs or other substances in schedule IV.
   (B) The drugs or other substance has a currently accepted medical use in the United States.
   (C) Abuse of the drug or other substance may lead to limited physical dependence or psychological dependence relative to the drugs or other substances in schedule IV.
   (c) Schedules I, II, III, IV, and V shall, unless and until amended pursuant to section 201, consist of the following drugs or other substances, by whatever official name, common or usual name, chemical name, or brand name designated.

Registration Requirements

Part C of this title describes the registration of manufacturers, distributors and dispensers of controlled substances. Generally, it authorizes the Attorney General to promulgate rules and regulations and to charge reasonable fees relating to the registration and control of the manufacture, distribution, and dispensation of controlled substances.

Every person falling into one or more of the above cited areas must obtain annually a registration issued by the Attorney General. Exempted from registering are the following:

1. An agent or employee of any registered manufacturer, distributor, or dispenser of any controlled substance if he is acting within the usual scope of the business or employment.
2. A common or contract carrier or warehouseman, or an employee thereof, whose possession of the controlled substance is in the usual scope of his business or employment.
3. An ultimate user who possesses such substance for his own use or for the use of a member of his household or for an animal owned by him or a member of his household.

Since the new law went into effect, the Internal Revenue Service and the Food and Drug Administration are no longer issuing a registration authorizing a person or firm to handle controlled substances. Registration with the Bureau of Narcotics and Dangerous Drugs (BNDD) became effecitve with the new law. (*See* footnote, p. 255.)

The registration fees are as follows:

Manufacturer (includes repackers and relabelers)	$50
Distributor (wholesalers)	25
Importer or Import Broker/Forwarder	25
Exporter or Export Broker/Forwarder	25
Foreign Firm (manufacturing for importation into the U.S.A.)	25
Retail Pharmacy	5
Hospital and Clinic	5
Practitioner	5
Researcher	5
Analytical Laboratory	5
Teaching Institution	5

The Attorney General may, in accord with the rules and regulations promulgated by him, inspect the establishment of a registrant or applicant for registration.

Registration may be granted to the applicant if the Attorney General determines that such registration is in the public interest. The following are some of the factors that are considered in determining the public interest:

1. Maintenance of effective control against diversion of the controlled substances into other than legal channels;
2. Compliance with applicable state and municipal law;
3. Prior conviction record of the applicant;
4. Past experience in the distribution of controlled substances;
5. Such other factors as may be relevant to and consistent with the public health and safety.

Registration Exemption for Hospital House Staff

When the Federal Controlled Substances Act became effective on May 1, 1971 every physician was required to register with the Bureau of Narcotics and Dangerous Drugs in order to prescribe, dispense and administer controlled substances. This policy applied to interns, residents, and foreign-trained physicians working in hospitals. The only exception allowed was where a person administered or dispensed controlled drugs as the employee of the registrant, such as a nurse or intern working with in-patients in a registered hospital.

The problem this policy caused soon became apparent in that interns, residents and foreign-trained physicians had to obtain BNDD registrations even though their occasion to use the registration was limited to the times they prescribed controlled substances in the emergency or ambulatory clinics. To alleviate this situation, an alternative procedure was developed which allowed the temporary or provisionally licensed doctor to prescribe controlled substances without an individual registration with BNDD.

Under the new policy, the intern, resident or foreign-trained physician does not have to register individually but may use the hospital's registration number for writing prescriptions, provided that the hospital complies with the following:

> First, the hospital has the responsibility for verifying that the intern, resident or foreign-trained physician may lawfully write prescription while working in the hospital.
> Second, the hospital must assign a code system which designates individual physicians using the hospital's registration number. This code serves as the intern's, resident's or foreign-trained physician's individual number in lieu of the DEA* registration number.
> Third, the hospital must assure that the individual physician uses the full number assigned to him and not merely the code num-

*A new agency, the Drug Enforcement Administration, was created under Reorganization Plan No. 2 of 1973 which assumed the functions of various enforcement arms of the Department of Justice, including the Bureau of Narcotics and Dangerous Drugs (BNDD), and the investigative functions of the Bureau of Customs. Effective date was July 1, 1973.

ber which the hospital added to its registration number to identify him. In addition, the physician should have his name stamped, or typed, or handprinted on the hospital's prescription form.

Fourth, upon the request of an outside pharmacy, law enforcement agency, or other registered person seeking to verify the authority of the prescribing individual practitioner, the hospital will determine whether or not the prescription is written by one of its staff by checking the name and code number of the physician as requested against a current list of internal code numbers and the corresponding individual practitioners.

Separate Registration for Independent Activities

The following eight groups of activities are deemed to be independent of each other:

1. Manufacturing (including repackaging and relabeling) controlled substances.
2. Distributing controlled substances.
3. Dispensing (including prescribing and administering) narcotic and non-narcotic, and conducting research with nonnarcotic, and conducting instructional activities with narcotic and non-narcotic controlled substances listed in schedules II through V.
4. Conducting research with narcotic controlled substances listed in schedules II through V.
5. Conducting research and instructional activities with controlled substances listed in schedule I.
6. Conducting chemical analysis with controlled substances in any schedule.
7. Importing controlled substances.
8. Exporting controlled substances listed in schedules I through IV.

Every person who engages in more than one group of independent activities must obtain a separate registration for each group of activities, with the following exceptions. Any person, when registered to engage in the group of activities described hereinafter shall be authorized to engage in the coincident activities, provded that, unless specifically exempted, he complies with all requirements and duties prescribed by law for persons registered to engage in such coincident activities: For example—

1. A person registered to manufacture or import any controlled substance or basic class of controlled substance shall be authorized to distribute that substance or class which he is not registered to manufacture or import.
2. A person registered to manufacture any controlled substance

listed in schedules II through V shall be authorized to conduct chemical analysis and preclinical research (including quality control analysis) with narcotic and non-narcotic controlled substances listed in those schedules in which he is authorized to manufacture.

3. A person registered to conduct research with a basic class of controlled substances listed in schedule I shall be authorized to manufacture such class if and to the extent that such manufacture is set forth in the research protocol filed with the application for registration.

4. A person registered to conduct chemical analysis with controlled substances shall be authorized to manufacture and import such substances for analytical or instructional purposes, to distribute such substances to other persons registered to conduct chemical analysis or instructional activities and to persons exempted from registration pursuant to Section 301.26, to export such substances to persons in other countries performing chemical analysis or enforcing laws relating to controlled substances or drugs in those countries, and to conduct instructional activities with controlled substances.

5. A person registered to conduct research with narcotic controlled substances listed in schedules II through V shall be authorized to conduct research with non-narcotic controlled substances listed in schedules II through V.

One or more controlled substances listed in schedules II through V may be included in a single registration to engage in any independent activity. Only one basic class of controlled substance listed in schedule I, and no controlled substances listed in other schedules, may be included in a single registration, except that a registration to conduct chemical analysis with basic classes of controlled substances listed in schedule I may include more than one basic class and also controlled substances listed in any other schedule.

Separate Registrations for Separate Locations

A separate registration is required for each principal place of business or professional practice at one physical location where controlled substances are manufactured, distributed, or dispensed by a person. An office used by a practitioner (who is registered at another location) where controlled substances are prescribed but neither administered nor otherwise dispensed as a regular part of the professional practice of the practitioner at such office and where no supplies of controlled substances are maintained shall be deemed not to be places where controlled substances are manufactured, distributed or dispensed by a person.

Exemption of Agents and Employees

The requirement of registration is waived for any agent or employee of a person who is registered to engage in any group of independent activities, if such agent or employee is acting in the usual course of his business or employment. An individual practitioner who is an agent or an employee of another practitioner registered to dispense controlled substances may, when acting in the usual course of his employment, administer and dispense (other than by issuance of prescription) controlled substances if and to the extent that such individual practitioner is authorized or permitted to do so by the jurisdiction in which he practices, under the registration of the employer or principal practitioner in lieu of being registered himself. For example, a pharmacist employed by a hospital need not be registered individually to fill a prescription for controlled substances if the hospital pharmacy is so registered.

Time for Application for Registration

Any person who is required to be registered and who is not so registered may apply for registration at any time. No person required to be registered may engage in any activity for which registration is required until the application for registration is granted and a Certificate of Registration is issued to him.

Expiration of Registration

Any person who is registered may apply to be re-registered not more than sixty days before the expiration date of his registration.

At the time any person is first registered, he will be assigned to one of twelve groups, which shall correspond to the months of the year. The expiration date of the registrations of all persons within any group will be the last day of the month designated for that group. In assigning any person to a group, the DEA may select a group the expiration date of which is less than one year from the date such person was registered. If the person is assigned to a group which has an expiration date less than three months from the date on which the person is registered, the registration will not expire until one year from that expiration date; in all other cases, the registration will expire on the expiration date first following the date on which the person is registered.

Application Forms

Individuals seeking registration under the Act are required to file special forms. A person applying for registration:

1. To manufacture or distribute controlled substances shall apply on DEA Form 225.
2. To dispense narcotic or non-narcotic, or to conduct research with non-narcotic, or to conduct instructional activities with narcotic or non-narcotic controlled substances listed in schedule II through V, shall apply on DEA Form 224.
3. To conduct research with narcotic controlled substances listed in schedule II through V, shall apply on DEA Form 225.
4. To conduct research with a controlled substance listed in schedule I, shall apply on DEA Form 225, with two copies of a research protocol describing the research project attached to the Form.
5. To conduct instructional activities with a controlled substance listed in schedule I, shall apply as a researcher on DEA Form 225 with two copies of a statement describing the nature, extent and duration of such instructional activities attached to the Form.
6. To conduct chemical analysis with controlled substances listed in any schedule, shall apply on DEA Form 225.
7. To import or export controlled substances listed in any schedule, shall apply on DEA Form 225.

Applications for registration must include all of the information called for in the form, unless the item is not applicable, in which case this fact must be indicated. In addition, each application, attachment, or other document filed as part of an application, shall be signed by the applicant, if an individual; by a partner of an applicant, if a partnership; or by an officer of the applicant, if a corporation, corporate division, association, trust or other entity. Another person may be authorized to sign for the applicant, if proof of authority (e.g. general power of attorney) accompanies the application.

Modification in Registration

Any registrant may request a modification of his registration by submitting a letter of request to the Registration Branch, Drug Enforcement Agency, Central Station, Washington, D.C. 20005. Each letter of request for modification must be signed and dated by the same person who signed the most recent application for registration or reregistration.

Inventory Requirements

Every registrant, other than an individual practitioner, must on the day he is first registered and every two years thereafter, make a complete and accurate record of all stocks of controlled substances under his control. The record must indicate the date on which the inventory was taken and whether taken at the close or opening of business; be signed by the person responsible for the taking of the inventory; and be maintained at the location appearing on the registration for a period of two years.

The term "individual practitioner" means a physician, dentist, veterinarian, or other individual licensed, registered, or otherwise permitted by the United States or the jurisdiction in which he practices, to dispense a controlled substance in the course of professional practice, but does not include a pharmacist, a pharmacy, or an institutional practitioner.

Under the law, a registered individual practitioner is not required to keep records with respect to narcotic controlled substances listed in Schedules II through V which he prescribes or administers in the lawful course of his professional practice. However, he must keep records with respect to such substances that he dispenses other than by prescribing or administering. A registered individual practitioner is not required to keep records with respect to non-narcotic controlled substances listed in Schedule II through V which he dispenses in any manner unless he regularly charges his patients, either separately or together with charges for other professional services, for such substances so dispensed (e.g. when he substitutes his services for those of a pharmacist).

In addition to the above, Section 307 (a) through (3) requires that, after inventory, every registrant shall maintain, on a current basis, a complete and accurate record of each substance manufactured, received, sold, delivered or otherwise disposed of by him. A perpetual inventory is not required.

Furthermore, records to be kept must be in conformity with the regulations of the Attorney General; they must be maintained separately from all other records of the registrant; the records of the non-narcotic controlled substances must be in such form that information required by the Attorney General is readily retrievable from the ordinary business records of the registrant; and all records pertaining to this law must be maintained for a period of two years.

Prescriptions

In studying the contents of Section 309 which follows, the reader is urged to make constant reference to the Federal Food, Drug, and Cosmetic Act Section 503 (b).

Section 309 provides the following requirements:

1. Except when dispensed directly by a practitioner, other than a pharmacist, to an ultimate user, no controlled substance in Schedule II, which is a prescription drug as determined

under the Federal Food, Drug, and Cosmetic Act, may be dispensed without a written prescription of a practitioner.

2. Drugs may be dispensed on an oral prescription in an emergency situation.
3. Prescriptions shall be retained in conformity with the requirements of this law.
4. No prescription for a controlled substance in Schedule II may be refilled.
5. Controlled substances in Schedule III or IV may not be dispensed without a written or oral prescription in conformity with Section 503 (b) of the Federal Food, Drug, and Cosmetic Act.
6. Such prescriptions may not be filled or refilled more than six months after the date thereof or be refilled more than five times after the date of the prescription unless renewed by the practitioner.
7. No controlled substance in Schedule V which is a drug may be distributed or dispensed other than for a medical purpose.

Prescriptions filled with controlled substances in Schedule II must be written in ink or indelible pencil and must be signed by the practitioner issuing them.

No prescription for a controlled substance in Schedule II may be refilled and such prescriptions, as well as prescriptions for narcotic substances in Schedules III, IV and V, must be kept in a separate file.

Prescriptions for controlled substances in Schedule II or IV may be issued either orally or in writing and may be refilled if so authorized. These prescriptions may not be filled or refilled more than six months after the date issued, or be refilled more than five times after the date issued. After five refills or after six months the practitioner may renew any such prescription. A renewal should be recorded on a new prescription blank and a new prescription number should be assigned to that prescription.

Offenses and Penalties

Part D concerns itself with a listing of prohibited acts, most of which are familiar to the pharmacist. Examples include:

1. Dispensing controlled drugs without first becoming registered.
2. Removing, altering or obliterating a symbol or label required by this title.
3. Refusing or failing to make, keep or furnish any record, report, notification, declaration, order or order forms, statement, invoice or information required under this title.
4. Refusing an entry into any premises or inspection authorized by this title.

Finally, the section provides for various penalties to be assessed for the various violations and range from fines, imprisonment or both depending upon the seriousness of the violation.

Labeling and Packaging Requirements

Labeling and packaging requirements under this law are cited in Section 305 (a), (b), (c) and (d). Generally, they require that containers of controlled substances must meet the labeling requirements of the Federal Food, Drug, and Cosmetic Act or the regulations to be promulgated by the Attorney General.

Each controlled substance manufactured after December 1, 1971 must have on its label a symbol designating to which schedule it belongs. The symbol will be a letter C with the Roman numeral I, II, III, IV or V. This symbol will appear in the upper right hand portion of the label. Manufacturers and other registrants will be given adequate time, to be specified by regulations, in order to comply with the symbol requirements.

A Model Set of Hospital Controlled Substances Regulations

The Controlled Substance regulations here set forth comply with Title II of the 'Comprehensive Drug Abuse Prevention and Control Act of 1970' and subsequent amendments or proclamations concerned with the implementation of the Federal Law. The law is administered by the Drug Enforcement Agency. This regulation deals specifically with Schedule II Substances which include drugs formerly known as Class A narcotics, amphetamines, methamphetamines, and any subsequent additions.

Definitions:

1. "Order": The direction for the drug, strength and frequency of administration as written on the Doctor's Order Sheet of the patient's Medical Record.
2. "Prescription": The direction for the drug, strength, quantity, and frequency of administration as written on a prescription blank by a doctor for dispensing by the Pharmacy.
3. "Administer": The word "administer" is employed when a nurse or other properly qualified individual gives medication to a patient, pursuant to the order of a qualified practitioner.
4. "Dispense": The word "dispense" is employed when a pharmacist gives medication to a nurse of other properly qualified individual in accord with the directions of a properly written prescription.
5. "Doctor": This term is herein employed to indicate an individual who has qualified for and has received a number from the Drug Enforcement Agency.

6. *Controlled Drugs Reqisition* (Fig. 66) is used by the head nurse to order drugs from the Pharmacy.
7. *Daily Controlled Drugs Administration Form* (Fig. 67) serves three purposes: a 24-hour administration record for all Schedule II Substances administered, allows space for inventory count for each nursing shift, and a section which serves as a record of losses and as a basis for review of errors.
8. *Monthly Controlled Drug Inventory* (Fig. 68) serves as a monthly dispensing record for each nursing unit and receipt for Schedule II Substances dispensed directly from Pharmacy.

Registration

A. HOSPITAL
The hospital is registered with the Drug Enforcement Agency.

B. DOCTORS
Doctors (Practitioners), in order to prescribe narcotics for or order administered (dispensed) to their patients in the hospital, must be licensed to practice under the laws of the state and must be duly registered with the DEA.

C. INTERNS and RESIDENTS
Interns and Residents who are attending patients in the hospital or hospital clinics must obtain a license to practice medicine in this State. According to the *Federal Register,* Vol. 36, No. 140, p. 13390, registration requirements were waived to allow interns and residents to dispense and prescribe controlled substances under the registration of the hospital by which they are employed, provided that:

a. Such dispensing or prescribing is done in the usual course of professional practice.
b. Such individual practitioner is authorized or permitted to do so by the jurisdiction in which he is practicing.
c. The hospital which employs him has determined that the individual practitioner is so permitted to dispense or prescribe drugs by the jurisdiction.
d. Such individual practitioner is acting only within the scope of his duties within the hospital.
e. The hospital authorizes the intern, resident, or foreign physician to dispense or prescribe under the hospital registration and designates a specific internal code number for each intern, resident, or foreign physician so authorized. The code number shall consist of numbers or letters, or a combination thereof and shall be a suffix to the hospital's DEA registration number. Example: AM1901176-WH2.

A Hospital House Staff Identification card may be obtained from the Medical Staff Registrar and the DEA number will be issued by the Pharmacy upon request.

Hospital Control Procedures

A. *RESPONSIBILITY for CONTROLLED SUBSTANCES in the HOSPITAL*

The administrative head of the hospital is responsible for the proper safeguarding and the handling of controlled substances within the hospital. Responsibility for the purchase, storage, accountability and proper dispensing of bulk controlled substances within the hospital is delegated to the Pharmacist-in-Chief. Likewise, the Head Nurse of a nursing unit is responsible for the proper storage and use of the nursing unit's controlled substances.

B. *PREPARATION of ORDERS*

All controlled substances orders and records must be typed or written in ink or indelible pencil and signed in ink or indelible pencil.

PETER BENT BRIGHAM HOSPITAL PHARMACY

REQUISITION FOR WARD STOCK NARCOTICS

Ward _____ Code _____ Date _____

Each floor is entitled to 2 containers of each of the following tablets and 2 units of the injectables. Empty bottles except tubex, along with narcotic or barbiturate accounting sheets must be returned to the pharmacy. All other narcotics and barbiturates must be ordered for and charged to the patient. These special narcotic and barbiturate orders must be accompanied by a prescription.

No. of Tabs-Caps mls.	(√)	Check item needed	Price
25		Codeine Sulfate Tablets 15 mg.	
25		Codeine Sulfate Tablets 30 mg.	
10		Codeine Sulfate 30 mg. Tubex	
10		Codeine Sulfate 60 mg. Tubex	
10		Hydromorphone (Dilaudid) 2 mg. Tubex	
10		Hydromorphone (Dilaudid) 4 mg. Tubex	
10		Meperidine HCl 50 mg. Tubex	
10		Meperidine HCl 75 mg. Tubex	
10		Meperidine HCl 100 mg. Tubex	
25		Meperidine HCl Tablets 50 mg.	
10		Morphine Sulfate 8 mg. Tubex	
10		Morphine Sulfate 10 mg. Tubex	
10		Morphine Sulfate 15 mg. Tubex	
10		Methadon HCl Ampul 10 mg./1 ml.	
15		Methadon HCl Tablets 5 mg.	
15		Percodan Tablets	
25		Chloral Hydrate Capsules 500 mg.	
1		Pentobarbital Injection 50 mg./ml. 20 ml.	
25		Pentobarbital Capsules 50 mg.	
25		Phenobarbital Tablets 15 mg.	
25		Secobarbital Capsules 50 mg.	

FORM 107 REV.

FIG. 66.   Requisition form for ward stock controlled substances.

C. *ORDERING WARD STOCK CONTROLLED SUBSTANCES from the PHARMACY*

1. A requisition for ward stock controlled substances is completed by placing a check mark opposite the name, strength, form of the controlled substance desired. The completed form is then sent to the pharmacy along with the empty containers and the nurse's inventory sheet. Figure 66 is an example of this type of form.
2. Before any new controlled substances are issued to a ward, the previous supply must be fully accounted for. Therefore, each request for a new supply must be accompanied by the Daily Controlled Drugs Administration Form shown in Figure 67. Whenever a new supply of drug is issued, it is accompanied by one of these forms. This form serves three purposes: a 24-hour administration record for all Schedule II Substances administered, allows space for inventory count for each nursing shift, and a section which serves as a record of losses and as a basis for review of errors.
3. Whenever a dose of a drug is lost or wasted on the war, the nurse in charge must prepare a report to cover the incident.

PETER BENT BRIGHAM HOSPITAL
DAILY CONTROLLED DRUGS ADMINISTRATION FORM

DATE ______ FLOOR ______

PATIENT'S NAME	Specific Description of Drug Ordered and Strength	Number of Tabs or ml	Strength Used	Ordered By–Doctor	Administered By–Nurse	Time Given

N-179 REV. 12/71

SIGNATURE OF NURSE ______

SUMMARY OF DAILY REPORT

	On Hand at Beginning of This Report	Received	Total	3 p.m. Count	11 p.m. Count	7 a.m. Count	Used	Balance at End of Shift
Codeine TBX 30 mg								
60 mg								
Codeine Tabs 15 mg								
30 mg								
Hydromorphone TBX (Dilaudid) 2 mg								
4 mg								
Meperidine TBX 50 mg								
75 mg								
100 mg								
Meperidine Tabs 50 mg								
Morphine TBX 8 mg								
10 mg								
15 mg								
Methadone Tabs 5 mg								
Methadone 10 mg/ml								
Percodan Tabs								
Deod. Tr. Opium								

3 p.m. Signature ______ / ______

11 p.m. Signature ______ / ______

7 a.m. Signature ______ / ______

FIG. 67. Daily Controlled Drugs Administration Form.

This is accomplished by using a special report form shown in Figure 69. This report is prepared in duplicate and sent to the pharmacy along with the nurse's account sheet and a request for a new supply of drug. The original is filed in the pharmacy and the duplicate is forwarded to the Nursing Office.

D. DOCTOR'S ORDERS FOR ADMINISTRATION of CONTROLLED DRUGS

The doctor's orders for the administration of ward stock controlled drugs must be written on the doctor's order sheet of the patient's chart. However, if the desired controlled drug is not on ward stock a complete controlled drug prescription must be written on a hospital prescription blank. The signed prescription must be sent to the pharmacy. A notation must then be made on the patient's chart by the doctor or nurse indicating that the doctor's signature for the order is in the pharmacy.

A *controlled drug order* must be *written* by a *licensed physician or a registered intern or resident.*

E. INFORMATION WHICH MUST APPEAR ON THE DAILY CONTROLLED DRUGS ADMINISTRATION SHEET

The full information required on the Daily Controlled Drugs Administration Sheet (Fig. 67) is as follows:

1. Date
2. Amount given
3. Patient's full name
4. Patient's hospital number
5. Name of doctor ordering
6. Signature of nurse administering

The following information is requested for auditing purposes and is not required by Federal law:

1. Number of tablets or ml. administered
2. Filling out inventory column (to be retained for Pharmacy).

F. DOCTOR'S SIGNATURE

The doctor's full name or initials are required on the doctor's order sheet.

The doctor's full name is required on a controlled drug prescription.

In each of the above, the signature must be by the doctor's own hand.

G. PRO RE NATA (p.r.n.) or SI OPUS SIT (s.o.s) ORDERS

A p.r.n. or s.o.s. order for controlled drugs must be discouraged except under special circumstances.

H. TELEPHONE ORDERS

A doctor may order a controlled drug by telephone in case of necessity. The nurse will write the order on the doctor's order sheet, stating that it is a telephone order and will sign the doctor's name and her own initials. The controlled drug may then be administered at once. The order must then be *signed by the doctor* with either his signature or his initials within 24 hours.

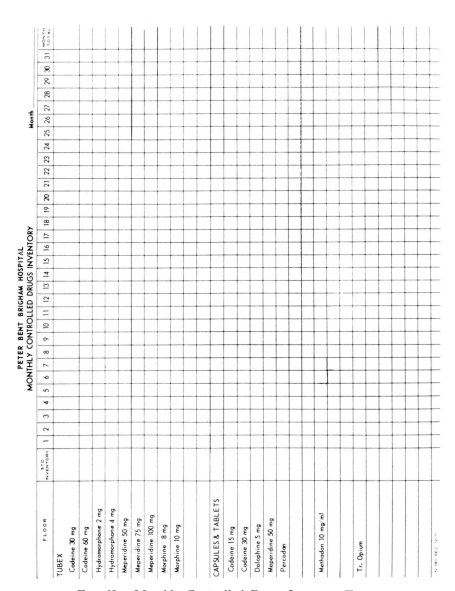

FIG. 68. Monthly Controlled Drugs Inventory Form.

PETER BENT BRIGHAM HOSPITAL
REQUEST FOR REPLACEMENT
OF NARCOTIC LOSS OR WASTE ON WARDS

Date_____

Send Original and One Carbon
TO PHARMACY

                                                                      ml.
Name of Drug_____Quantity_____Tab.

Bottle No._____   Narcotic Sheet No._____

Explicit statement of what happened:

_____
Signature of Nurse Making Report

Attested by Head Nurse or
          Nursing Supervisor _____

Reviewed by Pharmacist _____

This report must be prepared in duplicate and sent to the Pharmacy. The
signed report is brought to the Pharmacy along with a requisition for a new
supply of the lost narcotic. The report will be signed by the Pharmacist on
duty. The reports will be retained in the pharmacy.
Form 248

FIG. 69. Narcotic Loss or Waste Form. Although originally designed for
use with formerly classified "narcotic drugs," this form may be used for recording loss of any of the controlled substances.

I. VERBAL ORDERS

A verbal order may be given by a doctor in an *extreme emergency* where time does not permit writing the order. The nurse must write the order on the doctor's order sheet. The doctor must sign the order with either his signature or his initials within 24 hours.

J. ORDERING NON-WARD STOCK CONTROLLED DRUGS FROM PHARMACY

Drugs which are not stocked on the nursing stations may be ordered from the Pharmacy on written prescription only.

The amount of drugs sent to the nursing unit is the amount covered on the prescription by the doctor's signature. If more is needed a new signed prescription must be obtained. The prescription must have the following information:

1. Patient's full name
2. Patient's address or hospital number
3. Date
4. Name and strength of drug prescribed
5. Total amount of drug to be dispensed
6. Registration number of the licensed physician

The prescription must be written in ink or indelible pencil. It shall not bear erasures, or alterations of any kind.

A doctor may not write a prescription for controlled drugs for his own use.

K. PRESCRIBING CONTROLLED DRUGS IN THE OUT-PATIENT DEPARTMENT

Prescriptions for Schedule II and other controlled substances drugs may be dispensed from Pharmacy and must include the following information:

a. Patient's full name
b. Patient's address or hospital number
c. Date
d. Name and strength of drug prescribed
e. Quantity of drug to be dispensed
f. DEA number and signature of physician
g. Frequency and route of administration.

The prescription must be written in ink or indelible pencil and shall not bear cross outs or erasures. Discharge prescriptions for Schedule II drugs must be picked up by a registered nurse.

L. DISPENSING CONTROLLED DRUGS FOR HOME USE WHEN PHARMACY IS CLOSED

Occasionally patients who require drugs for use at home are discharged from the hospital or released from the Emergency Ward during hours when the Pharmacy is closed. Whenever possible, a prescription signed by a member of the staff who has a License to practice medicine and a DEA number should be obtained.

A staff physician whose DEA number is issued to an outside office should use his own prescription blank. If this is not available, then he must insert his office address on the hospital prescription blank. This will permit the patient or his relative to purchase the drugs at an outside pharmacy.

If no physician is available, or during hours when the local pharmacies are closed, the following procedure is allowed, but only as an EMERGENCY MEASURE:

The attending doctor will calculate the smallest amount of the drug necessary to treat the patient until the Pharmacy opens. He will write a prescription for this amount and the nurse may dispense the medication from her stock supply. The prescription will be presented to the pharmacy the following morning for replacement of stock.

M. PROCEDURE IN CASE OF WASTE, DESTRUCTION, CONTAMINATION ETC.

   1. *Aliquot Part of Narcotic Solutions Used for Dose:*

The nurse shall use the proper number of tablets or ampuls from nursing unit stock. She shall record the number of tablets or ampuls used and the dose given in the proper columns on Daily Controlled Drugs Administration Form (Fig. 67). She shall, in arriving at the proper aliquot part, expel into the sink that portion of the solution that is not used.

   2. *Prepared Dose Refused by Patient or Cancelled by Doctor:*

When a dose has been prepared for a patient but not used, due to a refusal by the patient or because of cancellation by the doctor, the nurse shall expel the solution into the sink and record why the drug was not administered. Example: "Discarded" "Refused by patient" or "ordered cancelled by Dr.—." The head nurse of the unit shall countersign the statement.

   3. *Accidental Destruction and Contamination of Drugs:*

When a solution, ampul, tablet etc., is accidentally destroyed or contaminated on a Nursing Unit, the person responsible shall indicate the loss on Figure 69.

Miscellaneous Regulations

1. Ward supplies of narcotics are to be used only for patients on the ward. They may not be given to patients to take home (except as an emergency measure as noted above) and are not for the treatment of employees.
2. Narcotic prescriptions may not be refilled.
3. A nurse, though the agent of a hospital or doctor, as such, may be partially or wholly responsible for the violation of any of the regulations described above or any others under the Federal Narcotic Act as amended, but not included here.
4. Federal regulations do not allow for a shortage from a vial of injectable narcotic.
5. A physician may not prescribe narcotics for his own personal use.

EIGHT HOUR NURSE AUDIT RECORD

DATE	7 A. M.		3 P. M.		11 P. M.	
	SIGNATURE ON-COMING NURSE	INITIALS OFF-GOING NURSE	SIGNATURE ON-COMING NURSE	INITIALS OFF-GOING NURSE	SIGNATURE ON-COMING NURSE	INITIALS OFF-GOING NURSE

RETURNED TO THE PHARMACY BY _____

DATE _____

FIG. 70

Control of Narcotics on the Pavilion by Nurses

Once the narcotics for the pavilion have been dispensed from the pharmacy, the nursing service assumes the responsibility for the administration, control and auditing of the inventory.

The auditing of the narcotic inventory takes place with each change of nursing shift. At this time, both the nurse coming on duty and the nurse going off duty take a physical count of the narcotics then on the nursing station. If the tally is correct both sign the audit record (Fig. 70). If the tally is incorrect, then a check of the medications ordered for the day by the physicians is in order so that the omission of recording is immediately corrected. On the other hand, if the error cannot be explained, then a narcotic loss report must be executed and forwarded to the department of pharmacy.

Narcotics—Delivery to Floor

The delivery of narcotics from the pharmacy to the nursing station may be assigned to any reliable person in the hospital's employ. It is usually entrusted to a member of the messenger staff since it is presumed that sufficient control records are maintained so that any narcotics that are diverted for illegal use would be immediately detected and appropriate measures taken for their recovery.

Charges to Patients for Narcotics

Charging for narcotics depends upon the policy of the individual hospital. Many hospitals make a charge for each dose received while others make a flat charge to cover all narcotics and hypnotics. In general, hospitals include narcotics along with other floor stock drugs for which no specific charge is made to the patient. Where there is a split policy in operation, the general plan is not to charge the patient for routinely used narcotics but to make a charge for those that must be obtained on special order.

Narcotics which commonly fall into the routinely used category are Codeine Phosphate Injection, Codeine Sulfate Tablets and Morphine Sulfate Injection.

One factor affecting the decision as to which narcotic drug should be included in the per diem charge is its cost. Accordingly, large teaching hospitals with a sterile products manufacturing section produce, at reasonably low cost, a large variety of injectable narcotic preparations and therefore make these available to the patient at no charge.

Smaller hospitals, who purchase their narcotics in ampul form find it necessary to charge for each dose administered.

The New Systems

Although the system herein described for the distribution of floor stock narcotics has been used by many hospital pharmacists and has been found to be dependable and satisfactory, some hospital pharmacists have developed modifications for which they claim the advantage of saving of personnel time and the reduction of the possibility of error.[1,2]

In addition, the pharmaceutical industry has developed new concepts in the packaging of narcotics for distribution in the hospital. One of these systems provides narcotic injectables in a single-dose ampul which is packaged in a space-saving, see-through dispenser of ten, which in turn is packaged in a carton of two floor-stock dispenser trays.

Narcotic tablets are being packaged in strip packs thereby permitting the pharmacist and the nurse to easily identify each individual tablet up to the time of its consumption as well as to "measure count" for inventory purposes.[3,4,5,6]

SELECTED REFERENCES

Regulations No. 5, I.R.S. Publication No. 428 (6-59), Superintendent of Documents, U.S. Government Printing Office, Washington 25, D.C.
HASSAN, WILLIAM E., JR.: Law for the Pharmacy Student, Philadelphia, Lea & Febiger, 1971.
A.Ph.A. Newsletter, Vol. 60 No. 6 March 20, 1971.
Ibid., Vol. 10 No. 20 October 9, 1971.
Ibid., Vol. 10 No. 23 November 20, 1971.
Ibid., Vol. 10 No. 24 December 4, 1971.
GERLACH, ALBERT J.: A Simple, Effective Narcotic Distribution and Control System. Am. J. Hosp. Pharm. 29:1:63, January 1972.

BIBLIOGRAPHY

1. DAVIS, NEIL M.: A Case Study in Narcotic Control, Hospitals, J.A.H.A., 36:56, 1962.
2. ECKEL, FRED M. and LATIOLAIS, CLIFTON J.: An Effective Narcotic Control System Using Electronic Data Processing, Am. J. Hosp. Pharm., 22:9: 519, 1965.

3. Mabol, Philip D.: Evaluation of a New Ready-to-Dispense System for Oral Narcotics, Am. J. Hosp. Pharm. 24:10:543, 1967.
4. ZELLERS, DARRYL, D. and DEREWICZS, HENRY J.: Twenty-Four Hour Narcotic Disposition Recording System, Am. J. Hosp. Pharm. 24:10:550, 1967.
5. WIRTH, BRADFORD P.: A Computerized System for Restricted Drug Control and Inventory, Am. J. Hosp. Pharm. 24:10:556, 1967.
6. AUSTIN, LEONARD H.: A Simplified Narcotic Distribution System, Am. J. Hosp. Pharm. 24:10:561, 1967.

Chapter

17

Tax-Free Alcohol—Its
Procurement and Control

BECAUSE the hospital is a prime user of tax-free alcohol which is commonly purchased, stored, dispensed and accounted for by the hospital pharmacist, it seems proper to devote a separate chapter to the technical procedures involved in the above processes.

The hospital pharmacist should obtain from the U.S. Government Printing Office the latest document[1] governing the distribution and use of tax-free alcohol. In addition, the local assistant regional commissioner will make available the appropriate "Industry Circular" a publication of the Office of the Commissioner of Internal Revenue, Alcohol and Tobacco Tax Division.

Although this chapter will deal with the various aspects of Part 213 of Title 26 (1954), Code of Federal Regulations, the reader is cautioned to make reference to the Federal publication and where questions arise to consult freely with the assistant regional commissioner.

In the following discussion, the various sections of Part 213 of Title 26 (1954) will be listed along with their subtitles. Where the section should be of particular interest to the hospital pharmacist, its content will be quoted and, where necessary, elaborated upon. Samples of all the forms discussed in the various sections may be obtained from the Assistant Regional Commissioner (Alcohol and Tobacco Tax) for study along with the appropriate section.

Those sections which are not of particular interest to the hospital pharmacist *per se* are listed in the text along with their subtitles. In this way, the pharmacist will have a ready reference to the total contents of Part 213 of Title 26 (1954) and should the occasion arise may then refer to the Federal publication (No. 44) for the detailed content or he, at least, may provide the exact reference to the administrator or the hospital's counselor where the situation dictates such action.

Subpart A—Scope

Sections 213–1 (General) and 213–2 (Territorial extent) provide that the regulations published under Title 26 Part 213 relate to tax-free alcohol and cover its procurement, storage, use, and recovery in the several states of the United States and the District of Columbia.

Subpart B—Definitions

Section 213–11 defines a number of terms which are used throughout the code. Because of the specific nature of the definitions, those having application to the hospital use of tax-free alcohol are quoted verbatim.[1]

Alcohol. "Spirits having a proof of 190 degrees or more when withdrawn from bond, including all subsequent dilutions and mixtures thereof, from whatever source or by whatever process produced."

Gallon or wine gallon. "The liquid measure equivalent to the volume of 231 cubic inches."

Industrial use permit. "The document issued—authorizing the person named therein to use tax-free alcohol, as described therein."

Permittee. "Any person holding an industrial use permit on Form 1447."

Proof. "The ethyl alcohol content of a liquid at 60° F., stated as twice the per cent of ethyl alcohol by volume."

Proof gallon. "A gallon at 60° F. which contains 50 per cent by volume of ethyl alcohol having a specific gravity of 0.7939 at 60° F. referred to water at 60° F. as unity, or the alcoholic equivalent thereof."

Spirits or distilled spirits. "The substance known as ethyl alcohol, ethanol, or spirits of wine, having a proof of 190 degrees or more when withdrawn from bond, including all subsequent dilutions and mixtures thereof, from whatever source or by whatever process produced."

Withdrawal permit. "The document issued—authorizing the person named therein to withdraw tax-free alcohol, as specified therein, from the premises of a distilled spirits plant."

Subpart C—Administrative Provisions

Section 213–21 (Forms prescribed) authorizes the Director of Internal Revenue to prescribe the necessary forms for the procurement of tax-free alcohol.

Section 213–22—(Alternate methods or procedures) provides the Director of Internal Revenue with the necessary authority to accept alternate methods or procedures as well as emergency variations from the requirements. The pharmacist is here reminded that no variations from the official procedure may be employed prior to the specific approval of the Director.

Section 213–23—(Allowance of claims) authorizes the assistant regional commissioner to allow claims filed with him concerning the loss of tax-free alcohol.

Section 213–24—(Permits) deals with permits and states that the Director shall issue permits to the Federal Government for the use of tax-free alcohol, whereas the assistant regional commissioner is authorized to issue permits to all other users.

Section 213–25—(Bonds and consents of surety) authorizes the assistant regional commissioner to approve all bonds and consents of surety.

Section 213–26—(Right of entry and examination) authorizes any internal revenue officer to enter, during business hours, any premises housing tax-free alcohol for the purpose of inspecting the required records. The officer is also authorized to take samples of the tax-free alcohol to which the records relate.

Section 213-27—(Detention of containers) authorizes any internal revenue agent to detain any container containing or supposed to contain tax-free alcohol when he has reason to believe that some facet of this code has been violated. The period of detention may not exceed seventy-two hours without due process of law, intervention by the assistant regional commissioner or an execution of a waiver by the owner of the detained container.

Section 213-28—(Persons liable for tax)

Section 213-29—(Responsibility and liability of carriers)

Section 213-30—(Time of destruction of marks and brands) states that all marks and brands required to be placed upon containers of tax-free alcohol shall not be removed, destroyed or altered until all of the alcohol contained therein has been removed.

Section 213-31—(Execution under penalties of perjury)

Section 213-32—(Filing of qualifying documents)

Subpart D—Qualification

Section 213-41 (Application for industrial use permit)

This section provides that every person desiring to use tax-free alcohol shall, prior to commencing use, obtain an industrial use permit, Form 1447.

Application, Form 2600, must be filed with the assistant regional commissioner.

This section further provides that a state, municipal subdivision thereof or the District of Columbia may file an application for and receive a single permit on Form 1447 authorizing the use of tax-free alcohol in a number of institutions under its control if all of the conditions are satisfactory to the assistant regional commissioner.

Section 213.41a Application, Form 4326, for Limited industrial use and withdrawal permit.

This section (added in 1970) provides that any person desiring to use not more than 120 proof gallons of tax-free alcohol during a calendar year may file application, Form 4326, for a limited industrial use permit and a limited withdrawal permit if (a) all such tax-free alcohol will be obtained from one supplier; (b) the maximum quantity of tax-free alcohol to be on hand, in transit, and unaccounted for at any one time will not exceed 14 proof gallons; and (c) tax-free alcohol will not be recovered.

A State or political subdivision thereof, and the District of Columbia, may file application on Form 4326 for a limited industrial use and withdrawal permit, regardless of the quantity to be procured or on hand provided that no alcohol is to be recovered, and all tax-free alcohol will be obtained from one provider.

Section 213-42 (Data for application, Form 2600)

This section deals primarily with the information required on Form 2600. Reference to Figure 71 will provide the reader with an idea of the type of information required.

Under number 11 of this form is a statement requesting the specific manner in which the tax-free alcohol is to be used in the hospital. The pharmacist is reminded that all *clinical* and *laboratory* uses of tax-free alcohol are permitted including the preparation of medicinal preparations which

FORM **2600** (REV. 7-60)	U. S. TREASURY DEPARTMENT - INTERNAL REVENUE SERVICE **APPLICATION FOR PERMIT TO USE ALCOHOL FREE OF TAX**	1. INDUSTRIAL USE PERMIT *(If amendment of industrial use permit)* TF –

This form shall be executed in duplicate and filed with the assistant regional commissioner of the region in which the premises are situated.

Applications on this form which are not executed in accordance with instructions and regulations or which do not contain all the information required by the regulations will be returned to the applicant or permittee for correction.

TO	ASSISTANT REGIONAL COMMISSIONER (ALCOHOL AND TOBACCO TAX) *(City and State)*	2. DATE OF APPLICATION

Application is hereby made for an industrial use permit to use alcohol free of tax, as described herein.

3. APPLICATION MADE BY *(If individual owner, give full name and address; if partnership, give full name and address of each person interested in enterprise; if corporation, give name of corporation, State under laws of which incorporated and address of principal office)*

4. TRADE NAME AND OFFICE WHERE REGISTERED	5. MAXIMUM NO. PROOF GALLONS WHICH WILL BE ON HAND, IN TRANSIT, AND UNACCOUNTED FOR AT ANY ONE TIME 1/

6. SERIAL NUMBER	7. PURPOSE FOR WHICH FILED *("For original industrial use permit," "For amendment of industrial use permit to authorize (state privilege desired)," etc.)*

8. PERMIT IS FOR ☐ USE OF ALCOHOL FREE OF TAX ☐ RECOVERY OF TAX-FREE ALCOHOL	9. *(If application is made by central authority, as a State, municipality, university, etc., for use of alcohol by an agency, institution, department, etc., thereof, the name of such agency, etc., shall be stated)*

10. PREMISES ON WHICH ALCOHOL WILL BE USED *(Number, street, city or town, zone, State)*

11. ALCOHOL TO BE USED IN THE FOLLOWING MANNER *(The specific use which will be made of the alcohol and resulting products (if any), that is, the purpose or purposes for which the alcohol will be used, shall be stated explicitly, and not in general terms. For example, when the alcohol is to be used at a hospital, the specific purposes for which the alcohol will be used shall be stated, such as clinical use, treatment of patients, compounding medicines for use of patients in the hospital, preserving specimens of anatomy, etc. If alcohol so used is recovered, state that fact) 2/*

12. SIZE AND COMPLETE DESCRIPTION OF THE ALCOHOL STORAGE FACILITIES

CONDITIONS

The applicant fully understands that any permit that may be issued pursuant to this application will be subject to the following conditions:

1. That this application contains no misrepresentation of fact; that he and all persons employed by him in any connection with such permit privileges, and all persons employed by him while on the permit premises, will in good faith observe and conform to all the terms and conditions of said permit, the laws of the United States relating to the manufacture, taxation, and control of and traffic in, intoxicating liquors, and all regulations issued pursuant to such laws which are now, or may hereafter be, in force; and he will pay the tax, together with penalties and interest, on all alcohol diverted while being transported to him, and on all alcohol withdrawn, transported, used, or disposed of by him in violation of laws and regulations now or hereafter in force; and that he and all persons interested in the business to be conducted under said permit are duly qualified, under the law and regulations pertaining thereto, to receive the permit privileges herein applied for.

2. That all data, written statements, evidence, affidavits, and other documents, submitted in support of this application, or upon hearing thereon, shall be deemed to be included in the provisions and conditions of this application and any permit issued pursuant thereto the same as if set out at length therein.

I declare under the penalties of perjury that this application has been examined by me and to the best of my knowledge and belief is a true, correct, and complete application.

13. SIGNATURE OF APPLICANT 3/	14. BY *(Name and capacity)*

FORM **2600** (REV. 7-60)

FIG. 71

will not be sold to the patient. Examples of these categories of use are preparation of sterilizing solutions, sponging lotions, tincture of iodine, operating room arm-dips, preparation of laboratory stains and reagents, pathological specimen preservatives, mouth wash, or any pharmaceutical which is considered as ward stock and not directly charged to the patient.

Examples of products for which tax-free alcohol may not be used are the preparation of any extracts to be used in the flavoring of food or beverage such as tincture of vanilla and the preparation of any pharmaceutical or other preparation for which a direct charge is to be made to the patient.

The pharmacist will also avoid any problems in his application for a permit to use tax-free alcohol or during an inspection if he will pay particular attention to the security measures provided for the storage of the bulk supply of tax-free alcohol. For example, the lock provided should be of durable, tamper-proof construction and should be on a separate strictly controlled key system; the door itself should be of sturdy construction with hinges of the type which fit on the inside of the door thereby preventing easy access by merely unscrewing the bolts or the lifting out of the hinge pin.

When building new facilities, consideration may properly be given to the construction of a fire protected vault, special time recording lock systems and built-in burglar alarm system.

Section 213–42a Data for Applications, Form 4326

Each application on Form 4326 shall include the following information:

    (a) Serial number and purpose for which filed.

    (b) Name and principal business address of the applicant.

    (c) Location(s) where tax-free alcohol is to be used, if different from business address.

    (d) Type of business organization.

    (e) Trade names.

    (f) Maximum quantity, in proof gallons, of tax-free alcohol to be withdrawn in calendar year.

    (g) Name and address of supplier.

    (h) List of the offices, the incumbents of which are authorized by the articles of incorporation, the bylaws, or the board of directors to act on behalf of the applicant or to sign his name.

    (k) On specific request of the assistant regional commissioner, furnish a statement of the persons interested in the business, supported by any of the information listed in Section 213.52, or such other information as may be necessary for the assistant regional commissioner to determine whether the applicant is entitled to the permit.

Section 213–43 (Exceptions to application requirements)

Section 213–47 Disapproval of application

This section provides for the disapproval of applications on Form 2600 and 4326 under certain specific conditions.

Section 213–48 (Correction of permits)

Whenever an error in an industrial use permit is discovered, the assistant regional commissioner may demand the return of the permit for correction.

Section 213–49 (Suspension or revocation of permits)

This section permits the assistant regional commissioner to institute proceedings for the suspension or revocation of the permit according to a specific procedure. The reasons upon which such action may be instituted are clearly set forth in this section.

Section 213–50 (Rules of practice in permit proceedings)

This section authorizes the regulations in Part 200 of this chapter to be used in the procedure of suspending or revocating of permits.

Section 213–51 (Trade names)

Permits the use of a trade name by the applicant or permittee if it is listed on Form 2600 and is officially documented to the satisfaction of the Internal Revenue Service.

Section 213–52 (Organizational documents)

This section provides a listing of the organizational documents referred to in Section 213–42. Examples of the type information requested are, where applicable, certificate of incorporation.

Section 213–53 (Powers of attorney)

This section provides the means whereby an applicant or permittee may grant power of attorney to any individual to act or sign on his behalf. Form 1534 must be filed with the assistant regional commissioner, where required.

Section 213–54 (Changes affecting applications and permits)

Any change relating to the information provided on Form 2600 or supporting documents must be reported to the assistant regional commissioner in writing according to the procedure set forth in this section.

Section 213–55 (Automatic termination of permits)

Section 213–56 (Adoption of documents by a fiduciary)

Section 213–57 (continuing partnerships)

Section 213–58 (Change in proprietorship)

An industrial use permit shall not be transferred and the successor shall qualify in the same manner as the proprietor of a new business.

Section 213–59 (Change in name of permittee)

If at any time there is to be a change in the individual, firm or corporate name, the permittee shall file such information on Form 2600 in order that the industrial use permit be amended.

Section 213–60 (Change in trade name)

Same procedure as in Section 213–59.

Section 213–61 (Change in location)

Where the permittee intends to move to a new location within the same region he shall seek an amendment to his industrial use permit by filing an application on Form 2600.

In addition, if a bond on Form 1448 has been given, a consent of surety Form 1533 must be filed or a new bond provided.

Section 213–62 (Registry of stills)

This section provides that the listing of the stills on Form 2600 and the issuance of the industrial use permit shall constitute registration of the stills.

Where the above does not apply, Form 26 must be completed and filed.

Section 213–63 (Notice of permanent discontinuance of use of tax-free alcohol)

This section provides the means whereby a permittee who permanently discontinues the use of tax-free alcohol may discharge his obligations to the Internal Revenue Service. The necessary letters, their contents, and forms to be completed and submitted to the assistant regional commissioner are listed.

Subpart E—Bonds and Consents of Surety

Section 213–71 (Bond, Form 1448)

Every person filing an application, Form 2600, shall, before issuance of the industrial use permit, file bond, Form 1488 with the assistant regional commissioner.

Bonds are not required where the applicant is a state or political subdivision thereof or the District of Columbia.

Bonds also are not required where the quantity of tax-free alcohol to be withdrawn does not exceed 120 proof gallons per year and the quantity which may be on hand, in transit, or unaccounted for at any one time will not exceed 10 proof gallons.

The penal sum of the bond on Form 1448 shall be computed on each proof gallon of tax-free alcohol, including recovered or restored tax-free alcohol, authorized to be on hand, in transit to the permittee, and unaccounted for at any one time, at the rate prescribed by law as the internal revenue tax on distilled spirits.

The penal sum on any bond shall not exceed $100,000 nor be less than $500.

Section 213–72 (Corporate surety)

Section 213–73 (Deposit of securities in lieu of corporate surety)

Section 213–74 (Consents of surety)

Consents of surety to changes in the terms of the bonds shall be executed on Form 1533 by the permittee and the surety.

Section 213–75 (Strengthening bonds)

Section 213–76 (Superseding bonds)

Section 213–77 (Notice by surety of termination of bond)

Section 213–78 (Termination of rights and liability under a bond)

Section 213–79 (Release of pledged securities)

Subpart F—Premises and Equipment

Section 213–91 (Premises)

This section requires that the permittee shall have premises suitable for the business being conducted and adequate for the protection of the tax-free alcohol.

Section 213–92 (Storerooms)

Storerooms or compartments used for the storage of tax-free alcohol must be sufficiently large to accommodate the maximum quantity of tax-free alcohol which will be on hand at any one time, shall be equipped for locking and shall be so constructed as to prevent illegal access to the tax-free alcohol.

Section 213–93 (Storage tanks)

Requires that each stationary tank be equipped for locking as well as the measuring of the contents.

Section 213–94 (Equipment for recovery of tax-free alcohol)

Section 213–95 (Storage tanks for recovered and restored alcohol)

Subpart G—Withdrawal and Use of Tax-Free Alcohol

Section 213–101 (Authorized uses)

Provides for the uses for which tax-free alcohol may be applied for.

Of interest to the hospital pharmacist are the provisions whereby tax-free alcohol may be used by any laboratory exclusively engaged in scientific research; for use at any hospital, blood bank or sanitarium or at any pathological laboratory exclusively engaged in making analyses, or tests for hospitals or sanitariums; or for the use of any clinic operated for charity and not for profit.

Section 213–102 (States and the District of Columbia)

Section 213–103 (Educational organizations, scientific universities and colleges of learning)

Section 213–104 (Hospitals, blood banks, and sanitariums)

"Tax-free alcohol withdrawn by hospitals, blood banks, and sanitariums shall be used only for medicinal, mechanical, and scientific purposes and in the treatment of patients. Such use includes making any analysis or test at such hospital, blood bank, or sanitarium. Medicines made with tax-free alcohol may not be sold, but a separate charge may be made for such medicines compounded on the hospital or sanitarium premises for use of patients on the premises. Where a hospital holding permit to use tax-free alcohol operates a clinic on the hospital premises, tax-free alcohol withdrawn under the permit of the hospital may be used in the clinic to the same extent as it may be used in the hospital: *Provided,* that in the case of a clinic operated for charity and not for profit, medicines compounded with tax-free alcohol may be furnished to patients for use off the premises if such medicine is not sold and no fee or other charge is exacted by reason of the furnishing of the medicine to the patient. Similarly, tax-free alcohol withdrawn by a hospital or sanitarium may be used in a pathological or other laboratory operated in connection with such hospital or sanitarium, on the hospital or sanitarium premises, to the same extent as it may otherwise be used by the hospital or sanitarium . . ."

Section 213–105 (Clinics)

In essence, this section makes the same provisions for the use of tax-free alcohol as does section 213–104 with the exception that any medicine prepared with tax-free alcohol, on the premises, for use by the patient on the premises may be charged for.

Section 213–106 (Pathological laboratories not connected with a hospital)

Section 213–107 (Other laboratories)

Section 213–108 (Prohibited usage of tax-free alcohol)

This section provides that tax-free alcohol shall not be—

1. Used for beverage purposes.
2. Used in the preparation of any food or food products.
3. Sold by the permittee.
4. Used in the manufacture of any product offered for sale.
5. Used in the manufacture of a by-product which is later sold.

Authorized exceptions are listed in sections 213–104 and 213–105.

Persons holding a permit under Form 1447 may not remove tax-free alcohol or products resulting from its use unless special permission is obtained from the assistant regional commissioner, provided that (1) products made through the use of such alcohol but which do not contain any alcohol may be removed from the premises for the sole purpose of further research, and (2) medications prepared with tax-free alcohol may be used outside of the charitable clinic if no charge is made for the medicine.

Section 213–109 (Application for withdrawal permit)

10

Every person, other than as provided for in Subpart I of this part, desiring to obtain tax-free alcohol shall file an application on Form 1450 with the assistant regional commissioner for a withdrawal permit.

On March 23, 1964, *Industry Circular* No. 64-4 was distributed to all users of tax-free alcohol for the purpose of informing this group of the revision of Form 1450 resulting from the amendment of 26 CFR Part 213 by Treasury Decision 6714, effective May 1, 1964.

In brief the amendments provide the following:

1. A revised Form 1450.
2. An applicant for a withdrawal permit shall specify in his application the estimated average quantity of tax-free alcohol he desires to withdraw in one month.
3. The requirement that the applicant specify in his application the total quantity of tax-free alcohol to be withdrawn during the term of the permit has been eliminated.
4. The withdrawal permit will authorize the withdrawal, during any calendar month of as much as twice the estimated average monthly quantity or one drum (55 gallons), whichever is larger, but withdrawals over the full term of the permit will still be held to a figure not greater than the product of the monthly figure and the number of months that the permit runs.

Section 213–110 (Issuance and duration of withdrawal permits)

If the application submitted in accordance with section 213–109 is approved, the assistant regional commissioner shall issue a withdrawal permit on Form 1450 and mail the original to the permittee.

Any permit issued less than six months before April 30 of any year shall remain in force through April 30 of the following year.

Section 213–111 (Application for renewal of withdrawal permit)

An application on Form 1450 for the renewal of withdrawal permit expiring on April 30 shall be submitted by the permittee to the assistant regional commissioner on or before January 10 of such year in order that the renewal permit may be issued and become available for withdrawals by May 1.

The user's report (Form 1451) which is required to be submitted on or before January 10 shall be submitted with the renewal application.

Section 213–112 (Denial, correction and suspension or revocation; changes after original qualification; and automatic termination of withdrawal permits)

Section 213–113 (Cancellation of withdrawal permit)

Section 213–114 (Withdrawals under permit)

Whenever the permittee desires to purchase tax-free alcohol, he shall forward the original of the withdrawal permit to the vendor of such alcohol. Shipments shall not be made without a withdrawal permit nor may the amount shipped exceed that so authorized.

On shipment, the consignor shall enter the transaction on the withdrawal permit and return it to the permittee, unless he has been authorized to retain it for future shipments.

Section 213–115 (Regulation of withdrawals)

A permittee must so regulate his withdrawals of tax-free alcohol so that the quantity on hand, in transit and unaccounted for at any one time shall not exceed the quantity authorized on his permit.

Section 213–116 (Receipt of tax-free alcohol)

Upon receipt from the consignor, tax-free alcohol shall be placed in the storage facility prescribed by section 213–91 and secured until used.

If the local fire regulations require the tax-free alcohol to be transferred to safety containers, it becomes the responsibility of the permittee to affix to the safety container the serial number of the container from which the tax-free alcohol was transferred, the quantity transferred, the date of transfer and the name and address of the vendor.

On receipt of tax-free alcohol by the permittee, he shall check and account for the shipment on the original and copy of Form 1473, forward the original to the assistant regional commissioner of his region and file the copy in chronological order, by months.

Section 213–117 (Alcohol received from General Services Administration)

Section 213–118 (Records and reports)

Users of tax-free alcohol shall keep records and render reports as required under Subpart L of this part.

Subpart H—Recovery of Tax-Free Alcohol

Section 213–131 (General)
Section 213–132 (Deposit in Tanks)
Section 213–133 (Shipment for restillation)
Section 213–134 (Notice of shipment)

Subpart I—Use of Tax-Free Spirits by the United States or Governmental Agency

Section 213–141 (General)
Section 213–142 (Application and permit Form 1444)
Section 213–143 (Procurement of tax-free spirits)
Section 213–144 (Receipt of shipment)
Section 213–145 (Discontinuance of use)
Section 213–146 (Disposition of excess spirits)

Subpart J—Losses

Section 213–151 (Losses by theft)

The quantity of tax-free alcohol lost by theft shall be determined at the time of the discovery of the loss.

If the loss occurred on the premises of the user the loss shall be recorded as provided for by section 213–171 and reported on Form 1451.

If the loss occurred in transit it shall be reported on Form 1473.

It is the responsibility of the permittee to immediately report and make claim for allowance for such loss to the assistant regional commissioner.

Section 213–152 (Losses in transit)

Tax-free alcohol lost in transit to the premises of a permitteee shall be determined at the time shipment or report of loss is received and shall be reported on Form 1473.

If the loss from containers (other than wooden) exceeds 1 per cent of their original aggregate contents, and the quantity lost is more than 5 proof gallons, claim for allowance of the entire quantity lost shall be filed by the permittee.

If the losses do not exceed the above stated amounts and circumstances do not indicate unlawful removal or use, then no claim for allowance is required.

Section 213–153 (Losses at user's premises)

Tax-free alcohol lost on the user's premises shall be determined and recorded at the end of each month when the inventory of tax-free alcohol is taken as required by section 213–172.

Casualty or other unusual losses shall be determined at the time of the loss as required by section 213–171.

All losses on the premises of the permittee shall be reported on Form 1451.

"If the quantity lost during any one month exceeds 1 per cent of the quantity of tax-free alcohol to be accounted for during the month, and and is more than 5 proof gallons, claim for allowance of the entire quantity lost shall be made by the permittee."

If the losses do not exceed the above stated limits and there is no evidence of illegal use or removal, claim for loss will not be required except in the case of losses under section 213–151.

Section 213–154 (Claims)

Claims for allowance of losses of tax-free alcohol shall be executed on Form 2635 and filed with the assistant regional commissioner within thirty days after ascertainment of the loss.

Subpart K—Destruction, Return, or Reconsignment of Tax-Free Alcoho₁ and Disposition of Recovered Alcohol

Section 213–161 (Destruction)
Section 213–162 (Return)
Section 213–163 (Reconsignment in transit)
Section 213–164 (Disposition on permanent discontinuance of use)
Section 213–165 (Notice of shipment)

"When tax-free alcohol is shipped in accordance with sections 213–162 or 213–164, the consignor shall prepare Form 1473, in quadruplicate (quintuplicate if the consignee is located in another region) and, on the day of shipment, forward the original and one copy to the consignee, one copy (two if the consignee is in another region) to the assistant regional commissioner of his region, and retain the remaining copy for his files."

Section 213–166 (Disposition after revocation of permit)
Section 213–167 (Disposition of recovered tax-free alcohol on permanent discontinuance of use)

Subpart L—Records and Reports

Section 213–171 (Records)

This very important section provides that Form 1447 permit holders must keep sufficiently detailed records—

    a. "To enable any internal revenue officer to verify all transactions in tax-free alcohol and to ascertain whether there has been compliance with the law and regulations, and

    b. To enable the permittee to prepare Form 1451.

The code further provides that these records shall—

    1. Identify the tax-free alcohol by proof

    2. Show the date of each transaction and the actual quantities of alcohol involved

    3. Include tax-free alcohol received from General Services Administration

    4. Show the recovery of alcohol and disposition thereof.

Records of receipt and authorized removals of tax-free alcohol shall—
1. Show the name, address, registry or permit number of each consignee or consignor,
2. The type, number, and serial numbers of the containers involved.
All of the above records are required to be kept current.

Section 213–172 (Monthly inventories)
This section requires the permittee to take and record an inventory of all tax-free alcohol in his possession each month.
A rather simple format to follow is the following:

1. Tax-Free Alcohol on hand
   First day of July, 1964................100 proof gallons
2. Received during the month.........110 "   "
   Total   210 "   "
3. Used during the month...............110 "   "
   Gross Balance   100 "   "
4. Quantity on hand, last day of the
   month as shown by inventory....... 99 "   "
5. Gain or (loss) during the month........(1) "   "

Section 213–173 (Reports)
All Form 1447 permittees shall file an annual report on Form 1451 with the assistant regional commissioner not later than January 10th of each year, together with the renewal application (Form 1450).

Section 213–174 (Time for making entries)
Provides that all transactions be recorded on the day that they take place with certain exceptions provided for which do not normally affect the hospital pharmacy operation.

Section 213–175 (Filing and retention of records and copies of reports)
This section requires that, unless otherwise ordered by the assistant regional commissioner, all records and reports pertaining to tax-free alcohol be filed and maintained for a period of three years after the date of the report covering the transaction.

Section 213–176 (Photographic copies of records)
Any hospital desiring to reduce storage space through the microfilming of records required to be preserved under section 213–175 must obtain permission to do so from the assistant regional commissioner.
The application for permission shall consist of a letter, in triplicate, describing:
a. The records to be reproduced
b. The reproduction process to be employed
c. The manner in which the reproductions are to be preserved
d. The provisions to be made for examining, viewing, and using such reproductions

Dispensing Alcoholic Liquors to Patients

In the Summer of 1965, the Internal Revenue Service division of Alcohol and Tobacco Tax issued **Industry Memorandum No. NA 65–7** to hospitals and similar institutions. The purpose of the memorandum was to advise hospitals and institutions regarding liability for special tax which may be incurred by dispensing alcoholic liquors to patients.

Memorandum No. NA 65–7 provides that:

> Internal Revenue laws impose special taxes on persons engaging or carrying on the business or occupation of selling, or offering for sale, any alcoholic liquors for use as a beverage whether or not such liquors are fit for such use.
>
> Regulations issued pursuant to Internal Revenue law provides that hospitals and similar institutions furnishing liquor to patients are not required to pay special tax, provided that no specific or additional charge is made for the liquor so furnished. This regulation is found at Section 194.187 of the Federal Liquor Dealer regulations. The words "no specific or additional charge" are interpreted as applying, for example, to those cases where a hospital or institution makes a fixed charge for treatment, subsistence, medicine, etc., and the over-all fee or charge remains the same regardless of whether alcoholic liquors are furnished to the patient.
>
> A hospital or similar institution incurs liability for special tax as a retail liquor dealer whenever it furnishes an alcoholic liquor to a patient, whether pursuant to a prescription or otherwise, under conditions constituting a sale. These conditions would include any manner of accounting for a specific or additional charge made to patient for alcoholic liquor furnished him. Totaling of charges for various items under a general heading, such as "Drugs and Dressings," would not give relief from special tax liability, if a charge for alcoholic liquors is one of the items included in the total.
>
> Any hospital or similar institution which dispenses alcoholic liquors under conditions constituting a sale will be required to pay special tax as a retail liquor dealer. Special tax is paid by filing a tax return on Form 11 with the District Director of Revenue in the district in which the hospital is located. The special tax rate for a retail liquor dealer is $54.00 for each fiscal year beginning July 1.

Alcohol Records and Automatic Data Processing

Industry Circular No. 65–5 was issued to advise users of tax-free alcohol, among others, of the provisions of **Revenue Procedure 64–35, I.R.B. 1964–37, 21.**

The revenue procedure requires that the methodology built into a computer's accounting program "must include a method of producing from the punched cards or tapes visible and legible records which will provide the necessary details required by the regulations covering the respective operations, or such details must be available in supplemental records."

In addition, the revenue procedure suggests that the Assistant

Regional Commissioner, Alcohol and Tobacco Tax, be notified in advance of the actual installation of an automatic data processing system in order to assure the adequacy of the system as it relates to the required records.

Drawback on Tax-Paid Alcohol

Tax-paid industrial alcohol is defined as pure ethyl alcohol which has been released from Federal bond by payment of a tax. Presently, the tax is $10.50 a proof gallon, equivalent to $21.00 per wine gallon of 200 proof alcohol or $19.95 per wine gallon of 190 proof alcohol. Payment of this tax entitles a hospital pharmacy to purchase same for non-beverage use without a Federal permit—subject to local State law.

Hospital pharmacy manufacturing units using tax-paid alcohol for the production of approved medicinal preparations, food products, flavoring extracts which are unfit for beverage purposes are entitled to a tax drawback, or partial refund of $9.50 per proof gallon of alcohol used in domestic products. There is no drawback on alcohol used in cosmetic products.

To obtain the drawback, the formula and process for the product must be approved by the Director of Alcohol and Tobacco Tax Division, and a special tax—graduated according to the amount of tax-paid alcohol used—must be paid. The special tax rate is $25.00 per year for annual use not exceeding 25 proof gallons; $50.00 per year for use not exceeding 50 proof gallons; and $100.00 per year for use of more than 50 proof gallons.

To qualify for and obtain the drawback, the hospital pharmacist must observe the following:

1. Execute Form No. 1687, *Formula and Process for Non-beverage Product* and file with the Director of the Alcohol and Tobacco Tax Division for approval.
2. Execute Form No. 11, *Special Tax Return* and send it with a check for the amount of the Special Tax to the District Director of Internal Revenue.
3. After the approval of Form No. 11, the District Director issues the Manufacturer of *Non-beverage Products Stamp,* valid for the fiscal year July 1 to June 30. The Stamp must be conspicuously displayed in the hospital pharmacy.
4. To file a claim, execute Form No. 843 Claim, and send it, with supporting data, to the Assistant Regional Commissioner. This claim applies only to alcohol used during any one quarter of the year, and must be filed within three months of the quarter during which the alcohol was used.

Every person qualified to apply for the drawback on tax-paid alcohol must keep accurate and detailed records for two years. The nature of the records to be kept will be found in Part 197 of Title 26, Code of Federal Regulations and Amendments.

Tax-paid industrial alcohol may be resold only by those having a Federal Wholesale Liquor Dealer's Stamp (fee $255) and/or a Federal Retail Liquor Dealer's Stamp (fee $54). In addition, most states require the acquisition of additional local licenses.

As with tax-free alcohol, the marks and brands placed on packages of tax-paid alcohol must not be destroyed or removed until all of the alcohol has been removed from the container. All of the marks and brands shall be removed, effaced or obliterated from the empty container.

Summary of Federal Regulations

The procedure to be followed to obtain permits to purchase and use tax-free alcohol may appear complex and burdensome to the beginners particularly if it becomes necessary to wade through all of the federal regulations concerning the subject. Thus, the following summary should prove helpful.

Execute and submit Form 2600, Application for Permit to Use, to the Assistant Regional Commissioner. Submit with Form 2600 the data described in Sec. 213.42 and 213.43.

If required, execute a Bond in duplicate on Form 1448 and send to the Assistant Regional Commissioner with Form 2600. The amount of the bond must be equivalent to $10.50 per proof gallon of tax-free alcohol (including recovered and restored tax-free alcohol) authorized to be on hand, in transit to the permittee and unaccounted for at any one time. The minimum bond acceptable is $500, and the maximum required is $100,000. No bond is required when the quantity of alcohol applied for does not exceed 120 proof gallons per annum and when no more than 10 proof gallons are on hand, in transit, or unaccounted for at any one time (Sec. 213.71-213.79).

When Form 2600 is approved, Form 1447, the Industrial Use Permit, will be issued. This permit continues until automatically terminated by its terms, suspended, revoked, or surrendered (Sec. 213.44-213.63).

Execute Form 1450, application for Permit to Procure, and file with the Assistant Regional Commissioner. The application must show the total quantity in proof gallons to be withdrawn during the term of the permit, and the quantity to be withdrawn during any calendar month. The quantity to be withdrawn must be no more than is actually needed. One-sixth of the annual allowance may be withdrawn in any one month.

The Assistant Regional Commissioner then issues the Withdrawal Permit on Form 1450 which grants the applicant permission to receive a specified quantity of tax-free alcohol. These permits expire on April 30 each year, and application for renewal must be submitted before January 10. The original of Form 1450 must be filed at the distilled spirits plant of the vendor before the alcohol can be shipped. To facilitate future shipments, it is customary for the vendor to retain the Permit (Sec. 213.114).

Every person holding a Use Permit (Form 1447) shall make annual reports on Form 1451, Report of Tax-Free Alcohol, showing quantity on hand, received, and used. It must be filed on or before January 10 with a renewal application Form 1450 to receive prompt renewal of the Withdrawal Permit. All records must be kept for a period of not less than three years after the date of this report (Sec. 213.171-213.176).

When the tax-free alcohol is received, it must be stored in accordance with regulations (Sec. 213.116 and 213.91). The user must then execute Form 1473, which is sent him by the shipper, reporting any losses in transit. File the original of Form 1473 with the Assistant Regional Commissioner and retain the duplicate in a chronological file (Sec. 213.116).

The marks and brands placed on packages of tax-free alcohol must not be destroyed or altered until all of the alcohol has been removed from the package. When the package has been emptied, the marks and brands shall be effaced and obliterated (Sec. 213.30).

SELECTED REFERENCES

All of the following publications can be obtained from the Superintendent of Documents, U.S. Government Printing Office, Washington, D.C., 20402.

Distribution and Use of Denatured Alcohol and Rum, Part 211 of Title 26, Code of Federal Regulations, I.R.S. Publication No. 443.

Formulas for Denatured Alcohol and Rum, Part 212, Title 26, Code of Federal Regulations, I.R.S. Publication No. 368.

Distribution and Use of Tax-Free Alcohol, Part 213, Title 26, Code of Federal Regulations, I.R.S. Publication No. 444.

Drawback on Distilled Spirits Used in Manufacturing Nonbeverage Products, Part 197, Title 26, Code of Federal Regulations, I.R.S. Publication No. 206.

Rules of Practice in Permit Proceedings, Part 200, Title 26, Code of Federal Regulations, I.R.S. Publication No. 289.

BIBLIOGRAPHY

1. Distribution and Use of Tax-Free Alcohol. United States Treasury Department Internal Revenue Service, Publication No. 44 (9-60).

Chapter

18

Dispensing During Off-Hours

AT one time, the major criticism of the small hospital was the lack of clinical ancillary services on a one hundred sixty-eight hour per week basis. Over the years, the clinical laboratories, radiology, blood bank and the emergency service have successfully coped with the demand. The one area which has not kept pace has been the pharmaceutical service. Many reasons have been offered for this dilemma, the major ones being the shortage of trained personnel and the prohibitive cost.

Much has been published relative to the various means whereby a hospital may provide twenty-four-hour a day pharmacy coverage[1,2] and the following represents a brief review of them.

Use of the Nursing Supervisor

The first and probably the commonest method employed today is to permit the evening and night nursing supervisor to enter the pharmacy and provide a limited type of service. Although this method is the most widely used, it is dangerous and in some areas an illegal practice. Those who advocate such a practice are prone to cite the argument that there exists a correlation between the nurse selecting a medicine from the drug cabinet on the pavilion and selecting the same item from the pharmacy. The fallacy of this view is the fact that medications which have been forwarded to the nursing station have already had the benefit of special packaging, handling and labeling by professionally competent and legally qualified individuals.

Therefore, if this is the only means available to the small hospital, it should be practiced with caution. Nursing personnel serving in this category should be specifically prohibited from compounding a mixture and restricted to dispensing from the selection of pre-labeled and pre-packaged items.

Emergency Boxes and Night Drug Cabinets

The literature is replete with data concerning emergency boxes and night drug cabinets. Since these two items serve a different purpose, we shall discuss them separately.

The *emergency box,* although an integral part of the twenty-four-hour a day pharmacy coverage, is necessary to expedite treatment in situations where time is of the essence. Therefore, the emergency, or as it is often called the "STAT" box, must be large enough to contain the necessary supplies and yet sufficiently compact to facilitate handling them. The box should be kept in a readily accessible place, known to all ward personnel, and should be ready for use at all times. In order to accomplish this goal, the pharmacy should have reserve boxes prepared so that the units may be handled on an exchange basis and thereby reduce the period of time a ward may be without a ready-to-use emergency box.

If it is the hospital's policy to make a charge for the supplies used from the emergency box, then the nurse should prepare a charge ticket and submit it to the pharmacy along with the "used" box.

Some of the larger teaching hospitals have expanded on the emergency box concept and have developed the "emergency cart" or "resuscitation cart." These mobile units have on them the same basic supplies contained in the emergency box plus facilities for the administration of oxygen, the application of suction, and a cardiac pacemaker.

For the convenience of those desiring to establish an emergency box, a list of the pharmaceuticals and ancillary supplies which should be in it is given in Chapter 4, p. 90. However, where the services of a Pharmacy and Therapeutics Committee are available, the pharmacist should consult with the Committee prior to the adoption of a specific list of supplies.

Once an emergency box system is put into effect, the hospital pharmacist is reminded that it should not be forgotten. Many of the drugs which may be placed in the unit may deteriorate if not used within a reasonable period of time, and therefore are useless in an emergency. Therefore, a system of checking all emergency boxes must be initiated and pursued on a regular basis.

One such system requires the hospital pharmacist to check each emergency box on a monthly basis in order to remove outdated and deteriorated medications. This system requires placing an inventory and product control card in the box (Fig. 72). First, it serves as an inventory of the emergency box; second, it shows when the unit was last checked; and third, it provides the nursing personnel with adequate directions for replenishing any item which may have been used.

EMERGENCY BOX INVENTORY & CONTROL CARD

Inventory	Product	Monthly Control Check											
		J	F	M	A	M	J	J	A	S	O	N	D
6 ampuls	Aminophyllin 250 mg. I.V.	√	√	√	√								
4 ampuls	Calcium Gluconate 10 ml. I.V.	√	√	√	√								
6 ampuls	Digitoxin 0.2 mg. I.M.	√	√	√	√								

FIG. 72

The *night drug supply cabinet* is basically an adjunct to the charge floor stock medications already on the pavilion. These units also range from a simple cabinet with drawers to large elaborate installations which include narcotic vaults and refrigerated compartments.[3]

The large cabinets are usually constructed in a wall of the pharmacy so that the unit may be serviced from within the pharmacy yet is accessible from the corridor side to authorized nursing personnel.

The night drug supply cabinet should be stocked with pre-packaged and labeled containers of the drugs listed in the hospital formulary which the Pharmacy and Therapeutics Committee deems advisable. In addition, many hospitals also store certain medical and surgical supplies such as Foley catheters, oxidized cellulose and elastic hosiery.

The nursing supervisor opening the unit is required to leave a properly identified charge ticket listing the item removed and to whom it was administered. The next morning, pharmacy personnel restock the unit and forward the charge tickets to the accounting office.

Although the cost of purchase and installation of a night service cabinet may seem high to those who have inquired about such a unit, it would seem to be reasonably safe to state that the control of inventory which such a unit provides will more than offset its initial purchase and installation. Any plans for the construction of a new pharmacy or the renovation of existing quarters should include such a unit.

Use of Physicians

Next to the use of registered pharmacists, a safe administrative and legal practice would be to prohibit nursing personnel from entering the pharmacy after hours and require that the physician enter the pharmacy and obtain any special medication not provided through the floor stocks, night cabinets or emergency box.

The major drawbacks to this method are first that the physician might waste a great deal of time searching for a product in unfamiliar surroundings and second, in these days of physician shortages, it is an unfair burden to place upon their already heavily taxed work hours.

This system does, however, possess one major advantage in that rather than enter the pharmacy, the physician may be influenced to use a drug which will accomplish the same purpose, yet is more readily available.

Pharmacist-On-Call

Like all professional personnel, the hospital pharmacist understands the necessity of providing twenty-four-hour coverage and, therefore, will not hesitate to accept his share of an on-call assignment. In order to encourage this type of coverage, many administrators have developed bonus or extra pay plans to compensate the pharmacist.

Where the hospital employs a number of pharmacists, the institution of a rotational plan of on-calls will not burden any single individual.

In communities where more than one hospital is in operation, it is recommended that the pharmacists join forces in providing twenty-four-hour on-call service. Under such a system, one pharmacist will be assigned to on-call duty for any one period of time and he, therefore, will answer the needs of both institutions. This type of cooperation will spread out the frequency of on-call duty and, at the same time, acquaint a second person with the routine of each hospital in case of an emergency or sick leave and vacation coverage.

Purchased Service

Hospitals employing only one staff pharmacist have found a practical solution to the dilemma by contracting with the local community pharmacy for night, holiday and vacation relief for the staff pharmacist.

This method is a safe and legal one which, while protecting the drug needs of the hospital and patient, establishes good will in the community and perhaps a better understanding of the efforts of the hospital to safeguard the health needs of the area on a round-the-clock basis.

Where there is more than one pharmacy in the community, care should be taken to avoid any claims of favoritism or politics. One method by which this may be accomplished is to develop a set of specifications and requirements concerning the desired service and request the local establishments to submit their bids. Obviously, the specifications should be so prepared that only the retail pharmacies with adequate staff, inventory, and delivery service can qualify to bid.

In recent years, much has been done to make drugs available on the pavilions in order to cope with every emergency. Some of these methods include the use of mechanical dispensing units, self-medication programs and centralized unit dose dispensing systems available around the clock.

Machine Dispensing

With the advent of the 'Age of Electronics,' many new devices have been developed for the storage and dispensing of pre-packaged drugs. Some of these units and systems have been previously discussed in Chapter 13.

Thus, through the judicious selection of the medications to be placed in these machines, a hospital or nursing home may provide a limited type of pharmaceutical service on an around-the-clock basis in spite of the shortage of professional pharmacists.

SELECTED REFERENCES

ARCHAMBAULT, G. F.: Providing Pharmacy Coverage After Normal Hours— Legal Considerations, Hospitals, J.A.H.A., *32*:56, May 16, 1958.

HASSAN, WILLIAM E., JR.: You Can Provide 24-Hour Pharmacy Service, Hospital Management, *86*:3:50, 1958.

HILL, DONALD E. and WOLFTHAL, ABRAHAM: Medications for Nursing Stations When the Pharmacy Is Closed, Am. J. Hosp. Pharm., *18*:10:596, 1961.

EBERSMAN, DONALD S.: A Look at the Legal View: The Nurse and Medications, Hosp. Pharm., *1* :13, 1966.

SUDLER, ALONZO, JR.: Pharmacy Service After Hours: A Review of the Current Methods for Satisfying this Problem, Hosp. Pharm., *1*:16, 1966.

STERN, MARY B.: Dispensing Drugs After Hours: The Nurse's Dilemma, Hosp. Pharm., *1*:18, 1966.

BIBLIOGRAPHY

1. HASSAN, WILLIAM E., JR.: Six Ways to Provide Pharmacy Coverage After Normal Hours, Hospitals, J.A.H.A., *32*:54, May 16, 1958.
2. JEFFREY, LOUIS P.: Around the Clock Pharmacy Service, Am. J. Hosp. Pharm., *15*:12:1064, 1958.
3. THOMPSON, RICHARD F. and FEELY, WILLIAM J.: A Pharmacy Night Cabinet, Hospital Pharmacy *6*:10:21, October 1971.

Chapter

19

Drug Charges in the Hospital

BECAUSE of the tremendous increase in enrollment in voluntary health insurance plans coupled with the rising costs of drugs, the hospital pharmacist must become familiar with prepaid plans in order to ascertain their effect upon the operation of the pharmacy. Therefore, a brief review of the plans most commonly available is in order.

The Blue Cross Plan

Established in the 1930's, the concept of the Blue Cross plan today boasts a membership of upwards of 60 million people. The importance of this plan is further emphasized when one learns that in some hospitals nearly 75 per cent of all admissions are covered by a Blue Cross plan.

Under this type of coverage the hospital is paid, in addition to a portion of the room and board charge, an amount for ancillary services which is determined by a "reimbursement formula" or published charges, whichever is the lower.* In arriving at the actual dollar rate of reimbursement, the Blue Cross auditors exclude the cost of teaching, research and capital expenditures.

Since the reimbursement rate for ancillaries includes the cost of drugs, the pharmacist should be aware of the fact that the drug portion of this reimbursement is arrived at by determining the average drug cost per patient day.

The average drug cost per patient day is calculated by dividing the actual cost of drugs issued by the hospital for the fiscal year by the total number of patient days for the same period. The average cost per patient day is also ascertained for all other ancillary services rendered by the hospital.

A state-approved reimbursement formula is then applied to the average cost per patient day figures which then results in a dollar rate

*Varies with plan.

which will be paid to the hospital for every Blue Cross patient day of service rendered to the plan's subscribers.

Commercial Insurance Plans

Present-day insurance plans are of the deductible and co-insurance type. The deductible portion of the policy is primarily intended to eliminate small nuisance claims. However, many individuals who have a Blue Cross plan paid for by their employer purchase a commercial policy with the deductible portion being the maximum allowed by the Blue Cross plan. One of the reasons advanced for this is the lower cost to the subscriber and yet it provides him with extremely broad hospitalization insurance.

Because the deductible and co-insurance type of policy often provides for a specific maximum aggregate benefit, insurance carriers imposed the co-insurance factor as a control on the quantity and type of medical care to be received by the policyholder. Under such plans, the insurance carrier will pay a stated percentage of the medical expense and the policyholder undertakes to pay the balance.

Under the commercial insurance plans, the insured, if he has no other type of coverage, pays the deductible amount of his policy and the co-insurance amount, the balance being covered by the insurance company.

From the above brief comparison of the Blue Cross Plan with that of a commercial type health insurance plan, it should be clear that the Blue Cross subscriber utilizing the hospital pays for his drugs and other ancillary services on the basis of actual cost to the hospital, whereas the patient without any form of coverage or with commercial health insurance may pay the hospital's published charges.

Pricing of Drugs

Much has been published concerning the pricing of prescriptions in the retail pharmacy.[1,2,3] In addition, various pricing schedules have been developed and made available to the community pharmacist.[4]

On the other hand, the problem of pricing policy has remained local in nature. That is, some state hospital pharmacy groups have undertaken pricing surveys and have published the data obtained.[5] This type of information, although of local comparative value, does nothing in the way of establishing a workable nation-wide hospital pharmacy prescription pricing formula from which each hospital may develop its own schedule of prescription prices.

At the present time, too many hospital pharmacists establish prescription prices blindly. That is to say, their prices are simply based on a percentage mark-up over cost. The percentage selected is usually that of a neighboring hospital or what is thought to be prevalent in the local community pharmacies.

In hospitals with low direct and indirect costs, the arbitrarily selected percentage mark-up figure may be high enough to permit a profitable operation. If, on the other hand, the direct and indirect costs are high, an operating loss seems a reasonable certainty.

Therefore, it behooves the hospital pharmacist to work closely with the comptroller in order to establish the departmental direct and indirect cost. Once ascertained, this figure when divided by the number of prescriptions filled will result in a unit prescription portion of the operational expense. From this, it should not be too difficult for the pharmacist to visualize the end of the spectrum in which he is operating. In this calculation, "the number of prescriptions filled" has been used as the denominator. For general purposes, "prescription" here is intended to mean out-patient prescription, take-home drug prescription and in-patient drug order since irrespective of how the medication is administered or where it is consumed, the *dispensing* aspect remains the same.

From the above discussion, it would seem that each hospital should, at least for the present time, develop its own pricing schedule based upon its own financial experience.

Of interest to note at this point, is the fact that some hospitals intentionally sell medications to their patients at cost or even below cost. These situations usually exist in heavily endowed hospitals, in purely charitable institutions operated by the city, state or county, or by hospitals that are owned and operated by religious groups.

To this point, discussion has been aimed at developing an equitable price for drugs to be charged to all categories of patient and yet to be in a position to fully protect the hospital's financial interests in any transaction involving the sale of drugs to patients who do not have any form of insurance, as well as those who are covered by a commercial carrier whose policy provides for the payment of posted charges. Therefore, nothing has been mentioned of those patients whose hospital and medical needs are paid for by third party payors, other than Blue Cross or commercial insurance companies. These third party payors may be welfare agencies, industrial accident groups, or various governmental bureaus providing aid to the blind, to families of dependent children, to crippled children or for vocational rehabilitation.

Patients admitted to the hospital under the sponsorship of these agencies are accepted for a specified all-inclusive per diem rate (includes room and board, drugs and all ancillary services). Therefore, any difference between the hospital's posted charges and the per diem rate is considered to be an allowance by the hospital.

However, when the patients of some of these agencies are seen in the hospital clinics and receive a prescription, an entirely different pricing policy may be put into effect. This special pricing schedule is usually prepared by the agency and becomes a part of the agency's contract with the hospital.

Because of the limited scope of this text, it is not possible to become concerned with the many possible types of drug-pricing agreements. However, for the sake of acquainting the student with a prototype, a drug fee schedule of the Massachusetts Department of Public Welfare is hereby presented.

Concentrated perusal of this schedule by the student will be rewarded with an understanding of a pricing concept and philosophy not usually advanced in any course offered in the pharmacy curriculum.

The Commonwealth of Massachusetts was one of the first states in the nation to adopt a statewide formulary and legislation requiring the use of formulary listed drugs when physicians prescribed for patients who were recipients under a medical assistance program.

The *Massachusetts Drug Formulary* contains an alphabetical list of commonly prescribed brand named drugs, each followed by its generic name (See Fig. 21).

Payment for medications is also unique. The system utilizes the medication cost listed in the latest editions of the *Red Book* and the *Blue Book* plus a dispensing fee of $1.85.

Of import, are the following excerpts from the Rules and Regulations for Pharmacy Program under Medical Assistance as promulgated by the Massachusetts Department of Public Welfare:

"5. When medication is dispensed by the prescriber, cost only of the drug may be reimbursable as listed in the Drug List. The prescriber must provide the same information as required of pharmacies. No dispensing fee is allowed a prescriber."

"6. Certain drugs require prior approval from the Department. Prior approval shall be obtained by the prescriber if a required drug does not appear in the Drug List. ——An emergency supply of any unlisted legend drug may be ordered by an authorized prescriber in an amount not to exceed 72 hours supply when service from the Department is unavailable. ——"

"15. Where drugs are prescribed by trade name only, the pharmacist shall price the drug in accordance with the applicable price as listed in the Drug List.

a. When a prescription is written using the generic name of the drug only, the pharmacist shall be reimbursed according to the price for that generic drug not to exceed the price listed in the Department Drug List. The regulation on generic drug pricing applies whether the drug dispensed was a trade name product or a generic product. If the generic product is not listed in the Drug List, the price of the trade named product dispensed as listed in the Drug list shall be the basis of billing.

b. When a prescription is written for a drug using both trade name and generic name, the Department shall reimburse not to exceed the generic price in the Drug List. If the generic drug is not listed in the Drug List, the price of the trade product dispensed as listed in the Drug List shall be the basis of billing."

The Professional Fee Concept

The fee concept has been defined[6] as:

". . . the exclusive use of a professional fee to meet all operating expenses, including overhead and compensation, but not the actual cost of drug and container."

Many hospital pharmacists have developed a professional fee system to be used in their hospitals.[7-10] These individuals report that the concept has found acceptance with both the public and medical staff.

One hospital pharmacist[11] states:

"This system incorporates two basic elements in the charge; the cost of the medication and an added fee that will recover the expense of operating the pharmacy and the share of the total hospital expense assumed by the pharmacy. These two elements are combined into one charge to the patient."

The professional fee concept should not be confused with the traditional retail theory of "mark-up" or "margin." These two terms generally imply that a per cent of the wholesale cost or selling price is used as the basis for recovering all direct and indirect expenses.

Many pharmacists are of the opinion that, as a professional member of the health team, the pharmacist should make a charge for his services which is separate and distinct from the cost of the medication and its container. It is further argued that the fee concept is more equitable to and better understood by the patient since he is accustomed to paying professional fees to doctors, dentists or lawyers.

The House of Delegates of the American Society of Hospital Pharmacists adopted the following resolution.[12]

> Whereas the professional fee concept is recognized as a project consistent with the objectives, basic truths and goals of the ASHP Statement on Goals for Hospital Pharmacy, now therefore be it
> RESOLVED that the Society urge the adoption of the professional fee concept by hospital pharmacists, and be it further
> RESOLVED that the Society assist hospital pharmacists in adopting the professional fee concept by providing information in the American Journal of Hospital Pharmacy, at continuing education programs, and through related sources.

In order to make use of the fee concept in the pricing of prescriptions, the hospital pharmacist should become acquainted with all aspects of his direct and indirect operating costs so that he may arrive at a "fee" which in fact will meet all operating expenses. The thought has been advanced, in some circles, that a professional fee should be the same for all pharmacists in any one locality. Although this concept of standardizing the professional fee rates highly when one considers the public relations aspect, it is not advisable according to sound business and legal principles.

Reimbursement for pharmaceutical services under Title XIX (Medicaid) programs is now based upon "actual acquisition costs of the drug plus a fixed fee." The "fixed fee" is the terminology used by the Federal government for "professional fee."

At the present time, there rages within the profession a controversy relative to the definition of the term "acquisition cost." The issue seems to center around the role to be given to free goods, special discounts and direct purchasing credits in ascertaining the actual acquisition cost.

Break-Even Point Pricing

A useful tool in the overall analysis of cost-volume-profit relationships is the break-even point which is defined as that level at which there is neither profit or loss.

Foulke[13] states that the existence of a break-even point is not a matter of theory but is a very practical analytical factor which is useful in the comparison of net sales, expenses and operating profits within a budget; to ascertain the necessary increase in net sales to justify expansion of plant or personnel and to determine the effect upon net profits by any changes in personnel or material costs.

The application of the break-even point principle has been applied to the pricing of drugs both in the in-patient and out-patient pharmacies.[14]

To adapt the break-even point to the pricing of drugs requires that the pharmacist be in a position to ascertain the fixed and indirect expenses of his department, and then be in a position to charge to the dispensing unit its fair share of these expenses.

In general, the costs of a department of pharmacy should include its proportionate cost of the hospital's administration, maintenance and housekeeping, depreciation of plant and equipment, and labor. These figures may be obtained from the hospital's comptroller since they are usually required of him in the preparation of the hospital's annual report to the department of public health's division of hospitals. If these figures are not available, then the pharmacist may, with the cooperation of the comptroller, determine them.

For example, the pharmacy's share of the maintenance and housekeeping costs may be determined by calculating the total cost of these services to the hospital and dividing this figure by the total number of square feet of floor space utilizing these services. The resulting figure is the maintenance and housekeeping costs per square foot. By taking the total number of square feet in the pharmacy dispensing unit and multiplying by the maintenance-housekeeping cost per square foot, the pharmacy dispensing unit thereby is charged with its fair share. The actual cost of these services divided by the number of prescriptions filled on an average day results in the cost of these services per prescription.

1. Total cost of maintenance and housekeeping to the hospital $100,000
2. Total number of square feet in the hospital 100,000
3. Maintenance-Housekeeping costs per square foot $1.00
4. Pharmacy dispensing unit in square feet 25
5. Maintenance-Housekeeping costs per sq. ft. of dispensing unit (#3 multiplied by #4) $25.00
6. Number of prescriptions filled daily 100
7. Maintenance-Housekeeping cost per prescription .... $.25

Other indirect overhead costs such as the unit's share of administration, heat, light, water (these are not usually metered to each department) may be similarly obtained by arriving at a common denominator such as square feet or space; total number of personnel employed or number of quota hours assigned to the department.

Depreciation of equipment and direct costs such as the pharmacist's time, cost of container and label, laundry, etc. are readily calculable.

Once the direct and indirect operational costs are determined, to them is added the cost of the container and the cost of the drug. The total of these factors represents the break-even point.

The Profit Aspect. If a profit is desired, it may be calculated into the price to the patient in either of two ways:

(*a*) a fixed fee per prescription, or

(*b*) a predetermined percentage of the break-even point cost figure is added.

Advantages.   By the use of this system, the possibility of price fluctuations to the patient are eliminated because the pricing formula is established and the costs precalculated.

In addition, the hospital will at no time suffer a loss because as the cost of labor and overhead increases from year to year, the break-even point is adjusted upwards.

The academic value of such a pricing system cannot be over-emphasized for it provides the neophyte pharmacist with the opportunity really to learn of the many factors which must necessarily enter into the determination of a price to be charged for a drug.

Disadvantages.   The most obvious disadvantage to this system of pricing is that it is used so seldom that it is misunderstood by many because the final price arrived at by the use of this system has no relationship to the price of the same drug obtained from another hospital or retail pharmacy.

Public Law 89–97 (Medicare)

This legislation provides three programs for health insurance and medical care under the Social Security Act.

The basic responsibility for administration of the insurance program is vested in the Secretary of Health, Education and Welfare. Within this authority, the administrative and operational responsibility will be in the Social Security Administration, with responsibilty for certain professional aspects in the Public Health Service.

The Social Security Administration will make use of State agencies and organizations to assist in the administration of the program.

In view of the fact that drugs will be an integral part of the care rendered under these programs, it is essential that the hospital pharmacist familiarize himself with the basic requirements of each in order that he may develop proper charge procedures for the drugs dispensed to the enrollees.

I.   Title XVIII (A)—Compulsory Hospital Program

The first of these programs, the "compulsory hospital program," became effective July 1, 1966, and provides the following basic benefits to about nineteen million persons aged sixty-five or older:

1. *In-patient hospital services*—For up to ninety days in semiprivate accommodations during an illness. The patient pays the first $72 of the costs. If he stays in the hospital for more

than a sixty-day period, he also pays $18 for each day between 61st and 90th days. Psychiatric hospital in-patient services are limited to one hundred ninety days during a lifetime.

2. *Posthospital extended care services*—For up to one hundred days, beginning January 1, 1967. The patient pays $8.50 for each day over twenty days.

3. *Posthospital home health services*—Nurses' or technicians' services for up to one hundred home visits after discharge from a hospital or extended care facility.

4. *Out-patient hospital diagnostic services*—Patient pays $20 deductible and 20 per cent of any charges in excess of $20 during a twenty-day period.

The "inpatient hospital services" benefit includes drugs and biologicals ordinarily furnished by the hospital for the care and treatment of inpatients. "Posthospital extended care services" include drugs and biologicals ordinarily furnished by the nursing home. Drugs and biologicals are presently excluded from coverage in the "posthospital home health services."

The term "drugs and biologicals" is specifically limited by the law to drugs included (or approved for inclusion) in *The United States Pharmacopeia, The National Formulary, The United States Homeopathic Pharmacopeia, New Drugs,* or *Accepted Dental Remedies,* and drugs approved by the Pharmacy and Therapeutics Committees of the furnishing hospitals.

This program will be financed by increased social security payments. Payments for benefits will be made directly by the Federal Government to the providers of services who have entered into an agreement with the Secretary of Health, Education and Welfare or by selected private insurance carriers who will act as intermediaries.

II. Title XVIII (B)—Voluntary Insurance Program

The second of the programs, the "voluntary insurance program," became effective on July 1, 1966, and provides medical insurance for persons sixty-five or over who elected to enroll under it at a cost of $3 each. It was financed from premiums paid by the enrollees and by funds appropriated by the Federal Government. The services provided under this program are:

1. Home health services for up to one hundred visits during a calendar year.

2. Medical and other health services including:
   a. Physicians' and surgeons' services, whether furnished in the hospital, office, or home.

   b. Diagnostic x-rays and laboratory tests, electrocardiograms, and other diagnostic tests.

   c. Surgical dressings and splints; casts and other devices for reduction of fractures and dislocations; braces and artificial limbs; prosthetic devices; rental of durable medical equipment such as iron lungs, oxygen tents, hospital beds, and wheelchairs used in patients' homes.

   d. Ambulance services.

Payment for these services will be made by the Federal Government directly to the provider of such services or by private insurance carriers. (The patient pays $50 toward the annual costs of covered services and supplies in addition to 20 per cent of the costs over $50.) Drugs and biologicals are specifically excluded from "home health services." They are only covered in the "medical and other health services" if they cannot be self-administered and if they are furnished either as an incident to a physician's professional service or as a hospital service incident to a physician's service rendered to outpatients.

III. Title XIX—Grants to States for Medical Assistance Programs

Basically, Title XIX is an extended Kerr-Mills type of program. As written, it will have the following effects:

1. Serve to foster the present "vendor payment" type of system by increasing the amount of Federal matching funds under a formula based on state per capita income (ranges from 55 to 83 per cent).
2. Consolidate all state programs under one state administrator.
3. Broaden the scope of state programs to include more people and more services for many of these people by providing at least the following services to those eligible:
   a. In-patient hospital services
   b. Out-patient hospital services
   c. Other laboratory and x-ray services
   d. Skilled nursing home service
   e. Physicians' services

Under this program the supply of drugs is optional, but it is felt that most states will elect to supply them.

Title XIX is potentially larger than the other two Medicare programs since it authorizes and encourages government-assisted medical care to *all* persons receiving public assistance and to many other persons in need of medical aid regardless of age. It has been estimated that this program could encompass as many as thirty-five million people.

Conditions of Participation for Hospitals

The rules governing the aspects of the Medicare program are known as the *Conditions of Participation for Hospitals.* These were issued by the Social Security Administration after extensive consultation with the Health Insurance Benefits Advisory Council—commonly referred to as HIBAC.

Accordingly, it is from this document[15] that the following information governing the participation of hospitals and allied health agencies is obtained.

General Hospitals

Since the Joint Commission on Accreditation of Hospitals has adopted a requirement for utilization review, any hospital accredited by this group would generally be conclusively presumed to meet all the conditions for participation in the program.

The regulations also provide that accreditation by the American Osteopathic Association, or any other national accrediting body, may also be accepted if it is reasonable to do so, as evidence that a hospital meets some or all of the conditions of participation.

Further stipulations require the hospital to be licensed, certified or approved by the State (local law equivalents to licensing meet this requirement) and it must substantially comply with regulations pertaining to medical records, medical staff by-laws, pharmacy and therapeutics committees to mention a few.

Further requirements necessary to the health and safety of patients may be imposed by the Government; however, these health and safety requirements cannot be more strict than the comparable conditions enforced by the Joint Commission on Accreditation of Hospitals.

The regulations also permit the State to establish stricter requirements if such are specified under its Federal-State medical assistance programs. These stricter requirements may be enforced by the sovereign state even if they are not used in its own programs.

Psychiatric and Tuberculosis Hospitals

In order to avoid paying for care that is merely custodial in nature, the conditions of participation require that the institution:

(1) be accredited by the Joint Commission on Accreditation of Hospitals;

(2) maintain clinical records which are adequate to ascertain the degree and intensity of treatment furnished to the insured; and

(3) meet staffing requirements commensurate with those needed for carrying out an active treatment program.

The regulations also dictate that a distinct part of the institution may participate as a psychiatric or tuberculosis hospital, if it meets the above conditions, even though the institution of which it is a part does not. Also, if the distinct part of the institution meets requirements equivalent to accreditation requirements, it may qualify under the program even though the institution is not accredited.

Conditions of Participation for an Extended Care Facility

An extended care facility is liberally defined as a skilled nursing home or a distinct part of an institution, such as a ward or wing of a hospital.

An institution which is primarily for the care and treatment of mental diseases or tuberculosis is excluded from the definition of an extended care facility.

In general, extended care facilities will be required to have an agreement with a hospital for the transfer of patients and interchange of medical records. This requirement may be waived where an extended care facility has attempted, in good faith, to arrange a transfer agreement but failed and the State agency finds that the facility's participation in the hospital insurance program is in the public's interest and essential to assuring necessary care to the insured inhabitants of the community.

It should be emphasized that the requirement for a transfer agreement does not mean that a patient would have to be transferred between a hospital and extended care facility which have such an arrangement between them. A transfer agreement with any hospital would qualify the facility so that the patient's extended care would be paid for if he was admitted upon transfer from some other hospital.

Since the extended care facility is expected to render high-quality convalescent and rehabilitative care, it must meet the following requirements. They include:

(1) around-the clock nursing services with at least one registered nurse employed full time;

(2) the availability of a physician to cope with emergencies;

(3) utilization review;

(4) proper methods for handling drugs; and

(5) the maintenance of adequate medical policies, governing the nursing care and related services.

Conditions of Participation for a Home Health Agency

Visiting nurse organizations, hospital-operated home-care services as well as agencies specifically established to provide a broad spectrum of home health services are examples of home health agencies which may qualify under the program. A private organization providing home care on a profit basis may qualify if it is licensed, where State law requires it, and if it meets specified standards.

In general, a home health agency in order to participate will have to be:

(1) publicly owned; or

(2) a nonprofit organization exempt from Federal taxation; or

(3) licensed and meet staffing requirements and other conditions and standards prescribed by regulation.

It should be recognized that not all institutions desiring to participate will be certified for this purpose. Therefore, it will be possible for an insured person to encounter a medical emergency and find that he is admitted to a hospital not participating in the hospital insurance program. In these situations, the law permits the payment of benefits for emergency hospital diagnostic services or in-patient care until it is no longer necessary from a medical point of view to care for the patient in a non-participating institution provided that the hospital agrees not to charge the patient amounts (except the deductibles and co-insurance) in addition to the program's payments for covered services.

Conditions of Participation for Hospitals:
VIII Pharmacy or Drug Room

Drugs and biologicals furnished to hospital patients for their use while in-patients will be paid for under the health insurance program provided that the conditions of participation applicable to the pharmacy or drug room are complied with.

The following are conditions of participation as they apply to the hospital pharmacy:

STANDARD A—PHARMACY SUPERVISION

There is a pharmacy directed by a registered pharmacist or a drug room under competent supervision.

Factor 1. The pharmacist is trained in the administration of hospital pharmacy.

Factor 2. The pharmacist is responsible to the administration of the hospital for developing, supervising, and co-ordinating all the activities of the pharmacy department.

Factor 3. If there is a drug room with no pharmacist, prescriptions are compounded by a qualified pharmacist elsewhere, and only storing and distributing are done in the drug room. A consulting pharmacist assists in drawing up the correct procedures, rules, and regulations for the distribution of drugs, and visits the hospital on a regularly scheduled basis in the course of his duties. Whenever possible, the pharmacist, in dispensing drugs, works from the prescriber's original order or a direct copy.

STANDARD B—PHYSICAL FACILITIES

Facilities are provided for the storage, safeguarding, preparation, and dispensing of drugs.

Factor 1. Drugs are issued to floor units in accordance with approved policies and procedures.

Factor 2. Drug cabinets on the nursing units are routinely checked by the pharmacist. All floor stocks are properly controlled.

Factor 3. There is adequate space for all pharmacy operations and the storage of drugs at a satisfactory location provided with proper lighting, ventilation, and temperature controls.

Factor 4. If there is a pharmacy, equipment is provided for the compounding and dispensing of drugs.

Factor 5. Special locked storage space is provided to meet the legal requirements for storage of narcotics, alcohol, and other prescribed drugs.

STANDARD C—PERSONNEL

Personnel competent in their respective duties are provided in keeping with the size and activity of the department.

Factor 1. The pharmacist is assisted by an adequate number of additional registered pharmacists and such other personnel as the activities of the pharmacy may require to insure quality pharmaceutical services.

Factor 2. The pharmacy, depending upon the size and scope of its operations, is staffed by the following categories of personnel:
(i) Chief pharmacist; (ii) One or more assistant chief pharmacist; (iii) Staff pharmacists; (iv) Pharmacy residents (where a program has been activated); (v) Non-professionally trained pharmacy helpers; (vi) Clerical help.

Factor 3. Provision is made for emergency pharmaceutical services.

Factor 4. If the hospital does not have a staff pharmacist, a consulting pharmacist has overall responsibility for control and distribution of drugs and a designated individual(s) has responsibility for day-to-day operation of the pharmacy.

STANDARD D—RECORDS

Records are kept of the transactions of the pharmacy (or drug room) and correlated with other hospital records where indicated. Such special records are kept as are required by law.

Factor 1. The pharmacy establishes and maintains, in cooperation with the accounting department, a satisfactory system of records and bookkeeping in accordance with the policies of the hospital for:
(i) Maintaining adequate control over the requisitioning and dispensing of all drugs and pharmaceutical supplies; (ii) Charging patients for drugs and pharmaceutical supplies.

Factor 2. A record of the stock on hand and of the dispensing of all narcotic drugs is maintained in such a manner that the disposition of any particular item may be readily traced.

Factor 3. Records for prescription drugs dispensed to each patient (inpatients and outpatients) are maintained in the pharmacy or drug room containing the full name of the patient and the prescribing physician, the prescription number, the name and strength of the drug, the date of issue, the expiration date for all time-dated medications, the lot and control number of the drug, the name of the manufacturer (or trademark) and (unless the physician directs otherwise) the name of the medication dispensed.

Factor 4. The label of each outpatient's individual prescription medication container bears the lot and control number of the drug, the name of the manufacturer (or trademark) and (unless the physician directs otherwise) the name of the medication dispensed.

STANDARD E—CONTROL OF TOXIC OR DANGEROUS DRUGS

Policies are established to control the administration of toxic or dangerous drugs with specific reference to the duration of the order and the dosage.

Factor 1. The medical staff has established a written policy that all toxic or dangerous medications, not specifically prescribed as to time or number of doses, will be automatically stopped after a reasonable time limit set by the staff.

Factor 2. The classification ordinarily thought of as toxic or dangerous drugs are narcotics, sedatives, anticoagulants, antibiotics, oxytocics and cortisone.

STANDARD F—COMMITTEE

There is a committee of the medical staff to confer with the pharmacist in the formulation of policies.

Factor 1. A Pharmacy and Therapeutics Committee (or equivalent committee), composed of physicians and pharmacists, is established in the hospital and serves as the liaision between the medical staff and the pharmacist.

Factor 2. The committee assists in the formulation of broad professional policies regarding the evaluation, appraisal, selection, procurement, storage, distribution, use, and safety procedures, and all other matters relating to drugs.

Factor 3. The committee performs the following specific functions:

(i) Serves as an advisory group to the hospital medical staff and the pharmacist on matters pertaining to the choice of drugs; (ii) Develops and reviews periodically a formulary or drug list accepted for use in the hospital; (iii) Establishes standards concerning the use and control of experimental drugs and research in the use of recognized drugs; (iv) Evaluates clinical data concerning new drugs or preparations requested for use in the hospital; (v) Makes recommendations concerning drugs to be stocked on the nursing unit floors and by other services; (vi) Prevents unnecessary duplication in stocking the same basic drug and its preparation.

Factor 4. The committee meets as least quarterly and reports to the executive committee and the medical staff.

STANDARD G—DRUGS TO BE DISPENSED

Drugs dispensed are included (or approved for inclusion) in the United States Pharmacopoeia, National Formulary, United States Homeopathic Pharmacopeia, New Drugs, or Accepted Dental Remedies (except for any drugs unfavorably evaluated therein), or are approved for use by the Pharmacy and Therapeutics Committee (or equivalent committee) of the hospital staff.

Factor 1. The pharmacist, with the advice and guidance of the Pharmacy and Therapeutics Committee, is responsible for specifications as to quality, quantity, and source of supply of all drugs.

Factor 2. There is available a formulary or list of drugs accepted for use in the hospital which is developed and amended at regular intervals by the Pharmacy and Therapeutics Committee (or equivalent committee) with the cooperation of the pharmacist (consulting or otherwise) and the administration.

Factor 3. The pharmacy or drug room is adequately supplied with preparations so approved.

SELECTED REFERENCES

BRODIE, DONALD C.: A Review of the Philosophy and Methodology of the Professional Fee Concept, Am. J. Hosp. Pharm., *23*:9:489, 1966.

APPLE, WILLIAM S.: Significance of the Professional Fee Concept to the Profession of Pharmacy, Am. J. Hosp. Pharm., *23*:9:493, 1966.

ARCHAMBAULT, GEORGE F.: Application of the Professional Fee Concept to Government Insurance and Funding Programs, Am. J. Hosp. Pharm., *23*:9:496, 1966.

PETRICK, ROBERT J. and LATIOLAIS, CLIFTON J.: Applicability of the Professional Fee Concept to Hospital Pharmacy, Am. J. Hosp. Pharm., *23*:9: 501, 1966.

ARCHAMBAULT, GEORGE F.: Professional and Economic Impact of Medicare on Hospital Pharmacy, Am. J. Hosp. Pharm., *23*:4:186, 1966.

HELLER, WILLIAM M.: Challenge of Medicare to Pharmacy and Therapeutics Committees, Am. J. Hosp. Pharm., *23*:4:201, 1966.

RODOWSKAS, C. A.: Determining a Dispensing Fee by Cost Accounting Methods, J. A. Ph. A. NS*13*:1:8, January 1973.

WERTHEIMER, ALBERT I.: Pricing Pharmaceutical Service—Art, Science, or Whim. J. A. Ph. A. NS*13*:1:11, January 1973.

BIBLIOGRAPHY

1. *Systematic Prescription Pricing Digest.* Syracuse, Bristol Laboratories, Inc.
2. *The Lilly Digest.* Indianapolis, Eli Lilly & Co.
3. *The American College of Apothecaries Operational Survey.* Philadelphia, American College of Apothecaries.
4. *The Universal Prescription Costing and Pricing Calculator.* Rutherford, N.J., Becton, Dickinson & Co.
5. NARINIAN, GEORGE: Pharmaceutical Pricing in Hospitals, Hosp. Mgt., *90*:2:83, 1960.
6. HARTLEIB, CHARLES J., FLACK, HERBERT L., and ABRAMS, ROBERT E.: A Rational Method of Prescription Pricing—The Professional Fee Concept, J.A.Ph.A. Pract. Ed., *21*:11:696, 1960.
7. LATIOLAIS, CLIFTON, J.: Experiences with the Profesional Fee System in Hospital Pharmacy Practice at Ohio State University Hospital, Am. J. Hosp. Pharm., *23*:9:511, 1966.
8. BUTLER, JOHN L. and PARKER, PAUL F.: Experience with the Professional Fee System in Hospital Pharmacy Practice at the University of Kentucky Medical Center, Am. J. Hosp. Pharm., *23*:9:516, 1966.
9. ROURKE, SR. MARY VERA: Experiences with the Professional Fee System in Hospital Pharmacy Practice at Mercy Hospital (Buffalo), Am. J. Hosp. Pharm., *23*:9:520, 1966.
10. ULAN, MARTIN S.: Experiences with the Professional Fee System in Hospital Pharmacy Practice at the Hackensack Hospital, Am. J. Hosp. Pharm., *23*:9:522, 1966.
11. KASHINO, MINORU: Experiences with the Professional Fee System in Hospital Pharmacy Practice at the Palo Alto-Stanford Hospital Center, Am. J. Hosp. Pharm., *23*:9:518, 1966.
12. PROVOST, GEORGE P.: An Opportunity for Hospital Pharmacy, Am. J. Hosp. Pharm., *23*:9:487, 1966.
13. FOULKE, R. A.: *Practical Financial Statement Analysis,* 5th ed. New York, McGraw-Hill Book Co., 1961.
14. PROVOST, GEORGE P. and HELLER, WILLIAM M.: How Break-Even Pricing of Drugs Works, The Modern Hospital, *94*:122, 1960.
15. Health Insurance for the Aged, Conditions of Participation for Hospitals, Publication HIM-1 (2–66), Social Security Administration, U.S. Department of Health, Education and Welfare, Washington, D.C.

Chapter

20

Pre-Packaging in the Hospital

PRE-PACKAGING of drugs is not a new concept to the profession of pharmacy. It has been in practice since the apothecary of old grew his own herbs and drugs and harvested and packaged them for sale. Many retail pharmacies purchase various over-the counter tablets and syrups in bulk quantities and pre-package the material in smaller-sized containers.

In the hospital pharmacy, the concept of pre-packaging is utilized in both the large and the small hospital for it is, oftentimes, the means of coping with the periods of peak demand for pharmaceutical service. In the small hospital, the pharmacist may pre-package only those items which he considers require too much time if filled only when called for. In some hospital pharmacies, items which fall into this category are narcotics, barbiturates, oily products, heavy syrups or magmas.

Most large hospitals have found it economical to pre-package all ward stock items as well as the often prescribed tablets, capsules, syrups, ointments and creams used both by the in-patients as well as the out-patient clinics. Because of the scope of this phase of a large hospital pharmacy operation, it often requires a separate work force, special equipment, and detailed control procedures to ensure against the possibility of errors.

Pre-Packing Policy—*Its Determination*

The decision as to what product and how much of it should be pre-packaged is one which can be made only after a comprehensive study of the local situation. No rule of thumb can be reasonably stated which would be applicable in a majority of the instances.

Some of the factors which must be considered are:

> *a.* Demand for the product.
> Is it a year 'round demand or is it a seasonal demand?
> Is the demand one which originates from the clinics or the pavilions?

Can this product be purchased in quantities to meet the demand, yet have it packaged in small units by the manufacturer at a price lower than the hospital cost to pre-package the same item in a similar container?

b. What size units should be packaged? How many of each size?

c. What type of containers and closures must be used in order to maintain therapeutic integrity?

d. What special labeling will be required?

e. Can the item be machine packaged or must hand counting be resorted to?

f. What is the stability of the product?
Is it dated?

g. What will the unit cost of pre-packaging amount to? Who should pay it?

Those experienced with the problem are convinced that almost every item in the pharmacy can be pre-packaged. This includes preparations considered to be free ward stock as well as the items prescribed as charge drugs.

The size of each container of drug can best be ascertained by consulting the nursing service as well as the Pharmacy and Therapeutics Committee. The nursing service can be most helpful in providing data concerning the quantities and rate of use of such items as ward stock hypnotics, sedatives, antitussives, antiseptics, mouth washes, back rub lotions, etc. On the other hand, the Pharmacy and Therapeutics Committee can establish a quota regarding the number of capsules and tablets or volume of liquid preparations which may be sent to the pavilions. This figure is usually included in the published formulary as the quantity to prescribe and is arrived at by a decision not to permit more than a specific number of days of therapy on any one drug order. In a majority of hospitals, 20 to 25 capsules or tablets are considered as adequate for hospitalized patients and are therefore the commonly pre-packaged sizes.

Insofar as pre-packaging for the out-patient clinic is concerned, the most important factor to be considered is the cycle for obtaining subsequent appointments. If it is accepted hospital policy to schedule patients for appointments every thirty or forty-five or sixty days, then the quantity of drug, if the therapy warrants it, should be sufficient to last until the date of the subsequent appointment. Failure to do this will result in burdening the patient by forcing him to return to the hospital for an unscheduled appointment for the purpose of obtaining authorization for a refill. Thus quantities of 50, 75 and 100 unit doses may be pre-packaged for clinic dispensing.

As has been previously stated, no set rule can be provided which

11

will be of universal value in determining the total volume of material to be pre-packaged. Some hospital pharmacists have developed a routine whereby items are pre-packaged in a volume estimated to last for a period of sixty days, whereas others vary from as little as thirty days to as much as one hundred and twenty days. In this regard, a word of caution must be interjected—namely, an extremely large volume of pre-packaging of a single item may be quite risky should the use fall off or be jeopardized by reports of adverse reactions resulting from its use. The pre-packaged items may not be returned to the manufacturer for credit and may become a total loss to the hospital.

The Pre-Packaging Operation

In the small hospital, the pre-packaging operation is usually accomplished by the staff pharmacist with the assistance of a part-time helper. This is a practical approach to the problem when the volume is not great for it permits the pharmacist to remain busy throughout the work week. Under these circumstances, no special area need be set aside nor is there the need for any special counting equipment other than manual tablet counters or moderately sensitive scales for weighing.

Hospitals requiring large scale pre-packaging operations have found it feasible to establish a separate unit for this facet of the total operation. Here, a separate lay work force is marshalled under the supervision of a pharmacist, and the monumental task is undertaken with the assistance of automatic filling machines for liquid preparations, automatic tablet and capsule counters and automatic labeling machines.

In between these two extremes lie the majority of the hospitals. That is, the volume is too great for a total hand operation, yet too small for a separate automated division within the department proper. Here, the pharmacy staff usually rotates the responsibility for maintaining a supply of pre-packaged goods. Oftentimes, the pharmacist may have available the assistance of lay personnel already on the pharmacy payroll, other staff pharmacists during off-peak hours, or members of the volunteer staff in the hospital.

The pre-packaging of drugs in this type of operation usually makes use of some semi-automatic packaging aids such as the various types of automatic and electronic tablet and capsule counters, automatic filling and capping machines, pipetting machines, and semi-automatic labeling equipment. Figure 73 demonstrates one such piece of equipment—the Vi-Count electronic tablet and capsule counter.

Although the above-mentioned equipment is intended for use in the larger hospital, there is on the market a number of units

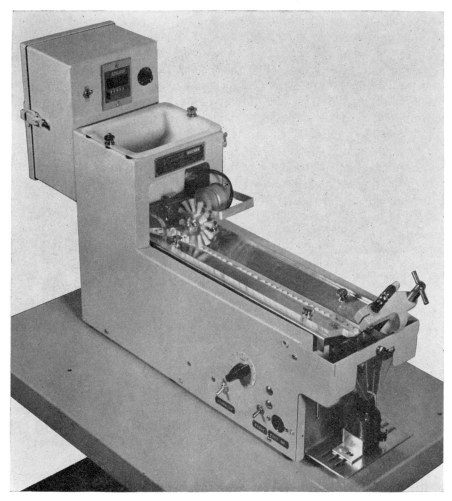

Fig. 73. The Vi-Count hospital pharmacy tablet and capsule counter. (Courtesy of the Lakso Co., Inc., Fitchburg, Massachusetts.)

intended for use in the small hospital. This is particularly true with the various tablet counters.

Types of Containers

The literature is amply documented[1,2] with the pros and cons associated with the choice of container for dispensing pharmaceuticals. This controversy was made possible by the advent of the plastic container, the plasticized paper or cardboard package, and the strip package. Those opposed to the use of these modern packaging aids often cite the requirements of the *United States Pharmacopeia* and *National Formulary* which direct that the official preparations be packaged, stored and preserved in air-tight, light-resistant containers.

The general claim is usually based upon the observation that some plastic containers do not meet the standards of moisture vapor transmission set for well-closed glass containers, that volatile oils and certain dyes migrate through the walls of polyethylene containers, and that "plastic containers" do not withstand heat sterilization.

A sophisticated study of the literature will quickly dispel many of these observations for, in fact, high density polyethylene containers do protect against migration of volatile oils, do measure up to high standards in the moisture vapor transmission tests, and can be subjected to heat sterilization.

Although plastic materials do all these things, it is the considered opinion of many that they still do not fully meet the requirements of the official compendia which provide as follows:[3]

"PRESERVATION, PACKAGING, STORAGE, AND LABELING

Containers.—The container is the device which holds the drug and which is or may be in direct contact with the drug. The immediate container is that which is in direct contact with the drug at all times. The closure is a part of the container.

The container does not interact physically or chemically with the drug that it holds so as to alter the strength, quality, or purity of the drug beyond the official requirements.

Light-Resistant Container.—A light-resistant container is designed to prevent deterioration of the contents beyond the official limits of strength, quality, or purity, under the ordinary or customary conditions of handling, shipment, storage, and sale. A colorless container may be made light-resistant by enclosing it in an opaque carton or wrapper. A multiple-dose container so protected bears a statement that the opaque covering is required for needed protection from light until the contents have been used.

Unless otherwise specified, a light-resistant container is composed of substance which in a thickness of 2 mm. does not transmit more than 18 per cent of the incident radiation of any wave length between 290 and 450 mμ. . . . A container for a preparation intended for injection and having walls less than 2 mm. in thickness is subject to the same limit.

The pharmacopeial requirement for the use of light-resistant containers does not apply to products when dispensed by the pharmacist unless so indicated in the individual monograph.

Well-Closed Container.—A well-closed container protects the contents from extraneous solids and from loss of the drug under the ordinary or customary conditions of handling, shipment, storage, and sale.

Tight Container.—A tight container protects the contents from contamination by extraneous liquids, solids, or vapors, from loss of the drug, and from efflorescence, deliquescence, or evaporation under the ordinary or customary conditions of handling, shipment, storage, and sale, and is capable of tight re-closure. Where a tight container is specified, it may be replaced by a hermetic container for a single dose of a drug."

Therefore, if the hospital pharmacist is to comply with all of the official standards, it stands to reason that any products which he pre-packages and dispenses must meet the above criteria. Clearly then, cardboard boxes, plastic vials, cellophane tape and the various combinations of paper and plastic should not be used in place of glass containers which are purchased to meet the specifications stated in the *Pharmacopeia.*

Some pharmacists have advanced the argument that the pharmacopeial standards do not apply to preparations not considered U.S.P. or N.F. nor to containers used by the pharmacist in dispensing a preparation on a prescription. Whether or not this contention can be supported is of no consequence for, in my opinion, the pharmacist is under a moral, ethical and legal obligation to dispense high-quality drugs of proven therapeutic value in such a manner as to preserve their quality, potency and curative value. In order to do this, a container meeting the standards set forth by the *Pharmacopeia* would appear to be mandatory.

Labeling

The labeling of the various pre-packaged drugs must be considered as one of the most important steps in the entire operation, yet, unfortunately, too many hospital pharmacists take this step for granted. Consider the following implications which may result from improperly labeled units.

1. If in the preparation of the label to be applied to a particular batch of pre-packaged drug is wrong, then every container in the lot, whether it be 50 units or 500 units, is also improperly labeled. This could lead to innumerable incidents on the pavilions and thereby cast reflections upon the accuracy of the pharmacy staff.

2. Insufficient information on the label may cause the nurse or physician or even the patient to make unnecessary and time-consuming telephone calls to the pharmacy.

3. Improperly or inaccurately labeled containers are an indication that the safety controls and checks are not functioning adequately.

4. In case of a drug recall by the manufacturer, it may be difficult to remove the affected containers from circulation due to the insufficient data on the label.

5. Labels which are ambiguous may lead to medication errors or may mislead the prescriber as to its contents.

One hospital pharmacist[4] utilizes a ¼ × 2-inch pressure sensitive label upon which is printed the following information:

Proprietary name	Pharmaceutical classification
Generic name	Description of the product
Strength	Control number

The finished label in this instance, is quite informative and in itself has a number of built-in checks against improper package contents and the possible administration of the wrong medication to a patient. Figure 74 is an example of this type of label.

Labeling a medication container with the generic name of the product is considered to be proper. However, the use of a brand or proprietary name other than the one which actually describes the contents is never

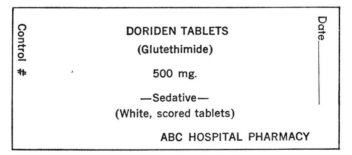

FIG. 74

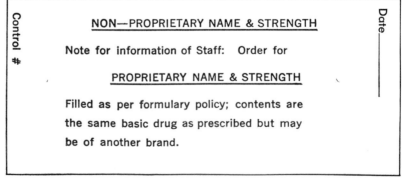

FIG. 75

proper; as a matter of fact it may be considered to be fraudulent. It is also considered to be improper if the proprietary name is used in such a manner as to imply that the contents are the same, although every one concerned knows that they are of a different make.

The format in Figure 75 has been recommended for the labeling of medication containers in the hospital in order to overcome the above situations.

Because many drugs which are pre-packaged in the hospital bear an expiration date, it is advisable to include this on an ancillary label. Although some hospital pharmacists feel that this is not needed because of the rapid consumption of drugs in the hospital and the fact that the proper control record will provide this information, it is suggested that the hospital pre-packaging operation should comply with the rules set for manufacturers or other pre-packagers of drugs.

In this regard, it is of interest to note that the regulations governing the location of expiration dates on labels of drug packages appeared in the *Federal Register of July 16, 1958* and reads as follows:

> "3.507 *Location* of *Expiration Date* in *Drug Labeling.* Drugs which require an expiration date should show the expiration date on the immediate container. When the immediate container is packaged in an individual carton, the expiration date should also be placed on the carton. When single dose containers are packed in single cartons, the expiration date may properly appear on the carton only. . . ."

For the benefit of the student or those who wish to, for the first time, establish a pre-packaging program the following is a program of labeling which when pursued will provide the safety and control needed in a successful operation.

Step One.—Using a marking or printing machine, prepare the proper number of self-adhering labels bearing the following information:

a. Date of pre-packaging by month and year.
   e.g. 8/64.
b. On the next line insert the name of the manufacturer.
c. On the third line insert the control number assigned by the manufacturer.
d. If the item is a dated product, place the expiration date on the far right of the first line. *e.g.* 8/64 (on left), 9/65 (on right).

Thus the completed tag will appear as shown in Figure 76.

This tag is then affixed to the container and is not to be removed by nursing or pharmacy personnel. Whenever dry goods are packaged, the label is placed on the inside of the cap of the capsule or tablet vial thus reducing the temptation to remove it.

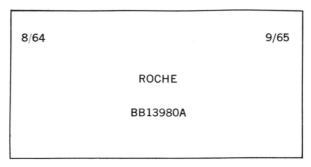

FIG. 76

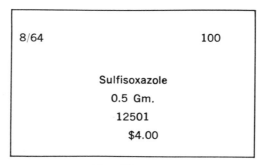

FIG. 77

Step Two.—Again using a marking or printing machine prepare the proper number of self adhering labels bearing the following information:

a. Date of pre-packaging by month and year.

b. Name and strength of the drug.

c. Unit cost—coded if desirable.

d. Unit selling price.

e. Number of capsules on far right of the first line.

Thus, the finished tag appears as shown in Figure 77 and is affixed to the outside of the container.

Step Three.—Affix any ancillary labels which are required, *e.g.* for the Eye; for the Nose; refrigerate, etc.

Step Four.—When the unit is dispensed, the tag described in Step Two is removed from the container and affixed to the prescription or to the medication order slip.

Many pharmacists have expressed the opinion that this final step is unnecessary and is burdensome; however it serves the purpose of affording the checking pharmacist another visible means (in addition to the characteristic color or shape of the dispensed product) of ascertaining accuracy.

HOSPITAL PHARMACY

PRE-PACKAGING CONTROL RECORD

PRODUCT: _____

FORM
(Check One)

Capsule _____   Elixir _____   Solution _____
Tablet _____   Syrup _____   Ointment _____
Powder _____   Tincture _____ Other _____

STRENGTH: _____

MFG.	MFG. LOT #	DATE OF PURCHASE	HOSPITAL PRE-PACK LOT #	UNIT OF PRE-PACK	DATE OF PRE-PACK	NUMBER PRE-PACKED	PACK'D BY	LABELED BY	CHECK'D BY

MISCELLANEOUS COMMENTS

FIG. 78

The Control Record

Besides accurate and comprehensive labeling practices, it is essential that the pharmacist maintain a written control record. Many different varieties of records may be kept; that is, sheets, cards, books, etc. What is important is the information which appears on these records.

Miller[5] recommends the use of a control card upon which is transcribed the following information:

a. Item packaged
b. Manufacturer's control number
c. Total number of units
d. Size of each unit
e. Identity of the pre-packer
f. Identity of the checker
g. Type of container and closure

Figure 78 is an example of one type of pre-packaging record. Of interest here is the fact that a separate sheet is used for each product pre-packaged and should be retained for a period of one year after the last entry.

Strip Packaging

In discussing the various methods of drug distribution in the hospital (Chapter 13), reference was made to the commercial availability of many drug products in strip packages. The pharmaceutical industry has made many drugs available to the hospital pharmacy in pre-packaged strips of five tablets or capsules, rolls of twenty-five and rolls of one hundred. Each strip of five is then placed in a bulk dispensing carton, whereas the rolled strips are packaged in cardboard reel-type dispensing packages.

In spite of industry's good intentions, there still remains a large number of drugs, in common hospital use, that are not strip packaged. Thus, some hospital pharmacists have, in cooperation with industrial packagers, sought to develop a practical yet inexpensive means of strip packaging within the hospital. One such study at the University of Kentucky Medical Center[6] has resulted in the development of both a machine and a program.

In describing the project, the authors state that the operational principles of the machine are very basic:

> Two strips of packaging material are fed through the machine from reels mounted on each side. As this packaging material is pulled into the meshing crimp rollers: (1) the packaging material is labeled where the pocket is to be formed; (2) the tablet or capsule is placed in position to be entrapped in the pocket; (3) the two strips of packaging material are sealed around the tablet or capsule to form the pocket and are then pulled from the heated crimp rollers. Thus, the three phases of the packaging operation are completed.

The packaging machine is known as the Una-Strip Packer and is shown in Figure 49.

Prior to undertaking such a program, the hospital pharmacist should undertake studies to ascertain the volume of drugs which must be pre-packaged. He must develop a satisfactory label to comply with all legal requirements, and finally he must select the proper packaging material to protect the product against air, moisture, and light.

A comparison of five hospitals to determine labor savings if single unit packaged medications replaced those now prepared and dispensed from bulk containers revealed the following figures:[7]

(a) Estimated labor cost per dose in the pharmacy for existing methods averaged 1.61 cents while the unit dose average was 1.33 cents. For nurses, the figures were 14.6 cents and 14 cents respectively. This represents a cost of 16.2 cents per dose for existing methods as opposed to 14.3 cents for unit dose.

(b) There was a direct labor savings of two cents per unit with single-dose dispensing over existing bulk methods, versus an average cost increase of one cent per single-unit of medication over conventional bulk containers.

Guidelines For Single Unit Packages of Drugs

In 1966, the American Society of Hospital Pharmacists approved *Guidelines for Single Unit Packages of Drugs.* As the art of packaging developed and newer materials for packaging became available, the Society, in 1970, revised the *Guidelines* in order that they might be useful guides to those who might need them. The following is a verbatim presentation of these *Guidelines*:[8]

Introduction

These guidelines have been formed with the hope that they will be sufficiently directive to be useful guides to pharmaceutical manufacturers and packagers. It is hoped that they will encourage the continued exploration of new packaging ideas and techniques.

Pharmaceutical manufacturers can package single unit packages more efficiently and economically than can hospitals; however, standardization of packages would provide even greater efficiency and greater economic savings. Even though manufacturers are not expected to package all items in all doses needed in the hospital, they should make an effort to package as many items as possible in single unit packages. The major premise of these guidelines is that a need continues to exist in the hospital for packaging materials and techniques which will provide the hospital a flexibility that permits available packages to fit into existing and future drug distribution systems.

A single unit package is one which contains one discrete pharmaceutical dosage form, i.e., one tablet, one capsule, one 2 ml quantity of a liquid, etc. A single unit package becomes a unit dose package when the physician happens to order that particular amount for a particular patient. In either case the package should be labeled and patient-ready so that the contents can be administered *directly from the package*.

General Considerations

1. *Packaging material*

   The characteristics of the packaging material which are essential in protecting the drug dosage form are the responsibility of the pharmaceutical manufacturer to determine and provide for each product. Comparable packaging material, equipment and devices should be commercially available to the hospital pharmacist to use in completing the hospital's packaging program.

2. *Shape and form*

   By definition, the contents must be deliverable directly to the patient without any repackaging into another container or device. In performing this function the single unit package should be easy to open and easy to use, and its use should require no additional education or experience.

3. *Label copy*

   Current Federal Government requirements for "Labeling" should be adhered to and particular attention given the following special considerations. The desired copy and format are as follows:

NONPROPRIETARY NAME   a.
(and proprietary name, if to be shown)
(dosage form, if special)   b.
STRENGTH   c.
CONTROL NUMBER   d.
(special notes, e.g., "Refrigerate")   e.

a. Nonproprietary (generic, official or established name) and proprietary (trade name) names: The nonproprietary name and the strength should be the most prominent part of the label. It is not necessary to have the proprietary name, if any, on the package. However, if one does appear, in compliance with requirements set forth in the Food, Drug and Cosmetic Act, the established name of any prescription drug or ingredient shall be printed in letters that are at least half as large as the letters comprising the proprietary name, and the established name shall have a prominence commensurate with the prominence of the proprietary name. The style of type should be chosen to provide maximum legibility, contrast and permanence.

b. Special characteristics of the dosage form should be a part of the label, e.g., extended release. Packages should be labeled as to the route of administration if other than oral, e.g., topical use. In a package containing an injection, the acceptable injectable route(s) of administration should be stated. The route of administration should appear on the innermost package.

c. Strength should be stated in accordance with terminology in the *American Hospital Formulary Service*. The metric system should be used, with dosage forms formulated to provide the rounded-off figures in the USP and NF tables of approximate equivalents and expressed in the smallest whole number.

Micrograms should be used through 999, then milligrams through 999, then grams. Thus,

300 mg. *not* 5 gr. nor 325 mg, nor 0.3 g;
60 mg, *not* 1 gr, nor 0.06 g. nor 64.5 mg, nor 65 mg;
400 mcg, *not* 1/150 gr, nor 0.4 mg, nor 0.0004 g;
ml (milliliters) should be used instead of cc (cubic centimeters).

d. The control number should appear on the label. The name of the manufacturer should be included if there is no proprietary name on the package.

e. Special notes such as conditions of storage (e.g., 2-10° C.; expiration date), preparation (e.g., shake well; moisten), and administration (e.g., not to be chewed) that are not obvious from the dosage form designation are to be included at the bottom of the label. When possible, all arbitrary expiration dates should become effective only during the months of January and July to simplify product location and recall.

f. The use of identification codes (that appear directly on the dosage form) for individual product identification is encouraged.

4. Minimum quantities of unit package products available from manufacturers should be within reason for hospitals of all sizes.

5. Each unit package should be so designed that it is evident

when the package is still intact, that it has never been entered or opened.

Specific Considerations

1. *Oral Solids*
    a. Blister package. A blister package should:
    —have an opaque and nonreflective backing (flat upper surface of package) for printing and be square in shape of the dimensions 1¼ × 1¼ inches;
    —have a blister (dome or bubble) of a see-through material that is a flat bottomed, round, nonangular cup with a top diameter of ⅞ inch tapering to bottom diameter of ⅝ inch with a depth of ⅜ inch;
    —be easily peelable;
    —peel from all sides and have opening tabs at multiple locations;
    —be in single cut units.
    b. Pouch package. A pouch package should:
    —have one of its sides opaque and nonreflective for printing and the other a see-through side;
    —be one of the following two outside dimensions: 1¼ by 1¼ inches or 1½ by 2 inches;
    —be easily deliverable (large tablets in large pouches, small tablets in small pouches);
    —tear from any point or multiple locations;
    —be in single cut units.
    c. The packages should be such that contents can be delivered directly to the patient's mouth or to the patient's hand.
2. *Oral Liquids*
    a. The unit package should be filled to deliver the labeled contents. It is recognized that over-filling will be necessary, depending on the shape of the container, the container material, and the formulation of the dosage form.
    b. The label should state the contents as follows:
    Delivers _____ mg (or g or mcg) in _____ ml
3. *Injectables*
    a. The device shall be appropriately calibrated in milliliters and scaled from the tip to the fill line. Calibrated space may be built into the device to permit addition of other drugs. The label should state the contents as follows:
    Delivers _____ mg (or g or mcg) in _____ ml
    b. An appropriate size needle should be an integral part of the device. The needle sheath should not be the plunger. The plunger should be mechanically stable in the barrel of the syringe.
    c. The device should be of such a design that it is patient-ready and assembly instructions are not necessary.
    d. The sheath protecting the needle should be a non-penetrable, rigid material to protect personnel from injury. The size of the needle should be indicated on the sheath.

e. The device shall be of such a design that easy and visible aspiration is possible. It should be as compact as possible and of such a size that it can be easily handled.

4. *Intravenous Solutions (large volume)*

   The pH of the solution and the amount of overfill in the intravenous infusion container should be stated on the label.

5. *Intravenous Additives*

   Drugs that are to be compounded into intravenous infusion solutions should be packaged so that the contents do not have to be withdrawn into a syringe in order to be added to an intravenous bottle. "Partial fills" (partially filled intravenous solution units) for intravenous additives should be made commercially available.

6. *Other Dosage Forms—ophthalmics, topical preparations, suppositories, etc.*

   Dosage forms other than those specifically discussed above should be adequately labeled to indicate their use and route of administration and should adhere to the above and other required labeling criteria.

Future Considerations

1. *Outpatient Dispensing*

   Dispensing packages for outpatient use should be developed. Packages should provide convenience and protect the integrity of the product regardless of the specialty or location or practice.

2. *Pediatric Packages*

   Packages for pediatric doses and for use in providing special pediatric doses should be developed.

3. *New Packages*

   In developing packages, concern for waste and for the eventual disposal of the package should be considered. Packages should be of lightweight, nonbulky materials that produce nontoxic fumes when incinerated. Materials that are reusable as raw materials should be considered. It is hoped that new lightweight packaging that is more patient acceptable, easily disposable and more economical will be developed, made available and released for use.

   The present and future use of computers and automation should be a consideration when developing new packages. It should be possible for hospital pharmacists to duplicate and process such packages themselves if necessary.

4. *Materials Available*

   Information should be available to practitioners indicating the stability, compatibility and possible drug interactions with various materials and films used.

Quality Control Guidelines for Single Packaging of Parenterals in the Hospital Pharmacy

The primary manufacturer of a product is liable for the quality and safety of his product until such time as another party assumes the responsibility from him. In the hospital pharmacy, the manufacturer may be relieved of his responsibility for the product whenever the hospital pharmacist undertakes to package it. Thus, to repackage and store these products without an adequate quality control program may result in a lawsuit for the hospital.

A good quality control program should concern itself with the details involved in container selection in order to eliminate stability and compatibility problems arising from a reaction with capping material or even the plunger tip. Contamination of the parenteral solution must be guarded against from such sources as personnel, environment, and containers. Vials and syringes should be checked for accuracy of calibration in order that the amount of overfill be ascertained.

The filling process should be performed under a laminar airflow hood and detailed records should be maintained.[9]

SELECTED REFERENCES

LIVINGSTON, B. P.: Proprietary Names and Labeling Under the Formulary System, Am. J. Hosp. Pharm., *17*:10:607, 1960.

AUTIAN, JOHN: Plastics—Uses and Problems in Pharmacy and Medicine, Am. J. Hosp. Pharm., *18*:6:329, 1961.

SCHWARTAU, NEAL and STURDAVANT, MADELYN: A System of Pre-Packaging and Dispensing Drugs in Single Doses, Am. J. Hosp. Pharm., *18*:9:542, 1961.

BARKER, KENNETH N., POLLOCK, DONALD R., MARTINEZ, DOMINGO R. and HELLER, WILLIAM M.: A Nurse Acceptance Evaluation of Some Pre-filled Disposable Injection Devices, Am. J. Hosp. Pharm., *23*:3:127, 1966.

BLUMBERG, M.: Packaging of Hospital Medications, Am. J. Hosp. Pharm., *19*:270, 1962.

HASSAN, WILLIAM E.: Quo Vadis Drug Packaging, Hospital Pharmacy, 4:7:9, July, 1969.

BIBLIOGRAPHY

1. ARCHAMBAULT, G. F.: Plastics and the U.S.P. Requirements for Tight, Light-Resistant Containers, Am. J. Hosp. Pharm., *15*:877, 1958.
2. ————: Standards for Prescription Containers, Am. J. Hosp. Pharm., *20*:538, 1952.
3. *Pharmacopeia of the United States of America,* 18th Revision, Easton, Mack Publishing Co., p. 9, 1970.
4. BENYA, THEODORE J.: Labeling Pre-packaged Medication, Am. J. Hosp. Pharm., *19*:1:20, 1962.
5. WEBB, JOHN W.: Methods of Promoting Safety and Control in Hospital Pharmacy, Am. J. Hosp. Pharm., *15*:11:977, 1958.
6. SAMUELS, TOM M. and GUTHRIE, DON L.: Unit Dose Packaging—a New Machine for Strip Packaging Tablets and Capsules, Am. J. Hosp. Pharm., *23*:1:4, 1966.

7. BLASINGAME, W. G., DREVNO, HAROLD, GODLEY, LEO F., KRATZ, RICHARD
L., VONA, JOSEPH P. and MINOTT, PAUL: Some Time and Motion Considerations with Single-Unit Packaged Drugs in Five Hospitals, Am. J. Hosp.
Pharm. *26*:6:310, June 1969.
8. Guidelines for Single Unit Packages of Drugs, Am. J. Hosp. Pharm. *28*:2:
110, February 1971.
9. PATEL, J. A., CURTIS, E. G. and PHILLIPS, G. L.: Quality Control Guidelines for Single Unit Packaging of Parenterals in the Hospital Pharmacy,
Am. J. Hosp. Pharm. *29*:11:947, November 1972.

Chapter

21

Manufacturing—Bulk and Sterile

STATISTICAL data on manufacturing or bulk compounding in hospitals[1] revealed that approximately 41 per cent of 1853 hospital pharmacies operate a manufacturing program. The survey further demonstrated that 78 per cent of the sample group prepared galenical pharmaceuticals; 74 per cent, products not commercially available; 42 per cent, sterile solutions for topical use; 33 per cent, sterile pharmaceuticals such as collyria, ointments etc.; and 30 per cent, small volume injectable solutions.

In addition, the same survey[2] showed that hospital pharmacists were also active in the preparation of sterile products such as surgical irrigating fluids, large volume injectable solutions, and special sterile products for investigational use.

This volume of hospital manufacturing may surprise the neophyte pharmacist particularly when viewed in the light of the magnitude of the American pharmaceutical industry. Obviously, there must be some explanation to this paradox. Those knowledgeable in the ways of the profession have advanced a number of reasons the more important of which are (a) that there exists a close relationship between doctors and pharmacists in hospitals, (b) that commercially available products are not often suited for the treatment of certain unusual illnesses which the physician with a hospital practice is expected to cope with, and (c) that, because of the physician-pharmacist relationship in the hospital, doctors feel at ease in requesting the pharmacist to prepare a special pharmaceutical form either for clinical or experimental use.

Also worthy of consideration here is the fact that hospital pharmacists engaged in this type of practice often encourage and promulgate its expansion and growth because they are of the consensus that such an activity promotes economy within the hospital, compliments the operation of the formulary system, increases the prestige of the hospital pharmacist, and provides the research clinician with the opportunity to develop new pharmaceutical formulations.

Those responsible for the education and training of future hospital pharmacists consider a manufacturing or bulk compounding program to be an extremely useful endeavor which draws together the classroom concepts of courses in product development, physical chemistry, instrumental methods of analysis, and preservation and stabilization of pharmaceutical products.

A manufacturing program within the department of pharmacy is also of interest to trustees and administrators because of its ability to reduce the cost of pharmaceuticals to patients and is, therefore, encouraged by them, whenever the pharmacist shows the desire and the ability to undertake such an endeavor.

For the purposes of this chapter, a manufacturing program for the hospital pharmacy shall be deemed to encompass both bulk compounding of pharmaceuticals and the preparation of sterile products. The same meticulous standards and principles should apply to the preparation of both classes of products.

Control, in General

The word "control" is defined[3] as

"To test or verify (a statement or experiment) by counter or parallel evidence or experiment."

"To exercise directing, guiding or restraining power over."

Klemme[4] has suggested that hospital pharmacists should consider control of their manufacturing program from two vantage points—"quality control" to govern the quality, purity and strength of the manufactured product and "budgetary control" to regulate the economic aspects of the program. All too often, the hospital pharmacist devotes a great deal of thought and effort to the quality control aspect of the manufacturing program only to learn that he has a technically and professionally sound program but at the same time one which is in economic distress.

Accordingly, the principles of budgetary and quality control will be discussed under separate sections within this chapter.

Budgetary Control

In order to develop adequate budgetary control over the manufacturing program, the hospital pharmacist is required to give lengthy consideration to his *inventory* and *consumption rate* for the *finished product, raw materials requirement, manufacturing capacity, available personnel* and *operating costs.*

Manufacturing Requirements

Probably the most difficult task lies in prognosticating, with reasonable accuracy, the consumption rate for each item to be included in a manufacturing program. This can be done by reviewing the records of the previous year or two and comparing this figure with the staff's present prescribing pattern. Since the figure to be arrived at is, at best, an educated guess, the pharmacist should not become too alarmed if, at the end of the first quarter, he realizes that he has overestimated or underestimated his requirements. Whichever the case may be, corrective measures may be put into effect for the second quarter, namely, increase the rate or volume of production or reduce the batch quantity or frequency of manufacture or eliminate one batch of the product which is considered to be above desirable inventory limits.

Material Requirements

Once the hospital pharmacist has determined what products he intends to manufacture and in what volume and quantity, he must next arrange for the procurement of the necessary supplies. These supplies should include, in addition to raw materials, such items as containers, labels and ancillary materials such as filter paper, filter pads, boxes, and labels.

The first step in this direction is to take each formula and determine the quantity of chemical or other material which will be required to produce the annual supply. This is done by taking the quantities of raw materials from the working formula and packaging specifications of each item and multiplying these quantities by the number of times the formula must be produced to satisfy the estimated annual requirement.

The second step is to enter these quantities on a *summary sheet* because the same drug, chemical or container may be required by many different formulas.

By totaling the quantities under each item on the summary sheet, the pharmacist will now have available to him his annual supplies and material needs to undertake the contemplated manufacturing program.

Since the budget period of the hospital is on a yearly basis, the purchasing agent or the purchasing pharmacist will divide the material and supply requirements into four quarters. This will allow the purchasing group ample time to utilize the basic principles of good purchasing technics and at the same time ensure against over inventory and shortage of materials in the pharmacy.

Manufacturing Capacity

Two important considerations in any bulk compounding program are first whether or not the pharmacist has available to him the kind of equipment necessary to produce the formulas selected and secondly, whether or not the machinery is capable of producing the desired quantity.

Because time is the costliest factor in any manufacturing program, it behooves the pharmacist to utilize the maximum capacity of his equipment. In addition, the selection of equipment should be made on the basis of the multiple or variety of uses to which a single piece of equipment can be put. This will prevent costly equipment from accumulating idle time.

Manufacturing Equipment and Its Sources

The kind and size of manufacturing equipment required in the hospital pharmacy will vary from institution to institution. Primary consideration must be given to the scope of the manufacturing program, the quantities to be produced during any production run as well as to the length of time that will be required to consume the product, the availability of personnel and the availability of physical facilities.

Modern technology has developed equipment to meet every production need. The available machinery can handle amounts that are considered to be of "practical volume or quantity" for a small or medium sized hospital. In addition, the larger hospitals have available to them automatic and semi-automatic heavy duty production equipment which is capable of handling large volume in a minimum of time.

In *Remington's Practice of Pharmacy*,[5] the student will find pictures and a brief description of the various pieces of equipment which may be useful in the formulation of pharmaceutical preparations.

As a means of assisting the pharmacist desirous of mechanizing his bulk compounding department, many producers of pharmaceutical manufacturing and packaging equipment have prepared excellent descriptive brochures and catalogues which are of value in assisting the pharmacist in selecting the most versatile equipment for his particular use and needs.

Manufacturing Staff

Next to equipment, personnel represent the most important consideration in a bulk compounding program. Too many personnel will raise the cost of a manufactured product to the point where it would be more economical to purchase it from a commercial supplier and too little help may mean the inability to maintain an adequate production schedule and potential errors—neither of which may be condoned.

Accordingly, production time must be determined for each formula in order that proper planning and scheduling be effected.

The manufacturing section of the pharmacy must be supervised by a technically competent, legally qualified pharmacist. In addition he must be supported with ancillary personnel who can be trained to carry on such non-technical pursuits as bottling, filtering, labeling, etc. Under no circumstances should a bulk compounding program be undertaken without the services of a pharmacist under the pretense that this is justified by the reduction in labor cost and that reasonably intelligent lay help can be trained to perform specific tasks with accuracy and dependability.

Operating Costs

A review of the literature pertaining to manufacturing programs in hospital pharmacies and central sterile supply rooms leads one to believe that many so-called "profitable ventures" are classified as such mainly because of an understated operating cost. In these instances, the operating cost was shown to consist of the direct costs only—direct labor and cost of materials.

Correctly used, operating costs should include both direct and indirect costs.[6] The terminology "overhead costs" is usually used interchangeably with "indirect costs" and, for the purpose of this section, is intended to include such items as the cost of supervisory personnel, space rental, insurance, equipment depreciation, maintenance, housekeeping, etc. In some hospitals, those items not directly connected with the pharmacy operation are included in a figure obtainable from the comptroller's office known as the *"overhead per square foot"* figure.

By whatever means obtainable, the indirect costs should be compared with the direct costs for the purpose of calculating a ratio of overhead dollars to direct labor dollars which may later be applied in ascertaining the true cost of the product.

An example of the above principle is best demonstrated as follows:
   a. Assume that the ratio of indirect costs to direct costs in hospital X is 100 per cent.
   b. Further assume that 5 gallons of product "A" require $4.25 in materials and $5.50 in direct costs. Therefore,

Direct Cost
    Materials ....$ 4.25
    Labor 5.50
Indirect Cost 9.75
—————
TOTAL COST ....$19.50 for 5 gallons

It is of importance to call the student's attention at this point to the fact that if the quantity of product "A" in the above example were doubled, only the cost of materials would double. The direct and indirect costs *do not* increase in direct proportion because it requires very little more time to manufacture 10 gallons than it does to manufacture 5 gallons. The packaging segment of the operation is where the direct labor cost will be in direct proportion to the batch size.

Since the increase in batch size will, to a point, reduce the unit cost, the student is cautioned that the cost curve does not decrease geometrically with the increase in batch size. Also, it is unwise to manufacture in a volume which will not be consumed within a reasonable period of time for this will now introduce problems in storage, long term product preservation, and reduced inventory turn-over.

Quality Control

The term "quality control" should not be confused with the term "statistical quality control" which involves the application of statistics for the control of sizes, weights and other physical characteristics of articles undergoing mass production. Statistical quality control plays a very important role in large scale pharmaceutical production plants but has very little value in the control aspect of hospital pharmacy manufacturing programs.

What is more important to hospitals, their staff and patients is a quality control that will ensure the integrity of the label. This can best be accomplished by developing a series of cross checks and laboratory analyses.

It should be clearly understood that no two hospitals develop control systems which are identical in every respect,[7,8] and therefore no system can here be recommended which will serve every purpose. Accordingly, it becomes the responsibility of the hospital pharmacist to make whatever modifications he deems necessary to ensure a product which will meet high pharmaceutical standards.

The Pharmaceutical Manufacturers Association has developed a policy statement entitled **General Principles of Control of Quality in the Drug Industry.*** Because this statement exemplifies the ultimate

*Adopted by the Board of Directors of the Pharmaceutical Manufacturers Association, May 3, 1961.

in a quality control program, it is presented here in order to permit the hospital pharmacists to compare his present quality control program with the specific considerations which ordinarily form the basis of a quality control program utilized by the pharmaceutical industry.

GENERAL PRINCIPLES OF CONTROL OF QUALITY IN THE DRUG INDUSTRY

Control of quality in the formulation, manufacture, and distribution of pharmaceutical, biological, and other medicinal products is the organized effort employed by a company to provide and maintain in the final product the desired features, properties and characteristics of identity, purity, uniformity, potency, and stability within established levels so that all merchandise shall meet professional requirements, legal standards, and also such additional standards as the management of a firm may adopt.

The large variety of substances used in this industry, the complexity of its products and the various types of company organizations make it impossible to design in detail a single universally applicable quality control system.

The adequacy of any control system is measured by its effectiveness in attaining its purposes.

The Quality Control and Production Functions

The quality of any medicinal product must be built into it during production. However, it is a basic principle of quality control that a production group should not be responsible for approving its final product for distribution. The person heading quality control should have the authority to approve satisfactory products, and to reject unsuitable products so they are not distributed. He should be responsible to a level of management which enables him to exercise independent judgment.

Quality Control Systems and Procedures

Quality control systems are designed to provide for the proper functioning of personnel, machines and operations, and encouragement of quality consciousness in all personnel. Quality control systems use many procedures, among them being checks and safeguards set up in a plant so that the integrity, strength, uniformity and purity of the finished products meet appropriate standards.

The control of quality by the manufacturer or by others in distribution involves such factors as the layout of the plant or other facilities, the procurement of raw materials, and all intervening operations up to the delivery of the products to the consumer. Among other things, the manufacturer should be concerned with proper receipt, identity, sampling and storage of raw materials, proper manufacturing and packaging facilities, and proper apportionment of raw materials to the manufacturing batches. Checks should be provided so that the specified amount of each ingredient, properly identified, is incorporated uniformly in the formula, and the materials should be handled in a manner which will safeguard against the loss of any component or ingredient or the introduction of any undesired substance.

Collateral and supplemental to the controls exercised in the manufacturing and packaging operations are appropriate observations, examinations, laboratory tests, and assays of samples of raw materials, in-process goods and finished products.

Control laboratories must possess competent personnel and have access to adequate facilities to make all the necessary tests for determining the identity, uniformity, strength, and purity of each product. They may employ, among others, chemical, physical, bacteriological, pharmacological and microbiological procedures according to the requirements of the particular product or process.

The maintenance of adequate records covering all appropriate areas of operation is a prime requirement of a well-designed quality control system.

Items Which May be Considered

The foregoing discussion covers the general principles of the control of quality in a manufacturing plant. In the following outline are mentioned some of the specific considerations which ordinarily form the basis of a quality control system. Certain items may, in some organizations, be the concern of individuals not directly responsible for the quality control function.

1. Buildings for manufacturing, testing, and storage operations are of adequate design, size and construction to:
   (*a*) provide for proper receipt and storage of raw materials.
   (*b*) allow proper segregation and identification of material during manufacturing and packaging.
   (*c*) provide for ease in maintaining cleanliness and for avoiding contamination.
   (*d*) provide suitable sampling facilities.
   (*e*) provide adequate laboratory facilities.
   (*f*) provide proper storage for final products.
2. Equipment is:
   (*a*) properly located.
   (*b*) adequate for the required operations.
   (*c*) constructed to facilitate cleaning.
   (*d*) properly maintained.
3. Raw materials are controlled by:
   (*a*) establishment of suitable specifications.
   (*b*) development of adequate test procedures.
   (*c*) specific identification markings.
   (*d*) proper storage conditions.
   (*e*) adequate sampling.
   (*f*) appropriate testing.
   (*g*) requiring compliance with specifications.
   (*h*) providing for quality control release.
   (*i*) maintaining records and samples whenever appropriate.

4. Manufacturing operations are controlled by:
   (*a*) use of a suitable batch numbering system.
   (*b*) preparation of formula or batch records.
   (*c*) checking of ingredients: identity, weight and measure.
   (*d*) maintaining identity during processing.
   (*e*) checking quality during processing.
   (*f*) checking yield against theory.
   (*g*) adequate sampling and testing.
   (*h*) requiring compliance with specifications.
   (*i*) maintaining appropriate records and samples.
5. Packaging and finishing are controlled by:
   (*a*) establishment of specifications for packaging and packaging operations.
   (*b*) a formal procedure providing for the inspection and issuance of packaging materials including labels and labeling.
   (*c*) providing for the proper disposition of unused labels and labeling.
   (*d*) use of suitable batch, lot or control numbers.*
   (*e*) maintaining identity of product before and during packaging.
   (*f*) checking yield against theory.
   (*g*) sampling and checking for compliance with specifications.
   (*h*) providing for release by quality control.
   (*i*) maintaining appropriate records and samples.
6. Finished stock quality is maintained by:
   (*a*) providing proper storage conditions.
   (*b*) collection and review of stability data.
   (*c*) investigating all significant complaints concerning quality of products.
   (*d*) providing for the disposition of returned goods.

The Work Sheet

The master formula card and work sheet must never be removed from the control of the pharmacy office. Therefore, a means must be devised whereby the manufacturing pharmacist will have available all of the necessary data for the production and packaging of the finished product, as well as having a form to record the necessary information obtained from the control laboratories.

---

*By "use of suitable batch, lot or control numbers" is meant a system of identifying each production lot, including marking the labeling of each package from each manufactured batch, whereby the manufacturer can establish the history of the batch, the source of each significant ingredient, the records of tests made on ingredients as well as on the final product, and the identity of the individual responsible for each of the steps in the manufacturing process. Such numbers shall likewise relate to records of the finishing operations, with the final audit accounting for the total number of packages produced. They also provide a means whereby recalls may be made if necessary.

This can be easily accomplished by the use of any of the modern day duplicating devices. A stencil can be cut, showing all the essential data on the master formula and work sheet, and readily duplicated within the hospital. These sheets when completed must be filed since they represent the detailed history of the manufactured product.

A good control system record will provide the hospital pharmacist with the following information on each product manufactured:

1. Name
2. Strength
3. Date of manufacture
4. Formula
5. Ingredients
   a. Manufacturer
   b. Lot number
6. Method of compounding
7. Person who prepared finished product
8. Person who checked the materials and process
9. The hospital lot number assigned to the product
10. Its disposition
11. Its packaging
12. Laboratory control data
13. Percentage yield
14. Time consumed in its preparation
15. Raw material cost
16. Packaging cost

In addition to the above, some authors recommend the use of a receiving number for all raw materials as a means of completely identifying each raw material container. In those hospitals where serially numbered receiving slips are utilized, the number on the receiving slip constitutes a suitable receiving number. (For information on the use of a receiving memo the reader is referred to Chapter 9 dealing with purchasing and inventory control.)

Also suggested as an additional means of control is a so-called "Identification Number" which is issued to each raw material, whether it be a chemical, bottle, cap, tube or drug.

If all these numbers are used, they should be attached to the raw material container and shown on the pharmacy inventory card. Although some hospital pharmacists write the numbers on the fiber drum containing the chemicals or on the label, if the material is in a glass bottle, the use of an ancillary colored adhesive label is suggested, one color to indicate the receiving number and a second color to identify the raw materials identification number.

Prior to the release of a manufactured product, it should be subjected to chemical or bacteriological analysis. In some hospitals, this control work is performed within the department of pharmacy by a group of pharmacists specifically assigned to the control laboratory. This, of course, is the ideal situation and those institutions with sufficient volume to support such a unit are strongly advised to do so.

On the other hand, small or medium sized hospitals who cannot afford this luxury are nonetheless not excused from the obligation of checking formulas for purity and accuracy produced in the pharmacy or central sterile supply room. This can be done through the close cooperation of the department of pathology (pyrogen testing), the chemistry laboratory (chemical analyses utilizing the spectrophotometer) and the bacteriology laboratory (for sterility determinations).

After all is said and done, none of the above described procedures will guarantee the purity and integrity of every product every time it is produced, unless the individuals concerned with the manufacturing program can be adequately supervised and trained.

With this in mind, it is of interest to present at this point the philosophy of Sr. Francis[9] on how to avoid troubles in the manufacture of parenteral solutions in the hospital pharmacy:

"1. *Pharmaceutical Supervision:*
   a. of the formulae prepared
   b. of the procedures
   c. of the cleaning process
   d. of controls

2. *Exacting cleanliness:*
   a. of the manufacturing room
   b. of flasks and other glassware
   c. of rubber tubings
   d. of flask closures
   e. of stored chemicals

3. Routine cleaning of water still

4. Careful selection of chemicals

5. Production of a pure, pyrogen-free distillate which is checked electrically before and after each operation of the still, and which is sterilized within 8 hours.

6. *Accurate measurements:*
   a. of original chemicals
   b. of the finished solution

7. Controlled sterilization process guided by exhaust line thermometer readings

8. Hermetically sealed flasks

9. Prompt and proper filling

10. Inspection and checking of finished products."

Maintenance of Manufacturing Equipment

Because of the hospital's high investment in pharmaceutical manufacturing equipment and the expense associated with frequent repairs, it behooves the pharmacist to develop an equipment maintenance program which will ensure maximum performance with the lowest possible repair cost.

HOSPITAL PHARMACY

EQUIPMENT MAINTENANCE RECORD

EQUIPMENT: _____   INITIAL COST $ _____

DATE OF PURCHASE	VENDOR	SERIAL NUMBER	EXPIRATION OF WARRANTY	SERVICE CONTRACT YES	NO	DATE OF REPAIR	TYPE OF REPAIR	COST OF REPAIR

MISCELLANEOUS DATA OR COMMENTS

					1964						1965														
	1	2	3	4	5	6	7	8	9	10	11	12	13	14	15	16	17	18	19	20	21	22	23	24	25
Grease																									
Oil																									

Fig. 79

This can be accomplished by establishing an Equipment Maintenance Record (Fig. 79) which may be kept by the pharmacist
or the plant engineer. In addition to identifying clearly the equipment as to name, vendor, serial number and cost, the Equipment
Maintenance Record provides the interested parties with a quick
history of the repairs required on the apparatus. Furthermore, the
routine or preventive monthly maintenance required by the equipment can be recorded and checked off when performed. Omission of
the monthly service can be easily detected by reference to this
record and corrected prior to the onset of mechanical difficulties.

Parenteral Hyperalimentation

Parenteral hyperalimentation is the intravenous administration of
sufficient nutrients above the usual basal requirements to achieve tissue
synthesis, positive nitrogen balance and anabolism.[10]

The preparation of parenteral hyperalimentation solutions must
be considered as an integral part of the pharmacy department's manufacturing program irrespective of its size. The procedures employed
are not unduly complicated and do not require extensive capital outlay for equipment.

Most hospital pharmacists prepare these solutions by using a technique described as the "wet method" through the extemporaneous compounding techniques of an intravenous admixture program.[10] This consists of mixing the dextrose solution from one flask with the fibrin hydrolysate solution in another flask utilizing a solution transfer set. In the "dry method" the pharmacist adds the appropriate amount of anhydrous glucose to the fibrin hydrolysate solution. Both methods must be carried out under a laminar flow hood.

Because of the nature of these product, the pharmacy must have available appropriate refrigeration equipment and the pharmacist must become familiar with membrane filtration processes in view of the fact that the heat associated with the normal sterilization process will cause caramelization of the dextrose contained in each formula.

Intravenous Additive Program

One writer has stated that an *intravenous additive program* and an *intravenous additive service* may not be the same.[11] The differentiation cited is that an IV additive program consists of policies and procedures for both the preparation and administration of intravenous fluids to which drugs are to be added under aseptic conditions, on an around-the-clock basis, and controlled as to location and person preparing the product. On the other hand, the IV additive service usually refers only to the preparation of the product by individuals who may not necessarily be the same as those who will administer them and assume the responsibility for the monitoring of its clinical effects. The conclusion arrived at is that an IV additive service is a part of an IV additive program.

Through the implementation of an IV additive service, the hospital pharmacist might be expected to achieve the following objectives:[11] (*a*) that the preparation of the final product be accomplished under aseptic conditions; (*b*) that drug interactions be avoided through the judicious choice of additive and mixing techniques; and (*c*) that the final product is appropriately labeled, dispensed and stored.

In the not too distant past, the preparation of intravenous solutions with their additives was a task performed on the nursing floor by nurses or interns and residents. The concept that the preparation of these product requires the skills of a pharmacist has raised many other questions not the least of which is availability of the product at odd hours particularly if the site of preparation is moved to the main pharmacy. Thus, has evolved the satellite pharmacy, staffed by a clinical pharmacist and pharmacy technicians (See Figs. 80, 81 and 82 for medication station for IV preparation.) On final analysis, it is irrelevant where the additives are added so long as definite policies are

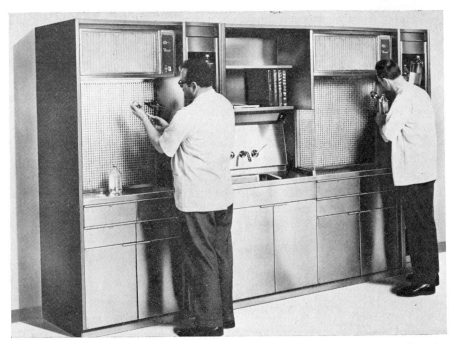

Fig. 80.   The Market Forge IV Prep Station. Units such as this offer the pharmacist and the nurse an area for the preparation of intravenous additives in a controlled environment. (Courtesy of Market Forge Co., Everett, Massachusetts.)

formulated which spell out responsibilities. In addition, it is imperative that the pharmacist become involved in the preparation of these products in an environment conducive to the efficient and safe preparation of them.[12]

Preparation of IV Additive Solutions

In the preparation of these solutions, the pharmacist should work from the physician's original order sheet or from a direct copy. Upon receipt of the order, a pressure-sensitive label must be prepared which provides the following information: (a) patient identification; (b) patient location; (c) physician's name; (d) name of drugs with quantities added; (e) date of compounding; (f) expiration date; and (g) identification of the pharmacist preparing the product. If necessary, any ancillary labeling should also be prepared at this time. When applying the label to the container, it must be positioned in an upside down position in order to facilitate reading when the container is hung from an intravenous solution pole on the patient's bed.

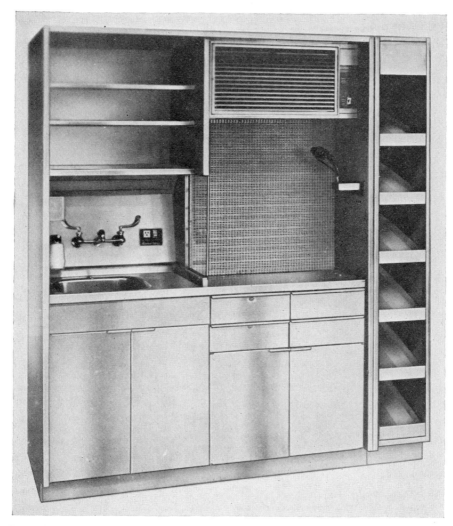

FIG. 81. The Market Forge IV Prep Station. (Courtesy of Market Forge Co., Everett, Massachusetts.)

Preparation of the solution should always take place under a laminar flow hood using sterile needles and syringes or double ended transfer needles. In some instances, a Cornwall syringe is useful in reconstitution procedures.

Once the transfer is made, the metal disc must be replaced and a new seal crimped on to the container. As a safety device, a different colored seal should be used in view of the fact that it warns individuals that drugs have been added.[13]

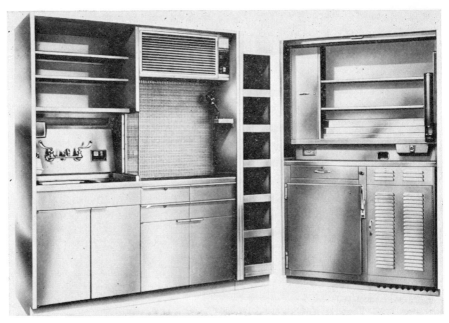

FIG. 82.   Combination installation of a Market Forge IV Prep Station and a Medi-Prep Unit. (Courtesy of Market Forge Co., Everett, Massachusetts.)

Before permitting the admixture to leave his control, the pharmacist must carry out a final inspection of the product. The inspection should include a review of the label, clarity of the solution, and the mathematics involved in the preparation.[14]

SELECTED REFERENCES

LOWE, REGINALD, and WORRELL, LEE F.:   Preparation, Assay and Standardization of Allergens, Am. J. Hosp. Pharm., *18*:6:351, 1961.

AVIS, KENNETH, CARLIN, HERBERT S., and FLACK, HERBERT L.:   Preparation of Injectables—Philosophy Master Procedures, Am. J. Hosp. Pharm., *18*:4:223, 1961.

GASDIA, SALVATORE D.:   Procedures Involved in Quality Control of Pharmaceuticals in Hospitals, Am. J. Hosp. Pharm., *18*:4:234, 1961.

BOGASH, R. C.:   Control Systems in Bulk Compounding and Pre-packaging, Hosp. Topics, *36*:3:39, 1958.

WILLIAMS, A. R.:   Small Scale Tablet Manufacture, Public Pharmacist (Great Britain), *16*:168, 1959.

HUGHILL, PHILIP R., OSHEROFF, BORIS J., and SKOLAUT, MILTON W.:   Equipment and Techniques for Sterile Dispensing of Ophthalmic Solutions, Am. J. Hosp. Pharm., *17*:9:535, 1960.

WEINBERG, STANLEY, and RAPPAPORT, HARVEY: Preparation of Small Volume Parenterals at the Delaware Hospital, Am. J. Hosp. Pharm., *21*:4:158, 1964.

BIBLIOGRAPHY

1. FRANCKE, DON, LATIOLAIS, CLIFTON J., FRANCKE, GLORIA N., and HO, NORMAN F. H.: *Mirror to Hospital Pharmacy*, Washington, D.C., American Society of Hospital Pharmacists, p. 122.
2. Ibid., p. 123.
3. *Webster's New Collegiate Dictionary*, 2nd ed. Springfield, Mass., G. & C. Merriam Co., p. 181.
4. KLEMME, CARL J.: Manufacturing Control Systems in Hospital Pharmacy, The Bulletin, A.S.H.P., 6:278, 1949.
5. MARTIN, ERIC W. and COOK, E. FULLERTON: *Remington's Practice of Pharmacy*, 12th Ed., Easton, Pa., The Mack Publishing Co., 1961.
6. EGOL, E., and BOGASH, R. C.: Hospital Mouthwash: An Examination of Direct and Indirect Costs, Hosp. Topics, 41:119, 1963.
7. SKOLAUT, MILTON W.: Quality Control Procedures for the Hospital Pharmacy, Hospitals, J.A.H.A., 38:83, 1964.
8. BOGASH, ROBERT C.: Why are Administrators and Physicians Reluctant and Sometimes Hostile to a Proposal for Making Sterile Solutions in the Pharmacy? Hosp. Topics, 41:75, 1963.
9. FRANCIS, SR. M. CLARA: Parenteral Fluids Prepared in the Hospital Pharmacy, The Bulletin, A.S.H.P., 5:114, 1948.
10. FLACK, HERBERT L., GANS, JOHN A., SERLICK, STANLEY E., and DUDRICK, STANLEY J.: The Current Status of Parenteral Hyperalimentation, Am. J. Hosp. Pharm. 28:5:326, May 1971.
11. RAVIN, R. L.: An IV Additive Program—Suggested Procedures, Hosp. Formulary Management 3:35, 1968.
12. DURGIN, J. M.: Developing Policies and Procedures for an IV Additive Service, Hosp. Topics, 48:47, 1970.
13. BROWN, R. G.: IV Additive Program Belongs in the Pharmacy, Hospitals, J.A.H.A., 43:92, 1969.
14. PULLIAM, C. C. and UPTON, J. H.: A Pharmacy Coordinated Intravenous Admixture and Administration Service, Am. J. Hosp. Pharm. 28:92, 1971.

Chapter

22

The Combined Pharmacy–Central Sterile Supply Room

THE Central Supply Department of a hospital has been defined as—

"... a centralized unit ... which provides professional supplies and equipment (sterile and non-sterile), to all specialized departments. ..."

A review of the literature will reveal that this specialized area of hospital operation is also known by other names, such as Central Sterile Supply Room, C.S.R., C.S.S.R. and Sterile Supply Room.

The "special departments" which are served include all nursing pavilions, clinics, certain specialized laboratories, such as the Cardiac Catheterization Laboratory, and the operating rooms.

In the early days of development, the majority of the items dispensed by the central supply room consisted of re-usable material. Today, with the advent of the age of plastics and disposables the reverse is true. Disposable drapes, syringes, tubing, urine collection sets, intravenous administration sets, needles, gloves and blood bags are an example of the inroads made by the plastic industry into the field of supplying hospitals with single use items.

In addition to the dispensing of the above mentioned items, the modern central sterile supply room may be involved in the cleaning, storage and dispensing of specialized equipment such as suction pumps, cardiac catheters, monitoring equipment, surgical dressing carts, resuscitation carts, as well as the preparation of intravenous fluids, surgical irrigating fluids, peritoneal dialysis fluids and a myriad of special kits and trays.[2]

The central sterile supply room is a relatively modern innovation in the hospital.[3,4] From its beginning as an equipment washroom with autoclaving facilities, it has adapted itself to modern production line technics with automatic control recording devices to insure sterility, modern washing, drying and powdering equipment for surgical gloves as well as taking an active role in developing the various gas and cold sterilization technics.

As to the management function of the central sterile supply room, there are three schools of thought. One group[5,6] is of the opinion that the procurement, storage and distribution of supplies as well as the preparation of the various sterile solutions lend themselves to the training of a pharmacist. In fact, the pharmacist is performing these very same functions within the department of pharmacy; therefore, if only from an economic point of view, it is feasible to incorporate into the pharmacist's duties the responsibility for the management of the central sterile supply room.

A second group contends that the majority of the items dispensed are ultimately used by nurses in the care of their patients and therefore since a nurse fully comprehends the intended use of the products, she logically should be responsible for the operation of the central sterile supply room.

The third group accepts the fact that the central sterile supply room has a dual function, namely, the cleaning, packaging and distribution of medical equipment and supplies as well as the manufacture of sterile fluids. Accordingly, it is the consensus that a nurse should be responsible for the former and a pharmacist should be responsible for the latter.

In actual practice, all three of these views are accepted and each can claim a representative number of hospitals which have adopted the respective ideology of each group.

The Central Sterile Supply Room in the Hospital Organization

Unlike the pharmacy which has been accorded full departmental status, the central sterile supply room is, in many hospitals, considered as a sub-department. In these institutions, the department may fall under the aegis of the Operating Room Supervisor or the Nursing Service. Under this type of organization, the director, supervisor or manager of the unit does not report to the administrator or his assistant but to some major department head.

In some hospitals, a division of surgical care is established as a section of the general nursing service. Within this division are the central sterile supply room, operating rooms, recovery rooms and intensive surgical care unit. Here again, the head of the central sterile supply room is again operating at a sub-departmental level.

In still other hospitals, the manufacture of sterile injectable or irrigating solutions are separated from the central sterile supply room and this "solution room" is placed within the administrative scope of the pharmacist. Under this arrangement, the pharmacist reports directly to the administrator or to one of his assistants. The same rung in the organizational structure of the hospital is retained if the pharmacy and central sterile supply room are considered as one unit.

It is of interest to note at this point that pharmacy and central sterile supply may have a joint responsibility. This situation is brought about when the pharmacy (1) prepares the solutions in bulk and transports the tanks to the central sterile supply room for bottling and sterilization, (2) prepares and packages the solutions for sterilization by the central sterile supply room, or (3) prepares a concentrated solution which is then diluted, packaged and sterilized in the central sterile supply room, or (4) prepares a mixture of the chemicals in the dry state which when dissolved in a specified volume of distilled water results in the desired product which is then packaged and sterilized by the central sterile supply room personnel.

Although it may seem strange to the reader to have the pharmacy prepare and bottle the various solutions and the central sterile supply room to assume the responsibility for their sterilization, it is, in effect, a very practical solution to the dilemma of whether or not identical sterilization equipment should be installed in both the pharmacy and the central sterile supply room.

Qualifications of the Hospital Pharmacist to Manage the Central Sterile Supply Room

Because the modern pharmacy curriculum provides the student with an exposure to bacteriology, the principles of sterilization, accounting and management, the hospital pharmacist is educationally better qualified to manage the central sterile supply room than is the nurse. Admittedly, the nurse has a better knowledge of the ultimate use of the products dispensed, and, in some instances, the experience required for an efficient operation. This is not a reflection upon the nurse who may be presently in charge of a central sterile supply room nor upon the nursing profession as a whole. It is merely a comparison of two different callings—one devoted to the direct care of the ill patient and therefore does not require training in the principles of procurement, packaging, storage and dispensing, whereas the other is a profession devoted to providing the various services associated with the needs of doctors, nurses and ill patients and therefore requires a thorough grounding in the above principles in addition to certain areas of scientific knowledge.

The pharmacist, as a part of his daily practice in the operation of the hospital pharmacy, performs many functions which are either identical to or closely resemble those which are performed by his counterpart in the central sterile supply room. These duties consist of:

a. Interviewing sales personnel
b. Purchasing of supplies
c. Meeting with and discussing procedures or specific problems with the medical staff
d. Dispensing of supplies in small lots
e. Distribution of supplies to pavilions
f. Receiving and storing of supplies
g. Charging, inventory and accounting procedures
h. Teaching or lecturing to various groups
i. Practices the principles of standardization
j. Manufactures in bulk
k. Manufactures in small lots, both sterile and non-sterile products.

Clearly then, it would appear that the pharmacist is qualified both by education and experience to supervise the activities of the central sterile supply room. It is also reasonable to state that such a consolidation of responsibility will result in more economical management as well as savings which result from a reduction in certain strata of personnel, fuller utilization of space and equipment and consolidation of inventories.

Location of the Central Sterile Supply Room

Ideally, the central sterile supply room should be centrally located in relation to the areas requiring the greatest utilization of its services. Consideration must also be given to the fact that the central sterile supply room must be able to receive large quantities of linen from the laundry, surgical dressings from the storeroom and large shipments of sterile intravenous and irrigating fluids if these are not manufactured by the hospital. If an ideal central location is not readily available, then resort must be made to utilize certain types of conveyor and pneumatic tube systems.

If the pharmacy and the central sterile supply room management are to be combined, then, where possible, the two units should be physically combined or at least adjacent to one another. By so doing, there can be closer supervision of the personnel as well as a consolidation of duties and coverage of both services on a twenty-four hour basis.

Planning the Central Sterile Supply Room

A close look at a modern central sterile room quickly reveals that it consists of a series of special work stations in a "dirty area" which is separated from the "clean area" by autoclaving and sterilizing equipment.

In effect then, we have all contaminated or non-sterile material and supplies entering one end of the room, passing through the various work stations and sterilizers and finally reposing in a sterile storage area ready to be dispensed from the clean side of the room. This concept is best illustrated by Figure 83.

The purpose of such a layout is to minimize the cross-flow of contaminated or non-sterile goods with those that are clean or sterile thereby eliminating the possibility of cross contamination or even the dispensing of a "dirty" kit for a clean one.

The number, type and size of work stations required will, of course, depend upon the size and nature of the hospital, the quantity of disposable materials used, the number of work shifts per day, the type of sterilization required, and whether or not the hospital purchases or manufactures sterile intravenous and irrigating fluids.

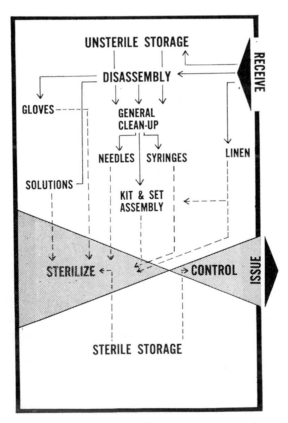

FIG. 83.   General concept of material flow in a central sterile supply room. (From *Macbick/CSR Equipment* brochure published by the Macbick Co., Wilmington, Massachusetts, 1963.)

Because the planning of a central sterile supply room's space requirements cannot be reduced to a square foot per bed formula, any hospital pharmacist who undertakes to assist in the development, planning and construction of a central sterile supply room should avail himself of the technical know-how and experience that can be provided by the design staff of a reputable producer of such equipment.

In order that the student and the pharmacist have an idea as to typical plans for central sterile supply rooms for various size hospitals, Figures 84, 85, and 86 are provided.

TYPICAL PLAN –
CENTRAL SUPPLY FOR THE SMALLER HOSPITAL

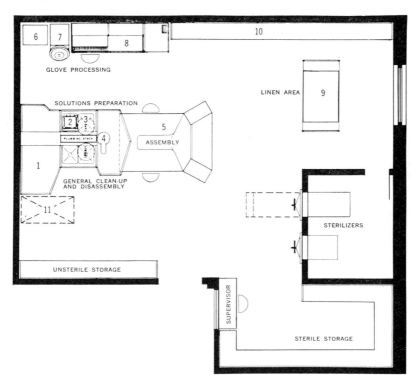

1 Clean-Up and Disassembly Station	6. Glove Washer-Drier
2. Flask Washer (set in sink)	7. Glove Powderer
3. Flask Rinser (set in sink)	8. Glove Packaging Station
4. Still	9. Linen Inspection and Folding Station
5. Kit Assembly Station	10. Linen Storage
	11. CSR Truck

FIG. 84. Typical plan of a central sterile supply room for a small hospital. (From *Macbick/CSR Equipment* brochure published by the Macbick Co., Wilmington, Massachusetts, 1963.)

TYPICAL PLAN –
CENTRAL SUPPLY FOR MEDIUM SIZE HOSPITAL

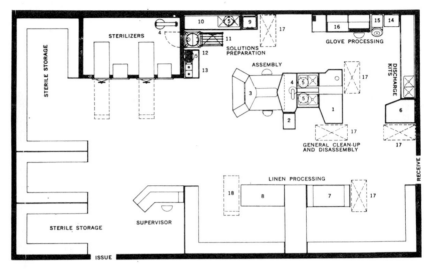

1. Clean-Up and Disassembly Station
2. Utility Washer
3. Kit Assembly Station
4. Still
5. Storage Tank
6. Clean-Up and Disassembly
7. Linen Inspection and Folding
8. Linen Packaging
9. Flask Washer

10. Solutions Clean-Up
11. Flask Drain Truck
12. Batch Tank
13. Flask Filling and Capping Station
14. Glove Washer-Drier
15. Glove Powderer
16. Glove Packaging Station
17. CSR Truck
18. Autoclave Truck

Fig. 85.   Typical plan of a central sterile supply room for a medium size hospital. (From *Macbick/CSR Equipment* brochure published by the Macbick Co., Wilmington, Massachusetts, 1963.)

TYPICAL PLAN
CENTRAL SUPPLY FOR LARGER HOSPITAL

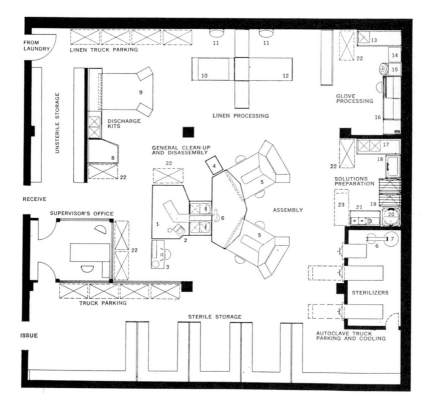

1. Clean-Up and Disassembly Station
2. Needle Washer
3. Needle Packaging Station
4. Utility Washer
5. Kit Assembly
6. Still
7. Storage Tank
8. Clean-Up and Disassembly Station (CD-0)
9. Kit Assembly Station
10. Linen Inspection
11. Linen Hamper
12. Linen Packaging
13. Accumulation Counter
14. Glove Washer-Drier
15. Glove Powderer
16. Glove Packaging Station
17. Solutions Clean-Up
18. Flask Washer-Rinser
19. Flask Drain Truck
20. Batch Tank (50 gal.)
21. Flask Filling and Capping Station
22. CSR Truck
23. Autoclave Truck

FIG. 86.   Typical plan of a central sterile supply room for a large hospital. (From *Macbick/CSR Equipment* brochure published by the Macbick Co., Wilmington, Massachusetts, 1963.)

Laminar Flow Hoods

Although many hospitals have abandoned the preparation of large volume, sterile intravenous fluids, a large number have commenced other programs, such as the intravenous solutions additive procedure, which require sterile technics to be performed in an atmosphere of microfiltered air.

In order to create such an atmosphere, various manufacturers of hoods have incorporated into them the laminar flow principle.

Laminar air flow is defined by Federal Standard No. 209[7] as:

> ". . . air flow in which the entire body of air within a confined area moves with uniform velocity along parallel flow lines, with a minimum of eddies."

By providing a constant outward flow of microfiltered air over the entire face of the hood's work area opening, dust particles may be kept from entering the work area from the ambient atmosphere.

Hospital pharmacists who plan to commence intravenous solutions additive programs or those who are called upon to produce special sterile research products should investigate the possibilities which such an installation offers.

Pharmacy-Central Sterile Supply Rooms that still produce parenteral fluids should install laminar flow hoods in order to ensure safe, sterile products.

The Standardization Committee

The Standardization Committee may be defined as that group within the hospital which is commissioned with the responsibility to investigate, to develop and to standardize procedures and equipment. In some institutions, this group is also known as the Current Practices Committee.

If such a committee is not in existence, it behooves the Director of Pharmacy and Central Sterile Supply Services to take the initial steps to have such a committee formed. By so doing, he will be assured of the creative thinking of a group of individuals who are intimately associated with the use of the supplies and products to be dispensed from the central sterile supply room. In addition, the Director of Pharmacy and Central Sterile Supply Services can then assure the hospital administration that a concerted effort is being made to reduce duplication of inventory and standardization of procedures.

Membership on this committee should be by appointment of interested staff members, the appointment being made jointly by the chief of staff and the Administrator of the hospital. Each major discipline in the hospital should be represented on the committee. Ideally, the following represents a good working group:

Administration (1)	Nursing Service (2)
Director of Laboratories	Nursing School (1)
Surgery (2)	Director of Pharmacy
Medicine (2)	and Central Sterile
Radiology (1)	Supply
Pathology (1)	

Other areas such as Dietary, Engineering and Maintenance should be invited to attend the meetings during which subjects pertaining to their services are discussed.

A chairman and a secretary should be appointed from the committee membership. Meetings should be held according to a set schedule throughout the year. The secretary of the committee should be assigned the responsibility of gathering all samples and prices of material as well as other pertinent data dealing with a particular procedure or type of equipment.

The chairman of the committee may then assign the responsibility for the investigation and development phases of the problem under discussion to a sub-group of the master committee. Once this smaller group has reached a decision as to equipment or developed a new procedure, the secretary should write up the material in accordance with a predetermined format and submit it to the master committee for approval. Once approved, the report should be distributed to the staff and pavilions.

To encourage proper filing of these documents, some hospitals provide each recipient with a binder and appropriate separators to demarcate the various divisions of the hospital—*i.e.* surgery, medicine, nursing, pharmacy, etc.

An index should be published periodically and distributed to all those on the mailing list. The bound volume of "bulletins" may then be referred to as the Standardization Manual or the Current Practices Manual and should serve as an authoritative procedural manual.

SELECTED REFERENCES

WALTER, CARL W.: *Aseptic Treatment of Wounds,* New York, The Macmillan Co., 1948.

LoBuGLIO, JEAN M. and PRICKETT, EDNA: Preparation of External Solutions in the Hospital, The Journal of Hospital Research, *1,* No. 1, 1963.

LLOYD, ROBERT S.: Ethylene Oxide Sterilization of Medical and Surgical Supplies, The Journal of Hospital Research, *1,* No. 2, 1963.

OWENS, T. B., PERKINS, J. J., IRONS, A. S., REICHERT, A. W., and MANNARION, S. J.:   Prevacuum High Temperature Steam Sterilization, The Journal of Hospital Research, *1*, No. 3, 1963.

BROWN, G. G. and PRICKETT, E. A.:   Processing Surgical Instruments, The Journal of Hospital Research, *2*, No. 2, 1964.

FLACK, HERBERT L., GREIF, ED E. and McDONNELL, JOHN A.:   A 'Space Age' Sterile Technics Laboratory, Am. J. Hosp. Pharm., *22*:8:446, 1965.

BIBLIOGRAPHY

1. TERESA, SR. M.:   Hospital Pharmacy and Central Supply Combination Service, Am. Prof. Pharm., *23*:4:358, 1957.

2. SKOLAUT, M. W.:   Pharmacy-Central Sterile Supply Services, Am. J. Hosp. Pharm., *17*:710, 1960.

3. ————:   Pharmacy-Central Sterile Supply Services—History, Am. J. Hosp. Pharm., *17*:11:244, 1960.

4. ————:   Pharmacy-Central Sterile Supply Services—Historical Background, Am. J. Hosp. Pharm., *17*:6:364, 1960.

5. PIERPAOLI, PAUL J.:   Some Administrative Considerations in Assigning Responsibility for Central Sterile Supply Service, Am. J. Hosp. Pharm., *20*: 8:370, 1963.

6. HASSAN, WM. E., JR.:   Who Should Manage Central Sterile Supply? Hosp. Management, *75*:5:76, 1963.

7. Clean Room and Work Station Requirements, Environment, Controlled Federal Standard 209 General Services Administration, December 16, 1963.

Chapter

23

The Pharmacist and Radioisotopes

WITH the increased use of radioactive isotopes in the hospital, many administrators and isotope users have felt the need to develop a means whereby there is a centralized responsibility for the dissemination of information, purchase, use, storage, disposal and monitoring of these potentially hazardous materials.

Hospital pharmacists have been quick to recognize this situation as one whereby they may fill the void and expand the professional services rendered by the pharmacy department. In addition, the American Society of Hospital Pharmacists in order to guide this movement established a Committee on Isotopes which was staffed by a group of hospital pharmacists who had already gained considerable experience in this new phase of hospital pharmacy.

In 1955 the committee submitted a comprehensive report[1] with a proposed outline for a course in isotope pharmacy. This report was followed by the report of the 1958 committee in which the following objectives were proposed.[2]

1. Develop suggestions for special courses for hospital pharmacists in the handling of isotopes in hospitals.
2. To determine the feasibility of an isotope section operated by the hospital pharmacy.
3. To determine layout and design for a radioactive branch of a pharmacy department.
4. To compile a bibliography on isotopes.

In the meantime, hospital pharmacists were publishing articles dealing with the fundamentals of radioactivity,[3] the various aspects of radiological health,[4] and descriptions of programs within hospitals having an established radioisotope pharmacy.[5]

Simultaneously the hospital literature began to publish articles concerning facilities and equipment for isotope programs[6] and data on the types of facilities required for the use of isotopes in the general hospital.[7]

Simultaneously, the American Hospital Association developed and distributed a *Manual on the Use of Radioisotopes in Hospitals*[8] with the stated purpose of:[9]

> ". . . for use by hospitals when setting up a radioisotopes program or when reviewing their current procedures for handling radioisotopes. It is intended to guide the administrator of the general hospital in the procurement procedures for radioactive materials, in the radiation protection measures necessary for their handling, in the allocation of space and equipment for isotopes laboratories, and in the organization and training of the hospital staff for the utilization of radioactive materials."

Thus, it becomes necessary to expose the student in hospital pharmacy to the licensing requirements of the Atomic Energy Commission, the radioisotope committee and its function and the role which the alert hospital pharmacist can assume in this rapidly developing phase of therapeutics and diagnosis.

Because of the limited scope of this text, and the highly technical nature of the equipment, no data concerning the various types of monitoring, handling or measuring devices in current use will be presented or the physical facilities needed to establish a radioisotope pharmacy.

A large number of hospitals and clinics in the United States are currently using radioisotopes for diagnostic, therapeutic and research purposes. The use of those potentially dangerous materials is subject to the control and supervision of the Atomic Energy Commission, a governmental agency established by the United States Congress under the **Atomic Energy Act of 1954.**

Jurisdiction of the AEC

The Act provides that the Atomic Energy Commission has jurisdiction over all "by-product material" which is further defined by the Act as—

> ". . . any radioactive material (except special nuclear material) yielded in or made radioactive by exposure to the radiation incident to the process of producing or utilizing special nuclear material."

Perusal of the Federal regulations reveals that jurisdiction of the AEC applies not only to radioisotopes produced in the United States, but also to those imported into this country.

Radioactive isotopes may be used only by duly licensed individuals who have complied with the statutory provisions of the Atomic Energy Act and the latest AEC regulations appearing in the *Federal Register*.

License Information

In order that the hospital pharmacist render a high quality, knowledgeable service with regard to isotope materials, it is necessary for him to have a general understanding of the basic requirements which must be met, by both individuals and institutions, before they may become licensed for the medical use of radioisotopes.

Accordingly, the following discussion relates to the types of licenses that can be issued, the types of applications which should be submitted to obtain the licenses, and the information which should be included in the application.

Licenses may be issued to institutions or to private practitioners. The type of licenses available and their characteristics are as follows:

Institutional License

This type of license is very specific in that it limits the use of the isotopes to those listed on the license. It also restricts the clinical use and the physicians who may use the material to those named on the license document.

In addition, the regulations require that an institutional licensee have a medical isotope committee to evaluate all proposals for research, diagnostic, and therapeutic uses of isotopes within the hospital.

One advantage of such a license is that it provides a means whereby physicians desiring licensure for the use of radioisotopes may obtain basic and clinical isotope training to meet the criteria required to qualify as an individual user.

Broad Medical Licenses Issued to Institutions

This type of license is issued to those institutions who meet the following criteria:

a. previous experience operating under a specific institutional license and,
b. are engaged in medical research, as well as routine diagnosis and therapy.

Although a medical isotope committee is required, no physicians are listed as individual users on the license, nor are the radioisotopes limited to specified users.

This type of license also permits physicians to obtain basic and clinical radioisotope training and experience.

Specific Licenses Issued to Physicians for Their Private Practice

This license is usually issued to the private practioner of medicine irrespective of whether or not his office is or is not located on the hospital premises. The license usually specifies the isotope and its clinical use. These licenses do not permit nor provide for other physicians to obtain basic and clinical radioisotope training and experience. In addition, the licenses are limited to well-established uses of by-product materials and require that the physician, so licensed, personally conduct the program.

Types of Application Forms

Form AEC 313 and Form AEC 313a are two application forms upon which information concerning a proposed medical radioisotope program may be submitted.

Form AEC-313MC may be appropriate for a specific institutional or for a specific private practice license. In addition, this form should be used only by physicians who are qualified to handle one entire category of uses. If the physician does not so qualify, application should be made upon Form AEC 313.

Form AEC 313a must be submitted for each physician who is to be listed on an institutional license or for each physician applying for a private practitioner's license.

Radioisotope Committee

The regulations of the Atomic Energy Commission require that a radioisotope committee be established for the supervision and control of the hospital isotope program. The committee should include a radiation physicist, a clinical radiologist, an internist, a hematologist and a surgeon. Other members or specialties to be represented on the committee should be determined by the type and scope of program being undertaken by the hospital.

In addition to the above, it is also suggested that a representative from nursing service, administration and pharmacy be included on the committee roster.

The reasons for the participation of nursing and administrative representatives are that the nurses will become familiar with the type of work carried out on the pavilions, the associated dangers and the means whereby the patient, doctor and nurse may protect themselves. The administrator can contribute to the development of the entire program through his efforts with the board of trustees and the pharmacist may be of assistance in the purchasing, receiving and storage of isotopes until such time as the theory of a centralized isotope pharmacy within the hospital materializes.

Generally the radioisotope committee should have the following responsibilities:[9]

1. Review, grant permission for, or disapprove the use of isotopes within the institution.
2. Prescribe special conditions as may be necessary, such as training of personnel, designation of limited areas of use, disposal methods and the like.
3. Receive reports from the radiation protection officer and review his records.
4. Recommend remedial action when an individual fails to observe protection recommendations, rules, regulations.
5. Keep a record of actions taken in approving the use of isotopes.

In order to acquaint the hospital pharmacist with the type of instructional and precautionary literature prepared by the committee, the following bulletin entitled *Protective Procedures for Personnel Caring for Patients Receiving Therapeutic Isotopes* is presented.[10]

"Radioactive isotopes are administered to patients for treatment of various conditions, *e.g.,* radioactive iodine for hyperthyroidism, radioactive gold for malignant effusions, radioactive phosphorus for malignant hematological conditions. These emit beta and gamma rays and exposure should be reduced to the minimum by:
   a. avoiding contamination of clothing and skin from body secretions of the patient.
   b. keeping the time close to the patient as short as possible.
   c. keeping as great a distance from the patient as possible when in the unit.

General Precautions
1. A radioisotope administration sheet (Fig. 87) is placed in the medical record by the isotope administrator at the time of treatment and is to remain there permanently. Particular precautions required by the specific isotope used will be listed on this sheet by the isotope administrator and called to the attention of the medical and nursing staff caring for the patient. These will be written in the Doctor's Order Book by the physician in charge of the patient.
2. An isotope sign is placed at the entrance of the room or unit by the isotope administrator.
3. The isotope administrator will provide the name of a substitute who may be contacted in case the administrator is not readily available.

RADIOACTIVE ISOTOPE ADMINISTRATION

TRACER ☐
THERAPY ☐

RADIOACTIVE ISOTOPE FORM

Addressograph Plate

PETER BENT BRIGHAM HOSPITAL

Isotope:_____ Effective Half-Life:_____

Dose _____

Route of Administration_____

The patient received_____mc. of radioactive

isotope_____at_____M on_____19_____

The following special precautions are to be meticulously observed.

All personnel responsible for the medical or nursing care of this patient must review and be familiar with the special procedures and requirements outlined in the Current Practice Manual, Peter Bent Brigham Hospital, Bulletin_____
In the event of spillage or isotopic contamination notify at once the undersigned and the Radiologic House Officer on duty. Make no attempt to clean the area or to remove any item touched by the isotope.

Signed_____M. D.
: _____Responsible Isotope Administrator_____

RADIOACTIVE
ISOTOPE FORM   Form 71

RADIOACTIVE
ISOTOPE FORM

FIG. 87. Radioactive Isotope Administration form which is placed in the medical record of each patient receiving radioactive isotopes at the Peter Bent Brigham Hospital, Boston, Mass. The sheet is a canary yellow in color and the Atomic Energy Commission insignia is printed in red ink.

Care of the Patient: for most patients, these precautions should be taken:

1. No nurse should care for more than one radioactive patient at a time.
2. The patient should be encouraged to do as much as possible for himself so that close bedside nursing can be reduced to the minimum.
3. Gloves are to be worn when the nurse handles the patient's linen, skin or excreta utensils.
4. A plastic apron or sheet of expendable plastic is to be worn for bedside nursing (to protect from spillage). If an apron is worn, it should be used for one patient only and marked clearly which is the inside of the apron.
5. Excreta utensils should be marked with a "radioactive" sign and reserved for one patient's use. These utensils should

be flushed clean with a superfluous amount of water; dilution is the best protection. If the radioactive element is difficult to flush, carrier solution (the ordinary substance such as iodine, not radioactive) will help and can be supplied by the isotope administrator.

6. The House Officer will notify the isotope administrator of any draining wound.
7. Anything soiled with body discharge is to be retained in a plastic bag until monitored and appropriate disposal directed by the isotope administrator. Linen is to be kept in large plastic bags. Dressings, tissues and small disposable articles in small plastic envelopes are to be placed in a yellow dump-lid waste container with radioactive marker provided by the isotope administrator and will be removed by him to the decay area properly labeled.

Visitors

No visitors are permitted for the first two weeks except by special dispensation by the isotope administrator. Children and pregnant women are not permitted at any time.

Therapeutic Procedures

Thoracentesis or paracentesis within fifteen days of isotope administration should be carried out only after specific approval of the isotope administrator and with his explicit direction for disposal of material and utensils.

Urine should be collected or sent to the laboratory only under the specific conditions imposed by the administrator.

Routine Post-operative Orders

1. Usual diet and medication may be resumed on return to the ward unless otherwise specified.
2. Patients receiving therapeutic isotopes are to be cared for in a specified radiation area and to be confined to this area unless bath room privileges are definitely assigned by the isotope administrator.
3. Soiled or wet dressings are to be brought to the attention of the House Officer immediately.
4. The Radiation Safety Officer should be contacted if the patient has a long distance to travel on discharge.
5. If any doubt arises about procedure for these patients, contact the isotope administrator whose name is signed on the yellow Form #71 or his deputy as indicated.

INCREASED DISTANCE AND REDUCTION IN THE TIME OF EXPOSURE ARE ALWAYS THE BEST PROTECTION. THE NEED FOR HANDWASHING CANNOT BE OVER-EMPHASIZED."

Responsibility of Permit-Holders

Those persons who are granted a permit to use radioisotopes have an obligation and a responsibility for the safe use of radiation sources by individuals under their control. Permit holders are therefore generally responsible for the following:[11]

1. Compliance with all rules and regulations for the safe use and handling of radioactive materials.
2. Insuring that employees under their control are instructed in the use of safety devices and procedures.
3. Adequate planning of an experiment, or procedure, to assure that the necessary safety precautions are taken.
4. Informing the Radiation Safety Officer of the hospital, of the names of all personnel involved in operational procedures, and of such changes in personnel; radioactive materials being used; procedures of handling; changes in the laboratory arrangement which could lead to changes in personnel exposure or contamination levels.
5. Direction of personnel under their control to comply with all recommendations by the Radiation Safety Officer relative to dosimeters, and other recommendations to control or to reduce exposure to radiation hazards.
6. Limitation of use of radioisotopes under their permit to those over whom they have direct supervision.
7. Maintenance of required current records of receipt, use, storage and disposal of radioisotopes.

Responsibility of the Individual Users of Radioisotopes

From the point of view of self preservation and moral obligation for the safety of others, each person who uses sources of ionizing radiation has the following responsibilities:[11]

1. To receive instruction in radiation safety as determined appropriate by the Radiation Safety Officer.
2. To keep his exposure to radiation at the lowest possible level and specifically below the maximum permissible exposure.
3. To wear recommended radiation dosimeters for personnel, such as film badges, pocket ionization chambers, and finger dosimeters.
4. To survey his hands, shoes, body, and clothing for radioactivity and remove all loose contamination before leaving the laboratory when appropriate.
5. To use all appropriate protective measures such as protective clothing, respiratory protection, remote pipetting devices, ventilated and shielded glove box and hoods.
6. To prohibit smoking and eating in radioisotopes laboratories.
7. To check working areas daily, or after each radioisotope procedure.
8. To maintain good laboratory practices, such as keeping work areas and equipment clean and orderly.

9. To use proper labels on equipment being used with radio-active materials.
10. To place all active waste in proper containers, equipped with proper labels.
11. To report immediately the details of a "spill" or other accident involving radioactive substances to the Radiation Safety Officer.
12. To conduct decontamination procedures as directed by the Radiation Safety Officer.

Role of the Pharmacist In the Hospital with an Isotope Pharmacy

In hospitals which have established a radioisotope pharmacy, the pharmacist purchases, stores and dispenses the various isotopes required by the medical staff licensed to use these materials.

In these institutions, the physician, upon deciding to prescribe radioactive material, calls the pharmacist and provides him with all of the necessary information.

The pharmacist then makes the necessary calculations in order to arrive at the required dosage, transfers same from the stock container, using a remote control pipette, places it in a paper cup within a lead container and transports it to the patient for administration.

From this point on, the responsibility for radiation protection, contamination, and disposal of waste products will fall under the aegis of the radiation safety officer.

Role of the Pharmacist in the Hospital without an Isotope Pharmacy

The mere fact that the majority of the hospitals using radioisotopes have not established, as yet, an isotope pharmacy is no criteria for the hospital pharmacist not to make some contribution towards the administrative aspects of the hospital's isotope program. In this regard, the hospital pharmacist may assume the responsibility for the ordering, receiving and storage of all isotopes in current use throughout the hospital. The purchasing phase of such a program is relatively simple and does not differ from the purchase of other pharmaceutical products. In fact, a number of the commonly used radioisotopes are usually purchased in pre-determined quantities for automatic shipment on a standing order basis.

The receiving aspect of radioisotopes differs from the receiving phase of purchased pharmaceuticals in that all packages coming to the pharmacy must be stored in a lead vault and a record maintained which indicates the date of receipt, the purchase order number, the ordering physician, the name of the isotope and the quantity of isotope received. Upon receipt, the appropriate physician or technician is notified to remove the material from the pharmacy vault.

The radiation safety officer monitors the pharmacy vault and the surrounding area as part of his safety program, therefore there is little possibility of harmful radiation within the environs of the pharmacy. All records of isotope materials received are to be maintained in the pharmacy office and are made available to the radiation safety officer and the Atomic Energy Commission inspector when necessary.

Sources of Information

Current copies of Atomic Energy Commission regulations may be obtained from the Division of Licensing and Regulation, U.S. Atomic Energy Commission, Washington 25, D.C.

SELECTED REFERENCES

BRINER, WILLIAM H.: The Preparation of Radioactive Chemicals for Clinical Use, Am. J. Hosp. Pharm., 20:11:553, 1963.
————: Radioactive Materials: New Dimensions for Pharmacy, Hosp. Topics, 43:6:79, 1965.

BIBLIOGRAPHY

1. LATIOLIAS, CLIFTON J., PARKER, PAUL F., HUTCHINSON, GEORGE, and STATLER, ROBERT A.: Radioisotopes in Hospital Pharmacy, The Bulletin, A.S.H.P., 12:4:372, 1955.
2. SOLYOM, PETER: Report of the Committee on Isotopes, Am. J. Hosp. Pharm., 15:8:712, 1958.
3. LATIOLAIS, CLIFTON J.: Fundamentals of Radioactivity, The Bulletin, A.S.H.P., 13:3:220, 1956.
4. BRINER, WILLIAM H.: Certain Aspects of Radiological Health, Am. J. Hosp. Pharm., 15:1:44, 1958.
5. SOLYOM, PETER: Pharmacy Service University of Chicago Clinics, Am. J. Hosp. Pharm., 15:1:52, 1958.
6. MORGAN, G. W.: Facilities and Equipment for Isotopes Program, Hospitals, 29:3:103, 1955.
7. INGRAHAM, S. C. and TAYLOR, W. R.: Radioisotope Facilities in the General Hospital, Hospitals, 26:12:74, 1952.
8. Manual on Use of Radioisotopes in Hospitals, American Hospital Association, Chicago, Ill.
9. Ibid. p. 12.
10. GREENE, ALLAN: Protective Procedures for Personnel Caring for Patients Receiving Therapeutic Isotopes, Current Practice Bulletin 6-1-3 of the Peter Bent Brigham Hospital, Boston, Mass.
11. Radioisotope Manual of the Peter Bent Brigham Hospital, Boston, Mass. January 1969.

Chapter

24

The Physical Plant and its Equipment

THE Minimum Standard for Pharmacies in Hospitals provides as follows:[1]

"Adequate pharmaceutical and administrative facilities shall be provided for the pharmacy department, including especially: (A) the necessary equipment for the compounding, dispensing and manufacturing of pharmaceuticals and parenteral preparations, (B) bookkeeping supplies and related materials and equipment necessary for the proper administration of the department, (C) an adequate library and filing equipment to make information concerning drugs readily available to both pharmacists and physicians, (D) special locked storage space to meet the legal requirements for storage of narcotics, alcohol and other prescribed drugs, (E) a refrigerator for the storage of thermolabile products, (F) adequate floor space for all pharmacy operations and the storage of pharmaceuticals at a satisfactory location provided with proper lighting and ventilation."

Accordingly, this chapter is presented for consideration of the student, as well as those seeking information which may be useful in developing plans either for the renovation of an existing department or the construction of a new facility, data concerning location, floor space, general equipment, refrigeration and storage facilities and general construction information relating to lighting, ventilation, plumbing and surface finishes.

Functional Planning

Many competent authorities have stated that before the architect's pencil touches paper, he must become thoroughly familiar with the hospital's objectives, plan of operation and operational policies relating to the area to be designed.

The architect may gather this information by attending various meetings with the hospital administrator, the department head and the Building Committee. During these sessions, many questions will be asked and at their conclusion it is possible that a special study or survey will be conducted to confirm or establish the need.

Because hospital pharmacists new to the field have seldom become involved in this aspect of the hospital planning, they are often frightened and confused at the prospect of having to meet with the architect and the trustees with regard to pharmacy construction or remodeling. This is especially so because they do not know what to expect during such sessions.

In order to acquaint these pharmacists with the type of information which they will be asked to present, the following questions, although not exhaustive on the subject, are abstracted from a U.S. Public Health Service publication[2] and are herewith presented.

PHARMACY

	Yes	*No*
1. Will the hospital operate a Pharmacy Department?	___	___
If not, what provision will be made for supervising the hospital pharmaceutical service? Specify _____		
2. Is pharmacy service to be provided for:		
a. Inpatient	___	___
b. Outpatient	___	___
3. Will the pharmacy carry out other functions in addition to compounding and dispensing individual prescriptions and other patient medications?		
a. Manufacturing pharmaceuticals		
(1) Bulk fluids	___	___
(2) Ointments	___	___
(3) Others (specify) _____		
b. Manufacturing sterile preparations		
(1) Small volume sterile solutions	___	___
(2) Small-medium volume sterile solutions, *e.g.,* antibiotic dilutions, collyria, etc.	___	___
(3) Large volume parenteral solutions	___	___
(4) Other sterile solutions for surgery, delivery room, and treatment purposes	___	___
c. Testing of fluids prepared (*e.g.,* simple determinations of dextrose, sodium chloride, etc.)	___	___
4. Will pharmaceuticals be distributed to nursing units on		
a. A floor stock basis	___	___
b. An individual prescription basis	___	___
c. A combination of a floor stock and an individual prescription basis	___	___

Yes   *No*

5. What provision will be made for emergency and after-hour dispensing?
   Specify _____

6. Will specifications for the purchase of drugs be a responsibility of the pharmacy?   ____ ____
   a. Will the final processing of purchase orders be done by the pharmacy?   ____ ____
   b. How many of the following items will be needed for purchasing and inventory control by the pharmacy: *Check*
      (1) Filing cabinets   ____
      (2) Card files   ____
      (3) Bookcase or shelving for:
         a. Reference books   ____
         b. Current literature   ____
         c. Catalogs   ____
      (4) Others (specify) _____

Number

7. Number of staff to operate these facilities   *Full time* *Part time*
   a. Chief pharmacist   _____ _____
   b. Staff pharmacist   _____ _____
   c. Pharmacy helper   _____ _____
   d. Secretary-stenographer   _____ _____
   e. Other (specify) _____

8. Which departments or services receive the bulk of the pharmaceutical service? _____
   _____
   _____

Yes   *No*

9. Will the pharmacy be centrally located to inpatient and outpatient services?   ____ ____
   a. If not conveniently located near the latter, is an outpatient department dispensary indicated?   ____ ____
   b. Will a "waiting area" be provided for outpatients?   ____ ____

10. What method will be used to distribute drugs to patient care units?   ____ ____
    a. Cart   ____ ____
    b. Dumbwaiter   ____ ____
    c. Pneumatic tube   ____ ____
    d. Other (specify) _____

11. Will bulk pharmacy stores be convenient to the pharmacy?   ____ ____

12. Indicate the functioning arrangement of the following areas: receiving, storage, compounding, issuing, and others:
    _____
    _____

13. What is the relationship of each function to work flow?
    a. Compounding and dispensing _____

  b. Prepackaging and inpatient medication filling _____

   (1) Floor and clinic basket filling _____
   (2) Filling and labeling floor stock units _____

   (3) Storage of finished pharmaceuticals _____

  c. Manufacturing
   (1) General pharmaceuticals _____
  d. Sterile preparation
   (1) Small-medium volume sterile solutions _____

   (2) Large volume parenteral solutions _____

   (3) External sterile solutions _____
 e. Office and library _____

14. Intercommunication is to be: *Yes*   *No*
  a. Only interdepartmental   ____ ____
  b. Intradepartmental   ____ ____
  c. With phone   ____ ____
  d. With extension   ____ ____
  e. With phone and extension ____ ____

15. The storage facilities to be provided will be:
  a. Separate bulk pharmacy stores ____ ____
  b. Active (work) storeroom in pharmacy ____ ____
  c. Special storage facilities
   (1) Alcohol vault   ____ ____
   (2) Narcotic safe   ____ ____
   (3) Refrigeration for thermolabile drugs ____ ____

16. The major equipment necessary will be
  a. Specialized pharmacy casework
   (1) Cabinets and drawers ____ ____
   (2) Carboy racks   ____ ____
   (3) Counters and cupboards ____ ____
   (4) Shelving   ____ ____
   (5) Sink assemblies   ____ ____
   (6) Work tables   ____ ____
  b. Manufacturing equipment
   (1) Filter press   ____ ____
   (2) Mixing and storage   ____ ____
   (3) Ointment mill and mixer ____ ____
  c. Specialized parenteral solution manufacturing equipment
   (1) Flask washer   ____ ____
   (2) Flask-filling apparatus ____ ____
   (3) Water still and meter ____ ____
   (4) Sterilizer (joint use if located nearby in central sterile supply department) ____ ____
   (5) Aseptic hood   ____ ____

17. What toilet and locker facilities will be provided?
  Specify _____

Although the foregoing list provides the hospital pharmacist with a reasonable check on the subjects and areas to be planned for, it is important for the planner to give consideration to the changes that have taken place within the practice of hospital pharmacy since the list was prepared. As a result of the changes made in the health care delivery system during the past ten years, consideration must now be given to the following subjects and areas in order that the end product be a modern hospital pharmacy.

1. Will the pharmacy have need for a quality control laboratory?
2. Will the hospital pharmacy become involved in the handling and dispensing of radioisotopes?
3. Will the hospital's Allergy Department require the hospital pharmacy to become involved in the preparation of allergenic extracts and subsequent dilutions?
4. Is there a need for a research laboratory?
5. Has consideration been given to providing space for certain specialized functions *i.e.* unit dose dispensing; I.V. solution additive program: drug information service; patient drug control system (patient profile): unit-dose packaging area and required equipment?
6. Will the pharmacy become involved with educational programs for the benefit of medical, nursing and pharmacy students; interns and residents; graduate physicians, nurses and pharmacists; cooperative clinical pharmacy programs with schools or colleges of pharmacy?
7. Will the pharmacy and its staff be an integral part of the local poison control center? If so, facilities planning should include space for information gathering, storage and a suitable communications system. Consideration must also be given to its location and staffing requirements.
8. With the improvements that have been made in electronic data processing systems, consideration should be given to the use of a computer by the pharmacy. If this is determined to be feasible, planning must include specialists from administration, pharmacy, nursing, medical staff and data processing in order to ascertain the extent of the program required as well as the selection and placement of appropriate equipment. In developing this system, all parties concerned should give consideration to building into it a system of inspections and checks as well as to provide for adequate back-up service in case of mechanical failure.
9. Consideration must be given to the means by which pharmacy supplies and requisitions will be carried between the pharmacy

and nursing stations. These mechanical systems may be any one or combination of pneumatic tube, vertical conveyor or horizontal conveyor.

10. Because of the nature of the modern practice of pharmacy, large medical center type operations may require that the planners provide space for direct writing intercoms, teletype, closed circuit television, printing and/or duplicating equipment.

In addition to the above cited questions, the hospital pharmacist should be prepared to furnish answers which pertain to such areas as pre-packaging, methods and statistics involving the volume of dispensing, the number of people who will be in any one sector of the pharmacy at any single time, the peak dispensing hours, the measurements of the various carts or trucks used in the pharmacy, the department's provisions for night emergency service, the number of nursing stations and other departments to be serviced and finally a plan which will outline the sequence of renovation (if such be the case) which will allow for a continuation of service to the hospital and yet permit forward progress for the construction crew.

Location

The hospital pharmacy should be located in an area which is convenient for providing service to the many departments and personnel who make daily use of such service. Therefore, since this is a primary consideration, it is irrelevant where the pharmacy is located in the hospital so long as it meets the test of convenience.

Milne and Taylor[3] in their article dealing with suggested plans for hospital pharmacies have stated:

> "In hospitals of less than 200 beds the pharmacy should be located on the first floor, in the center of the activities it is called upon to service frequently, easily accessible to the elevator, and near or adjoining the out-patient department, if such is maintained by the hospital. This will provide the most efficient service and conserve man-hours of work.
>
> Though it is recommended that the pharmacy be all located on one floor, it may be varied in larger hospitals when first floor space is at a premium.
>
> The basement is not desirable for a pharmacy."

Because most hospital pharmacies were designed and constructed during an era before out-patient clinic facilities had developed to their present status, many clinic administrators feel that they are poorly located insofar as the out-patient department is concerned. Since the majority of the hospital pharmacies serving clinic patients combine out-patient and in-patient facilities, the pharmacists concur with the observation made by the clinic administrative personnel.

The *Mirror to Hospital Pharmacy*,[4] in discussing this subject, states:

"If a hospital provides out-patient pharmacy service then, if possible, pharmacy facilities should be located either in or immediately adjacent to the out-patient department. It is not suitable for a cashier, nurse or other hospital personnel to accept the prescription from the patient and send it by pneumatic tube or by other means to the pharmacy located in some other section of the hospital and return the medication to this person for delivery to the patient. Although man-hours may be conserved by combining in-patient and out-patient dispensing units, this advantage should not take precedence over locating the out-patient pharmacy facility in the immediate area serving out-patients. If a low volume of work does not justify such a location, then it would seem best either to not offer out-patient pharmacy service or to have the patient carry his prescription to the in-patient pharmacy."

In general, the in-patient pharmacy appears to be reasonably well situated to render the services required of it. Where possible, all sections of the in-patient pharmacy—storage, dispensing, manufacturing, parenteral solutions, etc. should be contiguous. When these functions are separated from the main pharmacy, it is recommended that they be in a direct vertical relationship if possible. In addition, this concept of direct vertical relationship should be extended between the pharmacy and the various divisions of the hospital utilizing pharmaceutical services.

With the advent of clinical pharmacy programs, many hospitals have found it advisable to develop *satellite pharmacies* on the patient pavilions. In effect, these are sub-pharmacies that receive their supplies from the main pharmacy but have the advantage of being able to respond to the clinical needs of the patient on a current basis. In addition, such a system makes available to the patient, physician, and nurse the services of a pharmacist in a clinical capacity rather than as just a dispenser of medications. By being on the nursing floor, the pharmacist is available for the taking of patient drug histories, maintaining patient drug profiles, observing the patient for drug reactions and toxicity and dispensing unit-doses and intravenous products with additives.

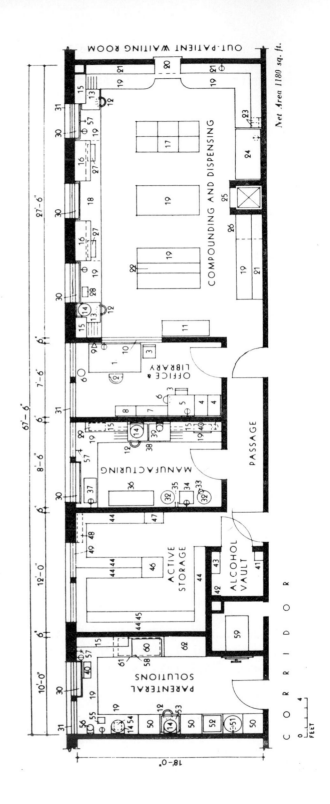

OUT-PATIENT WAITING ROOM

Net Area 1180 sq. ft.

COMPOUNDING AND DISPENSING

OFFICE & LIBRARY

MANUFACTURING

PASSAGE

ACTIVE STORAGE

ALCOHOL VAULT

PARENTERAL SOLUTIONS

CORRIDOR

FEET

374

1. Desk, executive
2. Chair, executive
3. Chair, straight
4. File, 4 drawer
5. Table, writing
6. Receptacle, waste paper
7. Case, book
8. Rack, magazine
9. Outlet, telephone
10. Glass panel
11. Rack, carboy
12. Can, sanitary waste
13. Sink, with goose neck spout and drainboard, graduate rack above, cabinets below
14. Tank, glass, distilled water, 12 gallon
15. Cabinets, adjustable shelves
16. Cabinet, drug, sectional type, with shelf above counter
17. Cabinets, drug, sectional type

18. Counter, prescription, cabinets and drawers below
19. Counter, cabinets and drawers below
20. Window, dispensing
21. Shelves, adjustable, open, starting 18 inches above counter
22. Shelf, above counter
23. File, prescription
24. Refrigerator, with biological drawers, 32 cubic feet
25. Dumbwaiter
26. Safe, narcotic, under counter
27. Scale, prescription, class A
28. Scale, prescription, heavy duty
29. Scale, counter
30. Heat outlet grill, inlet grill in base of cabinet
31. Guards, at all windows
32. Tank, mixing or storing, 20 gallons, mounted on stand with casters

33. Mixer, portable, electric
34. Filter press, suction-pressure type, mounted on casters
35. Outlets, hot and cold water
36. Rack, filter
37. Mill, colloidal
38. Sink, two compartment, with drainboard, goose neck spout, cabinets below
39. Still, 2 gallon per hour
40. Hot Plate, double element
41. Vent, outlet, 8 inches above floor to atmosphere
42. Vent, inlet, near floor to atmosphere
43. Shelves, starting 42 inches above, floor
44. Shelves, 12 inches wide, adjustable, open
45. Shelves, 24 inches wide, 36 inches high, adjustable

46. Rack, barrel
47. Locker, clothes
48. Radiator, above shelving
49. High windows
50. Rack, bottle
51. Cleaner, bottle, pressure type
52. Sink with goose neck spout
53. Sink, with distilled water rinser, omit hot & cold water supply
54. Drip pan with waste connection in counter top
55. Pump, suction and pressure
56. Still, 10 gallon per hour
57. Outlet, gas
58. Carriage, sterilizer, under counter
59. Sterilizer, 24 x 36 x 48 inches
60. Oven, hot air, 21 x 14 x 14 inches, on counter
61. Counter, open below
62. Cabinet, storage, open adjustable shelves

Pharmacy for a 200 bed general hospital

FIG 88. The above plan for a pharmacy for a 200-bed general hospital may still be found in a large number of hospitals. With slight modification it is adaptable to modern day dispensing practices. (From Public Health Service Publication No. 891, December 1961.)

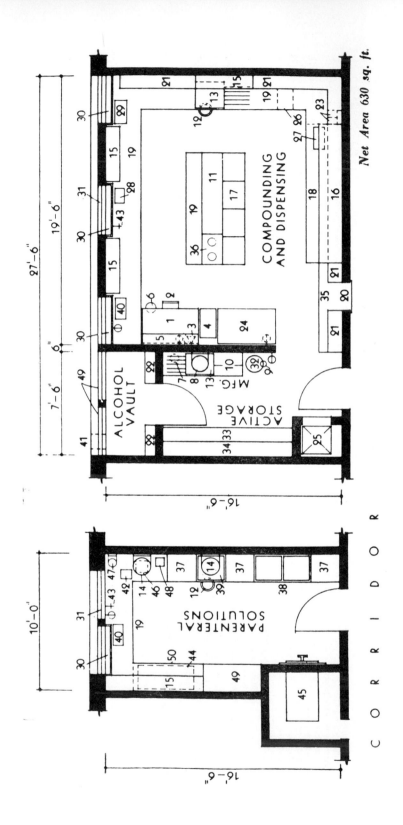

Net Area 630 sq. ft.

COMPOUNDING
AND DISPENSING

ALCOHOL
VAULT

ACTIVE
STORAGE

MFG.

PARENTERAL
SOLUTIONS

CORRIDOR

27'-6"

19'-6"

7'-6"

6"

16'-6"

10'-0"

16'-6"

376

Pharmacy for a 100 bed general hospital

1. Desk
2. Chair
3. Outlet, telephone
4. File, 4 drawer
5. Shelves, book, over desk
6. Receptacle, waste paper
7. Still. 2 gallon per hour. Required if parenteral solution room is omitted
8. Tank, glass, distilled water, 5 gallon
9. Mixer, portable, electric
10. Counter, cabinets below, shelves above
11. Rack, carboy, above counter
12. Cap, sanitary waste
13. Sink, with goose neck spout and drainboard: graduate rack above, cabinets below
14. Tank, glass, distilled water, 12 gallon
15. Cabinet, adjustable shelves
16. Cabinet, drug, sectional type, with shelf above counter
17. Cabinets, drugs, sectional type
18. Counter, prescription, cabinets, sectional type drawers below

19. Counter, cabinets and drawers below
20. Window, dispensing
21. Shelves, adjustable, open, starting 18 inches above counter
22. Shelves, starting 42 inches above floor
23. File, prescription
24. Refrigerator, 16 cubic feet, with biological drawers
25. Dumbwaiter
26. Safe, narcotic, under counter
27. Scale, prescription, class A
28. Scale, prescription, heavy duty
29. Scale, counter
30. Heat outlet grill, inlet grill in base of cabinet
31. Guards, at all windows
32. Tank, mixing, 20 gallons, mounted on stand with casters
33. Shelves, 24 inches wide, 36 inches high, adjustable, open
34. Shelves, 12 inches wide, adjustable, open

35. Counter, 18 inches wide, adjustable, shelves below
36. Rack, filter, above counter
37. Rack, bottle
38. Sink, two compartment, goose neck spout, cabinets below
39. Sink, with distilled water rinser, omit hot and cold water supply, cabinets below
40. Hot plate, double element
41. Vent, at ceiling and floor
42. Scale, metric, solution
43. Outlet, gas
44. Carriage, sterilizer, under counter
45. Sterilizer, 24 x 36 x 48 inches
46. Drip pan with waste connection in counter top
47. Still. 5 gallon per hour
48. Pump, suction and pressure
49. Cabinet, storage. open. adjustable shelves
50. Counter, open below

FIG. 89. The above design for a pharmacy for a 100-bed hospital was recommended by the Division of Hospital and Medical Facilities in the early 1950's. (From Public Health Service Publication No. 891, December 1961.)

13

Floor Space

Milne, Taylor and their Public Health Service Associates recommend the following floor space and its distribution within the pharmacy area:

AREA DISTRIBUTION FOR GENERAL HOSPITAL PHARMACIES

Areas in Square Feet	50 Bed	100 Bed	200 Bed
Compounding and Dispensing Laboratory	205	320	495
Parenteral Solutions Laboratory		185	200
Active Store Room		125	200
Manufacturing Laboratory			120
Office and Library			105
Circulation			60
TOTAL	205	630	1180

The areas shown in the above chart are net areas and do not include walls and partitions. Additional storage space of approximately 170 square feet per 100 beds is provided for bulk storage in an area directly beneath the pharmacy and separate from the main hospital storeroom.

Translating the above figures into a square foot per bed ratio, the following is noted:

AREA DISTRIBUTION—SQUARE FEET PER BED

Areas in Square Feet	50 Bed	100 Bed	200 Bed
Compounding and Dispensing Laboratory	4.1	3.20	2.48
Parenteral Solutions Laboratory		1.85	1.00
Active Store Room		1.25	1.00
Manufacturing Laboratory			0.60
Office and Library			0.53
Circulation			0.30
TOTAL	4.1	6.30	5.91

In contrast, Francke et al.[5] in their survey requested the survey participants to indicate the number of additional square feet of space they felt would be necessary for them to give the type of service the pharmacy should provide and obtained the following results which are compared with the Public Health Service recommendations for short-term hospitals.

# Beds	Public Health Service Recommendations	Survey Findings
100	6.3 sq. ft./bed	8.12 sq. ft./bed
200	5.9 sq. ft./bed	6.62 sq. ft./bed
300		5.39 sq. ft./bed
400		5.00 sq. ft./bed

Before utilizing the above figures, it should be remembered that the Public Health Service plans provide an additional 170 square feet per 100 beds for reserve storage of bulk pharmaceuticals outside the pharmacy and that the survey findings make no provisions for this additional storage facility.

Exclusive of the survey conducted by Francke *et al.*, little has been published relative to area distribution for general hospital pharmacies since the work of Milne and Taylor in 1950. Therefore, it is important to recognize the fact that in the intervening years pharmaceutical services in the hospital have expanded considerably thereby suggesting that, until more up to date information is developed, the recommendations of the Public Health Service for floor space in hospital pharmacies should be considered minimal for the construction of today's hospital pharmacy.

Furthermore, it is important to note that today's practice of pharmacy provides its practitioners the opportunity to perform variable functions ranging from standard type dispensing methods to unit dose dispensing methodologies. Involvement with intravenous additive programs, drug information centers and clinical pharmacy endeavors simply means that pharmacy floor space requirements must be determined by factors other than bed capacity and ambulatory clinic patient load. Also, no two hospitals should be compared for the purpose of determining the square footage requirements of the other in spite of the fact that both appear to have similar pharmaceutical involvement. It is not the similarity of involvement that determines space requirements but the degree or scope of involvement coupled with the type of equipment used in the programs.

Equipment Planner's Responsibility

The pharmacist, administrator, purchasing agent and architect, as a group, assume the responsibility for the planning and the subsequent purchase of the major equipment items to be located in the pharmacy. The less expensive items, commonly used in the daily practice of the profession, are usually purchased by the purchasing agent after he has consulted with the pharmacist.

In selecting the equipment, all parties must exercise extreme care in choosing those items which will provide good service, with minimal maintenance, at a price within the hospital's equipment budget. All too often, many pharmacists succumb to the temptation of equipping a particular section of the pharmacy with elaborate and expensive equipment and then purchase equipment of a lower quality for another division of the pharmacy in order to remain within the budgetary allowance.

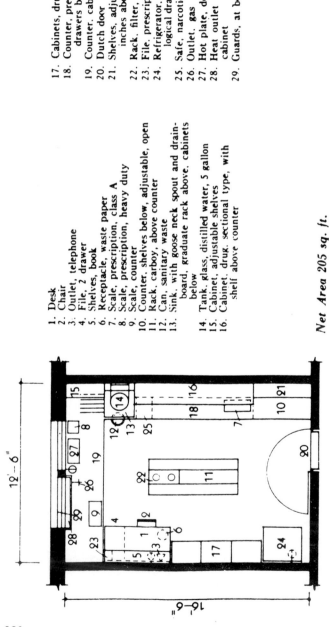

CORRIDOR

16'-6"

12'-6"

1. Desk
2. Chair
3. Outlet, telephone
4. File, 2 drawer
5. Shelves, book
6. Receptacle, waste paper
7. Scale, prescription, class A
8. Scale, prescription, heavy duty
9. Scale, counter
10. Counter, shelves below, adjustable, open
11. Rack, carboy, above counter
12. Can, sanitary waste
13. Sink, with goose neck spout and drain-board, graduate rack above, cabinets below
14. Tank, glass, distilled water, 5 gallon
15. Cabinet, adjustable shelves
16. Cabinet, drug, sectional type, with shelf above counter

17. Cabinets, drug, sectional type
18. Counter, prescription, cabinets and drawers below
19. Counter, cabinets and drawers below
20. Dutch door
21. Shelves, adjustable, open, starting 18 inches above counter
22. Rack, filter, above counter
23. File, prescription, on desk
24. Refrigerator, 8 cubic feet, with bio-logical drawers
25. Safe, narcotic
26. Outlet, gas
27. Hot plate, double element
28. Heat outlet grill, inlet grill in base of cabinet
29. Guards, at both windows

Net Area 205 sq. ft.

Pharmacy for a 50 bed general hospital

Fig. 90. The above design for a pharmacy for a 50-bed hospital was adequate for the type of pharmacy practiced in the period 1950-60. Many hospitals today still have similarly designed units. (From Public Health Service Publication No. 891, December 1961.)

0   4
FEET

The cost of equipment should not be estimated nor should a percentage of the building construction cost be used. Whenever such short cuts are taken, experience has demonstrated that insufficient funds are available for the purchase of the desired equipment. Clearly then, once the equipment list is prepared, it behooves the pharmacist to consult freely with the purchasing agent, manufacturer's representatives and vendors as well as to peruse through the latest editions of the catalogues.

Suggested Equipment Lists

Because the scope of service rendered by each hospital pharmacy will vary from one section of the country to the other or, for that matter, from hospital to hospital, it is an impossible task to attempt to prepare a standard list of equipment which will meet every need.

The Equipment Planning Branch of the United States Public Health Service has prepared a suggested equipment list[6] which may be used as a guide. For the convenience of the student and the hospital pharmacist who may wish to use the said equipment list as check list for the inventory of basic pharmaceutical equipment within the department, the suggested list is hereinafter published.

The symbols used in these lists have definite meaning as follows:[6]

1. " indicates that the item is required but the quantity is not determined. Quantity is dependent upon correlation of the schematic plans."
2. "– indicates the item is not applicable to the particular size group."
3. "Supplies are not included in the term 'equipment' as they are not participated in for hospital projects constructed under the 'Hospital and Medical Facilities (Hill-Burton) Program'."

	Suggested Quantity No. of Beds			Local Requirements		Unit	Total
PHARMACY DEPARTMENT*	50	100	200	Unit	No.	Price	Cost
Compounding and Dispensing Laboratory	1	1	1				
Group I Equipment							
Blinds, window							
Bookshelves	2	2	–				
Cabinet							
Adjustable shelves	1	1	1				
Below, sink	1	1	2				
Drug, sectional type	1	1	1				

* To this basic equipment list must be added the special equipment associated with unit dose dispensing programs or other specialized services offered by the pharmacy department.

PHARMACY DEPARTMENT	Suggested Quantity No. of Beds 50 100 200			Local Requirements Unit No.		Unit Price	Total Cost
Drug, sectional type with shelf above counter	1	1	1				
Clock outlet and electric clock	1	1	1				
Counter							
18 inches wide with open adjustable shelves below	–	1	–				
Cabinets and drawers below	1	1	1				
Open adjustable shelves below	1	–	–				
Prescription, cabinets and drawers below	1	1	1				
Dumbwaiter	–	1	1				
Dutch door	1	–	–				
Pneumatic tube station	–	1	1				
Rack							
Carboy	–	–	1				
Carboy, above counter	1	1	–				
Graduate, above sink	1	1	2				
Filter, above counter	1	1	–				
Shelf above counter	–	–	1				
Shelves, adjustable, starting 18 inches above counter							
Sink, gooseneck type spout, acid resisting drainboard	1	1	2				
Tank, resistant glass, distilled water, wall mounted							
Capacity 5 gallons	1	–	–				
Capacity 12 gallons	–	–	1				
Window, dispensing	–	1	1				
Group II Equipment							
Balance							
Counter, capacity 4½ kg.*	1	1	–				
Prescription							
Class A sensitivity 2 mg.†	1	1	2				
Heavy duty, sensitivity 15 mg.†	1	1	1				
Cabinet, filing							
Card size, 2 drawer, 3 × 5 inches	1	1	–				
Letter size							
2 drawer	1	–	–				
5 drawer	–	1	–				
Prescription	1	1	1				
Cart, to accommodate drug baskets	1	1	1				
Chair, office, swivel with arms	1	1	–				
Desk, office, single pedestal	1	1	–				
Filler, for sterile capped vials	1	–	–				
Homogenizer, hand	1	–	–				
Hot plate, electric, double element, 3 heat control, heavy duty	1	1	–				

*Must conform to state or city minimum requirements.
†Required if Parenteral Solution Laboratory is omitted.

PHARMACY DEPARTMENT	Suggested Quantity No. of Beds 50 100 200			Local Requirements Unit No. Price Total Cost			

PHARMACY DEPARTMENT	50	100	200	Unit	No.	Price	Cost
Lamp, desk	1	1	1				
Mixer, electric, portable, counter type	1	1	1				
Receptacle, waste, foot operated closed top	1	1	2				
Refrigerator, freestanding with biological drawers							
8 cubic feet	1	–	–				
16 cubic feet	–	1	–				
32 cubic feet	–	–	1				
Safe, narcotic	1	1	1				
Stool, operators, adjustable 19-25 inches	1	1	1				
Typewriter	1	1	2				
Weights							
Apothecary, ¼ grain to 8 drams, set	1	1	1				
Balance, lacquered brass, cylindrical body with knob, fractionals of aluminum, tolerance Class C., U.S. Bureau of Standards, Metric, 1 mg. to 500 mg., 1 gm. to 500 gm., set	1	1	1				

Active Storage Room and Manufacturing Area – 1 –

Group I Equipment

	50	100	200				
Blinds, window							
Cabinet, below sink	–	1	–				
Counter, cabinets below, shelves above	–	1	–				
Rack, graduate, above sink	–	1	–				
Shelves, adjustable, lower shelves 24 inches deep, upper shelves starting 36 inches from floor, 18 inches deep	–	1	–				
Sink, gooseneck type spout, drainboard	–	1	–				
Still, water, capacity 2 gallons per hour†	–	1	–				
Tank, resistant glass, distilled water, wall mounted, capacity 5 gallons	–	1	–				

Group II Equipment

	50	100	200				
Mixer, electric, portable, long shaft for tank	–	1	–				
Tank, mixing or storing, 20 gallons, mounted on stand with casters	–	1	1				

†Required if Parenteral Solution Laboratory is omitted.

	Suggested Quantity No. of Beds			Local Requirements			
PHARMACY DEPARTMENT	50	100	200	Unit	No.	Unit Price	Total Cost
Alcohol Vault	–	1	1				
Group I Equipment							
Shelves, metal, starting 42 inches above floor	–						
Vent, inlet and outlet	–	1	1				
Group II Equipment							
Pump, alcohol drum	–	1	1				
Parenteral Solution Laboratory	–	1	1				
Group I Equipment							
Blind, window							
Cabinet							
Adjustable shelves	–	1	1				
Below sink	–	1	1				
Below two compartment sink	–	1	–				
Storage, open, adjustable shelves	–	1	1				
Cleaner, bottle, pressure type	–	–	1				
Counter							
Cabinets and drawers below	–	1	1				
Open below	–	1	1				
Pan, drip with waste connection in counter top	–	1	1				
Rack, bottle	–	3	3				
Sink							
Distilled water rinser, omit hot and cold water supply	–	1	1				
Gooseneck type spout	–	–	1				
Gooseneck type spout, two compartments	–	1	–				
Sterilizer, pressure, corrosive resistant, 24 × 26 × 48 inches with loading carriage and cradle	–	1	1				
Still, water							
Capacity 5 gallons per hour	–	1	–				
Capacity 10 gallons per hour ..	–	–	1				
Tank, resistant glass, distilled water, wall mounted, capacity 12 gallons	–	2	2				
Group II Equipment							
Balance, metric solution with sliding poise and tare beam	–	1	–				
Cart, flask, draining	–	1	1				
Filler, for sterile capped vials	–	1	1				
Hot plate, electric, double element, 3 heat control, heavy duty	–	1	1				
Meter, conductivity							
Oven, sterilizing, counter type, 24 × 14 × 14 inches	–	–	1				

	Suggested Quantity No. of Beds			Local Requirements			
PHARMACY DEPARTMENT	50	100	200	Unit	No.	Unit Price	Total Cost
Pump, suction and pressure with gauges	–	1	1				
Receptacle, waste, foot operated closed top	–	1	1				
Stool, operators, adjustable, 19-25 inches	–	1	1				
Group III Equipment							
Burette, measuring for perenteral solutions							
1000 cubic centimeter	–	2	–	ea			
Standard set	–	–	5	set			
Bushing, rubber, for flask	–	144	200	ea			
Closures for flask	–	144	200	ea			
Filter, glass, fritted, 600 ml.	–	2	2	ea			
Flask, glass, heat resistant graduated							
Capacity 500 cubic centimeters	–	50	100	ea			
Capacity 1000 cubic centimeters	–	100	200	ea			
Holder, flask	–	12	24	ea			
Tag, flask, identification, stainless steel	–	48	96	ea			
Manufacturing Laboratory	–	–	1				
Group I Equipment							
Blinds, window							
Cabinet, below two compartment sink	–	–	1				
Cabinets, adjustable shelves	–	–	1				
Counter, cabinets and drawers below	–	–	1				
Outlet, hot and cold water	–	–	1				
Rack, filter	–	–	1				
Sink, gooseneck type spout, two compartments, drainboard	–	–	1				
Still, water, capacity 2 gallons per hour	–	–	1				
Tank, resistant glass, distilled water, wall mounted, capacity 12 gallons	–	–	1				
Group II Equipment							
Balance, counter, capacity, 4½ kg.*	–	–	1				
Filter press, suction pressure type, approximately 2-5 gallons per minute, mounted on casters	–	–	1				
Hot plate, electric, double element, 3 heat control, heavy duty	–	–	1				
Mill, colloidal	–	–	1				

*Must conform to state or city minimum requirements.

PHARMACY DEPARTMENT	Suggested Quantity No. of Beds 50 100 200	Local Requirements Unit Total Unit No. Price Cost
Mixer, electric, portable, long shaft for tank	− − 1	
Receptacle, waste, foot operated closed top	− − 1	
Tank, mixing or storing, 20 gallons, mounted on stand with casters	− − 2	
Active Storage Room	− − 1	
Group I Equipment		
Blinds, window		
Locker, clothes, steel, 15 × 18 × 60 inches	− − 1	
Rack, barrel	− − 1	
Shelves, adjustable, lower shelves 24 inches deep, upper shelves starting 36 inches from floor, 18 inches deep	− −	
Group II Equipment	− −	
Office and Library	− − 1	
Group I Equipment		
Blinds, window		
Panel, glass	− − 1	
Group II Equipment		
Bookcase†	− − 1	
Cabinet, filing		
Card size, 2 drawer, 3 × 5 inches	− − 1	
Letter size, 5 drawer	− − 2	
Chair		
Office, swivel with arms	− − 1	
Straight	− − 1	
Desk, office, double pedestal	− − 1	
Lamp, desk	− − 1	
Rack, magazine	− − 1	
Table, office, 24 × 36 inches	− − 1	
Pharmacy Department		
Group III Equipment		
Basket, drug, 6 compartments	2 4 8 ea	
Beaker, glass, low form with spout		
50 ml.	3 3 3 ea	
150 ml.	3 3 3 ea	
250 ml.	3 3 3 ea	
600 ml.	2 2 2 ea	
1000 ml.	2 2 2 ea	

†Built-in equipment, Group I, may be substituted.

PHARMACY DEPARTMENT

	Suggested Quantity No. of Beds			Local Requirements		
	50	100	200	Unit	No.	Unit Price	Total Cost

Books**

Essential

American Hospital Formulary Service, 1959 and supplements by American Society of Hospital Pharmacists, 4630 Montgomery Ave., Washington, D. C.* — 1 1 1 ea

Bureal of Internal Revenue Distribution and Use of Tax-Free Alcohol, No. 444, Government Printing Office, Washington 25, D.C. .... — 1 1 1 ea

Bureau of Internal Revenue Drawback on Distilled Spirits Used in Manufacturing Non-beverage Products, No. 206, Government Printing Office, Washington 25, D.C. .... — 1 1 1 ea

Copies of State and Municipal Pharmacy Laws Or Sanitary Codes, available locally.. — 1 1 1 ea

Federal Food, Drug and Cosmetic Act and General Regulations for Its Enforcement .... — 1 1 1 ea

Merck Index, Latest Edition.. — 1 1 1 ea

Merck Manual, Latest Edition — 1 1 1 ea

Modern Drug Encyclopedia and Therapeutic Guide, latest edition and quarterly supplements, by Marion E. Howard — 1 1 1 ea

National Formulary, Latest Edition, and supplements...... — 1 1 1 ea

New and Nonofficial Drugs, latest edition (published annually) .... — 1 1 1 ea

The Dispensatory of the United States of America, Twenty-fifth Edition, 1955, A. Osol and G. E. Farrar, Jr., Vol. I, Vol. II; *New Drug Developments* by A. Osol and Robinson Pratt .... — 1 1 1 ea

United States Pharmacopoeia, Latest Edition and Supplements .... — 1 1 1 ea

United States Treasury Department, Bureau of Narcotics, Regulation, No. 5, Washington 25, D.C. .... — 1 1 1 ea

**Books in this list must be supplemented by the newest publications in the field.

*Additional copies required for each nursing unit.

PHARMACY DEPARTMENT	Suggested Quantity No. of Beds 50 100 200	Unit	Local Requirements No.	Unit Price	Total Cost

Supplemental

Dorland's Illustrated Medical Dictionary, Twenty-fourth edition, 1965 .... 1 1 1 ea

or

Blakiston's New Gould Medical Dictionary, Second Edition, 1956, by H. W. Jones, N. L. Hoerr and A. Osol ...... 1 1 1 ea

Arithmetic of Pharmacy, Latest Edition, by Alvin B. Stevens .... 1 1 1 ea

Manual of Pharmacology, Latest Edition, by T. Solman.. 1 1 1 ea

Pharmacological Basis of Therapeutics, Latest Edition, by L. Goodman and A. Gilman .... 1 1 1 ea

Pharmaceutical Dispensing, Latest Edition, by W. J. Husa 1 1 1 ea

Remington's Pharmaceutical Sciences by E. W. Martin ..... 1 1 1 ea

The Art of Compounding. Latest Edition, by Glenn L. Jenkins, Edward Brecht, Don E. Francke, and Glen J. Sperandio .... 1 1 1 ea

Bottle, glass

2 gallon .... 4 6 10 ea

Carboy, 5 gallons .... 2 4 8 ea

Heat-resistant, 9-liter with two-way valve and clamp – – 1 ea

Brush, bottle .... 6 6 6 ea

Burner, Bunsen .... 2 2 2 ea

Dish, porcelain, evaporating with pour out

150 ml., diameter 100 mm. 2 2 2 ea

385 ml., diameter 145 mm. 2 2 2 ea

File, prescription, binder and box to hold 1000 .... 2 2 2 ea

Flask, glass, Erlenmeyer, narrow mouthed

125 ml. .... 2 2 2 ea

250 ml. .... 2 2 2 ea

500 ml. .... 2 2 2 ea

Heat resistant, graduated

500 cubic centimeter ...... – 50 100 ea

1000 cubic centimeter .... – 100 200 ea

Funnel

Glass

Plain

30 ml., diameter 50 mm. 1 1 1 ea

120 ml., diameter 90 mm. 1 1 1 ea

PHARMACY DEPARTMENT	Suggested Quantity No. of Beds				Local Requirements		
	50	100	200	Unit	No.	Unit Price	Total Cost
Ribbed							
Approximate capacity 2 ounces, diameter 2⅝ inches	1	1	1	ea			
Approximate capacity 4 ounces, diameter 3½ inches	1	1	1	ea			
Approximate capacity 8 ounces, diameter 4½ inches	1	1	1	ea			
Approximate capacity 32 ounces, diameter 7 inches	1	1	4	ea			
Metal							
Approximate capacity 4 ounces, diameter 3⅛	1	1	1	ea			
Approximate capacity 8 ounces, diameter 4 inches	1	1	1	ea			
Approximate capacity 16 ounces, diameter 6½ inches	1	1	2	ea			
Graduate, glass, conical double scale							
5 ml. and 60 minims	3	3	3	ea			
10 ml. and 120 minims	3	3	3	ea			
60 ml. and 2 ounces	3	3	3	ea			
125 ml. and 4 ounces	3	3	3	ea			
250 ml. and 8 ounces	2	2	2	ea			
500 ml. and 16 ounces	1	1	1	ea			
1000 ml. and 32 ounces	1	1	2	ea			
Holder, label, typewriter	1	1	1	ea			
Machine, numbering, repeat movement	1	1	1	ea			
Measure, metal, graduated, double scale							
500 ml. and 16 ounces	1	1	2	ea			
1000 ml. and 32 ounces	1	1	2	ea			
Moistener, label	1	1	1	ea			
Mold							
Suppository compressor	1	1	1	ea			
Tablet, triturate	1	1	1	ea			
Mortar and pestle, glass							
Capacity 2 ounces	1	1	1	ea			
Capacity 4 ounces	1	1	1	ea			
Capacity 8 ounces	1	1	1	ea			
Capacity 16 ounces	1	1	1	ea			
Mortar, wedgewood, and pestle, wooden handle							
No. 0000, capacity 60 ml.	1	1	1	ea			
No. 00, capacity 150 ml.	1	1	1	ea			
No. 1, capacity 300 ml.	1	1	1	ea			
No. 5, capacity 1650 ml.	–	1	1	ea			
Percolator, graduated, metric, 2000 ml.—4 pints	1	1	1	ea			

PHARMACY DEPARTMENT	Suggested Quantity No. of Beds 50	100	200	Unit	Local Requirements No.	Unit Price	Total Cost
Pipette, measuring, desired size	1	1	1	ea			
Punch, prescription	1	1	1	ea			
Rack, test tube, wood, 10 hole	1	1	1	ea			
Register, narcotic and exempt narcotics	1	1	1	ea			
Rod, stirring, glass or composition, assorted lengths	1	1	1	set			
Scoop							
No. 1, approximately 110 mm. × 65 mm.	1	1	1	ea			
No. 2, approximately 120 mm. × 70 mm.	1	1	1	ea			
No. 3, approximately 150 mm. × 95 mm.	1	1	1	ea			
Sieve, brass or copper wire cloth, diameter 8 inches							
No. 20	1	1	1	ea			
No. 40.	1	1	1	ea			
No. 80.	1	1	1	ea			
Slap, ointment, 12 × 12 inches ..	1	1	1	ea			
Spatula							
Flexible steel blade							
3 inches	1	1	2	ea			
4 inches	1	1	2	ea			
6 inches	1	1	2	ea			
8 inches	1	1	2	ea			
Hard rubber or composition blade							
6 inches	1	1	2	ea			
8 inches	1	1	2	ea			
Support stand, iron rectangular base, 6 inches × 9 inches, rod 24 inches with rings, diameter 3, 4, 5, 6 inches	1	1	1	ea			
Thermometer, general purpose							
ASTM, El (1C-39)—20 degrees to +150 degrees C.	1	1	1	ea			
ASTM, El (2C-39)—5 degrees to +300 degrees C.	1	1	1	ea			
Tripod, iron with ring, height 9 inches, outside diameter of ring, 6 inches	1	1	1	ea			
Tube, test, chemical, 125 mm. × 16 mm.	12	12	24	ea			
Water bath, round, copper with rings, diameter 6 inches	1	1	1	ea			
Wire gauze, asbestos center, 6 inches square	1	1	1	ea			

Supplies
Drugs, Chemicals, Biologicals, and Miscellaneous Supplies based on individual requirements. See "American Hospital Formulary Service."

Equipment Electrical Safety

Electrical safety within the hospital has become a topic of major interest amongst physicians, planners, engineers and safety experts. This has arisen because of the inherent danger involved in the use of some of the commonly used equipment in the hospital. At one time or another, articles have been written commenting on electrical hazards in electric beds, monitoring equipment, x-ray machines and cleaning equipment.

Thus it behooves the hospital pharmacist to select all equipment used in the pharmacy with care. In general compliance with the N.F.P.A. standards (National Fire Protective Association) is a start in the right direction.

Electrical safety in the hospital pharmacy could be improved if consideration is given to the following guiding principles:[8]

1. Keep electrical power cords as short as possible in order to eliminate electrical leakage.
2. Use equipment with proper ground lines. (Three-prong plugs)
3. Purchase equipment with power on-off switches which have clearly visible indication of power status (on or off).
4. Eliminate slow blow fusing whenever possible since this type of fusing increases the exposure time of the operator to the electrical hazard.
5. Before permitting personnel to operate new equipment, be sure that they are properly trained in its use. In addition, it is important that they read the instructional manual— particularly the section dealing with safe use and possible hazards.
6. Train operators to disconnect the power receptacle from the power source by pulling on the connector, not on the cable.
7. Avoid the use of extension cords.
8. Do not attempt to make repairs to the equipment.
9. Cooperate with in-house maintenance programs.

Refrigeration Facilities

Most hospital pharmacists and architects when developing plans for a new pharmacy are quite cognizant of the desirability and the need for air conditioning and large biological refrigerators in the hospital pharmacy. More often than not, little thought is given to the need of a freezer and a cold room.

A review of the storage requirements for drugs in the National Formulary XIII shows that the thermal storage requirements vary from "cold place" to "store in refrigerator" to "avoid excessive heat or excessive temperature."

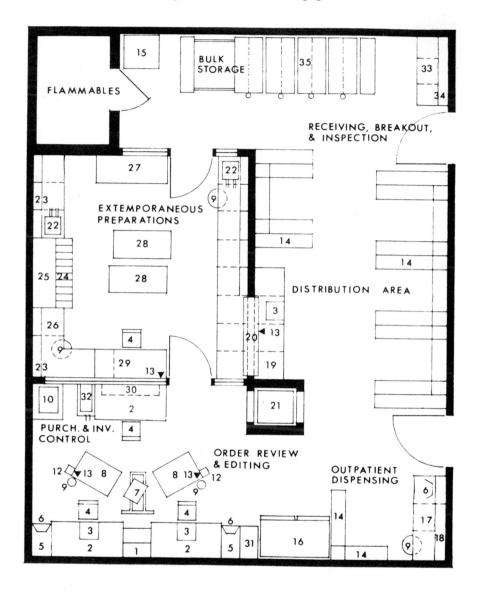

SCALE 5   0   5   10 FT

FIG. 91. Pharmacy Department in a 100-Bed Hospital. This plan is to be considered as one example of a modern pharmacy design. (From Planning for Hospital Pharmacies U.S. Dept. HEW, Health Services & Mental Health Administration, Health Care Facilities Services, Washington D.C. In press.)

Legend for Figure 91 on page 393.

The complete list of storage temperature terms and the definitions are as follows:

> Cold Place—A cold place is one having a temperature not exceeding 8° (46° F.).
> Refrigerator—A refrigerator is a cold place in which the temperature is held between 2° and 8° (36° and 46° F.).
> Cool Place—A cool place is one having a temperature between 8° and 15° (46° and 59° F.).
> Room Temperature—Room temperature is between 15° and 30° (59° and 86° F.).
> Excessive Heat—The expression "excessive heat" designates temperatures above 40° (104° F.).

Since many of the drugs, so described, are in common use in the hospital, the pharmacist should make every effort to see that proper storage facilities are made available. This is easily done in most hospitals by the purchase of a large biological refrigerator and a freezer. In the small hospital, these two units or, as is usually the case, the refrigerator with a built-in freezer compartment, provide adequate facilities. The problem which usually arises in the larger hospital is that the refrigerator is too small to accommodate the inventory requiring refrigeration. Some pharmacists have tried to solve this problem by purchasing additional refrigerators or by borrowing space in the large dietary walk-in "iceboxes."

Although both of these arrangements are workable, it would seem that a less expensive and a less inconvenient method of cold storage within the pharmacy could be had by the construction of a cold room.

For the purpose of this section, a cold room is defined as an artificially cooled room with a regulated temperature range of 12° to 15° C (53.6° to 59° F).

Legend

1. Pneumatic tube station
2. Desk
3. Typewriter, electric, nonmovable carriage
4. Chair
5. Files. intermediate height
6. Files, swinging panel, strip insert type
7. File, revolving on two levels
8. Table, movable, 2 feet by 3 feet
9. Waste receptacle
10. Photocopier
11. File, 2-drawer
12. Utility pole
13. Telephone
14. Shelving, adjustable, 12 inches
15. Safe
16. Refrigerator, with freezer
17. Counter, with file drawer, bins
18. Shelving, adjustable, 7 inches
19. Counter, dispensing
20. Two-shelf unit above counter
21. Dumbwaiter, open both sides
22. Cabinet, with sink, drain board
23. Cabinet, wall-mounted
24. Bins
25. Hood, laminar airflow, vertical or horizontal
26. Counter, with open adjustable shelving beneath
27. Cart, storage
28. Carts, utility
29. Desk, small
30. Bookcase, wall-mounted
31. File cabinet, 5-drawer
32. File, visible index type
33. Counter, with adjustable shelves beneath
34. Shelving, wall-mounted, 9 inches
35. Shelving, adjustable, rail-mounted

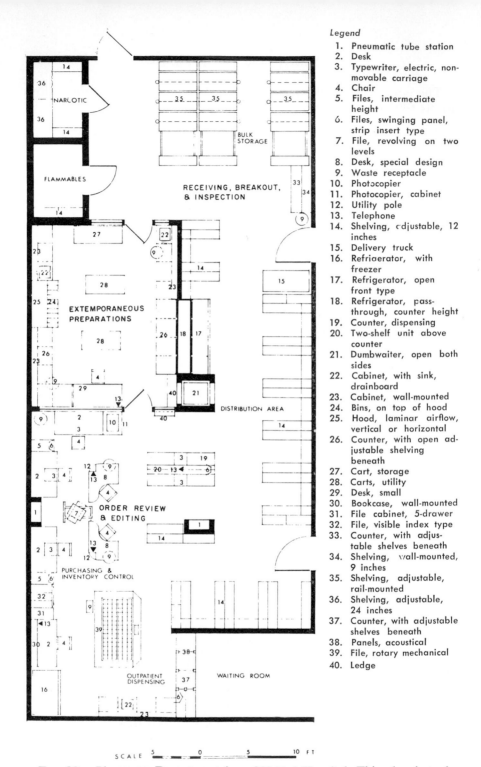

Legend

1. Pneumatic tube station
2. Desk
3. Typewriter, electric, non-movable carriage
4. Chair
5. Files, intermediate height
6. Files, swinging panel, strip insert type
7. File, revolving on two levels
8. Desk, special design
9. Waste receptacle
10. Photocopier
11. Photocopier, cabinet
12. Utility pole
13. Telephone
14. Shelving, adjustable, 12 inches
15. Delivery truck
16. Refrigerator, with freezer
17. Refrigerator, open front type
18. Refrigerator, pass-through, counter height
19. Counter, dispensing
20. Two-shelf unit above counter
21. Dumbwaiter, open both sides
22. Cabinet, with sink, drainboard
23. Cabinet, wall-mounted
24. Bins, on top of hood
25. Hood, laminar airflow, vertical or horizontal
26. Counter, with open adjustable shelving beneath
27. Cart, storage
28. Carts, utility
29. Desk, small
30. Bookcase, wall-mounted
31. File cabinet, 5-drawer
32. File, visible index type
33. Counter, with adjustable shelves beneath
34. Shelving, wall-mounted, 9 inches
35. Shelving, adjustable, rail-mounted
36. Shelving, adjustable, 24 inches
37. Counter, with adjustable shelves beneath
38. Panels, acoustical
39. File, rotary mechanical
40. Ledge

SCALE 5 ___ 0 ___ 5 ___ 10 FT

FIG. 92. Pharmacy Department in a 300-Bed Hospital. This plan is to be considered as one example of a modern pharmacy design. (From Planning for Hospital Pharmacies, U.S. Dept. HEW, Health Services & Mental Health Administration, Health Care Facilities Services, Washington D.C. In press.)

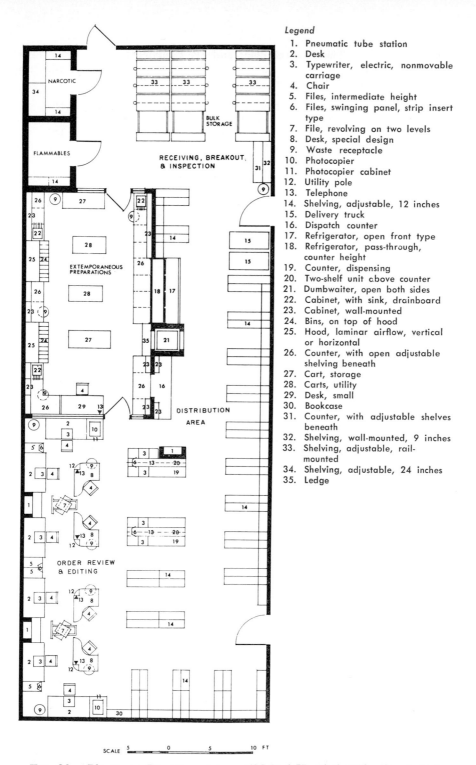

Legend

1. Pneumatic tube station
2. Desk
3. Typewriter, electric, nonmovable carriage
4. Chair
5. Files, intermediate height
6. Files, swinging panel, strip insert type
7. File, revolving on two levels
8. Desk, special design
9. Waste receptacle
10. Photocopier
11. Photocopier cabinet
12. Utility pole
13. Telephone
14. Shelving, adjustable, 12 inches
15. Delivery truck
16. Dispatch counter
17. Refrigerator, open front type
18. Refrigerator, pass-through, counter height
19. Counter, dispensing
20. Two-shelf unit above counter
21. Dumbwaiter, open both sides
22. Cabinet, with sink, drainboard
23. Cabinet, wall-mounted
24. Bins, on top of hood
25. Hood, laminar airflow, vertical or horizontal
26. Counter, with open adjustable shelving beneath
27. Cart, storage
28. Carts, utility
29. Desk, small
30. Bookcase
31. Counter, with adjustable shelves beneath
32. Shelving, wall-mounted, 9 inches
33. Shelving, adjustable, rail-mounted
34. Shelving, adjustable, 24 inches
35. Ledge

SCALE 5 0 5 10 FT

FIG. 93. Pharmacy Department in a 500-Bed Hospital. This plan is to be considered as one example of a modern pharmacy design. (From Planning for Hospital Pharmacies, U.S. Dept. HEW, Health Services & Mental Health Administration, Health Care Facilities Services, Washington D.C. In press.)

Constructing a Cold Room*

In existing facilities, a cold room may be inexpensively constructed if the parties involved will use a little imagination. A little-used corner of the basement storage area should be selected and the necessary area marked off. If windows are present, they should be bricked-up or at least double-paned and sealed against the outside atmosphere with caulking compound.

An electric light fixture and the required number of electrical outlets should be installed with the switch controlling the light fixture being on the outside wall nearest the entrance to the room.

The necessary additional walls of the room may be constructed of concrete, cinder block, concrete blocks, or brick. Where the use of the above building materials is not feasible, a similar result may be had by the use of wood studs with aluminum foil insulation. The inner side of this type of wall should be cement plastered and the outer side "finished-off" by covering with masonite or other inexpensive material. The door should fit tightly, be no larger than necessary, and be provided with a good automatic door closer.

An electric motor-driven air cooled Freon compressor unit with a remote blower-type cooling coil will provide the necessary refrigeration. This unit should be installed with the necessary thermostat and expansion valve required to maintain the desired temperature range. The blower is mounted in the cold room. To it, a small waste line is installed to drain away the condensate which collects on the refrigerator coil. The compressor may be installed outside of the cold room in order to conserve space within.

Obviously the size of the cold room to be constructed will determine the capacity of the refrigeration unit to be installed. In general, a room approximately $10' \times 10' \times 10'$ would require one ton of refrigeration to maintain a temperature range of 50° to 60° F.

Once constructed, the room may be equipped with the necessary shelving, storage bins, cabinets, and work bench.

Built-In Equipment

One of the most important aspects of a pharmacy modernization or construction program is that which involves the planning and selection of the built-in cabinets, counters and other types of casework. Due consideration must be given to such details as the height of the bench or cabinet, the size of the shelving or drawers, the types of handles on drawer and cabinet doors, whether or not the shelving is to be fixed or adjustable as well as the type of material which will be installed on the counter top.

*Adapted from an article entitled "A Cold Room for the Hospital Pharmacy" by William E. Hassan, Jr., and George Stilgoe, Am. J. Hosp. Pharm., 16:3:120, 1959.

The materials used in the construction of built-in equipment must be reviewed by the hospital pharmacist in the light of the activity to which the equipment will be subjected. Thus it is not sufficient to specify that the equipment will be constructed of stainless steel. One should specify whether it is expected to be constructed of mild, cold rolled, annealed furniture steel; the gauges of the metal to be used; the gauge of the metal to be used in the shelving and whether or not the face of the shelf should be turned back up under the shelf and brought into contact with it in order to provide additional support; and details relative to the doors, adjustability of the shelving, etc. Much of this type of detail is available from the manufacturer's catalogue and specification sheets.

Special attention should be given to the counter tops. All too often, excellent base cabinets are provided but the counter tops do not offer resistance to corrosion and abrasion. Accordingly, it is of importance for the pharmacist to inquire about the physical properties of the counter finishes. Some guidelines are the following:

1. To what degree can it be bent without cracking or breaking down?
2. How much of an impact will it withstand without flaking or peeling?
3. What effect will a high relative humidity have upon it?
4. Is it sufficiently hard to resist erosion?
5. If the material is colored, is the color retention quality sufficient to resist appreciable discoloration?
6. Is the finish coat abrasion resistant to the degree that prevents premature wearing through?
7. Is the finish coat reagent resistant? Bear in mind that it must resist acids, alkalies, oils and solvents.

Many of these units are available from the several manufacturers who specialize in the development and construction of such components.

Electric Lighting and Service

The availability of good electrical lighting and a sufficient number of grounded electrical outlets is mandatory for a smoothly functioning pharmacy.

Accordingly, sufficient lighting must be provided for the various work areas as well as the library and the offices. Although the present literature indicates that 30 foot candles are adequate for general illumination, and 50 foot candles for special areas, such as the prescription dispensing area, it is recommended that in any new construction the services of a lighting engineer be utilized. This is important because each hospital, or unit within the hospital, has particular needs based upon many factors some of which are characteristic of the operation, whereas others may be due to location and environment.

In selecting the type of lighting and light fixture, care should be given to the selection of a unit which will not become a housekeeping problem. That is to say that, when possible, a fixture which can be mounted in the ceiling is highly desirable since it will not gather dust and dirt. Fluorescent light is recommended, however, recent studies by the various manufacturers of lighting equipment seem to indicate that a combination of fluorescent tube and standard bulb in the same fixture provides a better light.

Grounded electrical outlets should be provided in all areas in which the use of electrical equipment may be indicated. In addition, thought must be given to the requirements of voltage in the range of 220 volts for some of the ovens or mixers in the manufacturing area.

If volatile solvents are used in the manufacturing areas or are stored in the pharmacy, consideration must be given to the installation of explosion proof fixtures and outlets.

Ventilation

Air conditioning of the pharmacy is desirable for a number of reasons. First, it obviates the need for the opening of windows and doors through which dirt, dust and other environmental contaminants may enter the pharmacy. Second, the use of the various autoclaves, ovens and steam jacketed kettles may render the working environment too hot. Third, air conditioning permits the maintenance of a temperature which is compatible with the official storage requirements for drugs on a year round basis irrespective of the climatic conditions. Fourth, adequate ventilation is essential for the removal of the strong odors which are characteristic of the chemicals used in the manufacture of the various galenicals, preservative fluids and reagents. Fifth, because doors and windows can be kept closed, there can be effected a saving in the cost of housekeeping service in the pharmacy.

Conveyor and Pneumatic Tube Systems

Modern engineering technology has made available a means of transporting nearly every item from the pharmacy to its hospital destination. Accordingly, in order to conserve pharmaceutical manpower, thought should be given to the installation of dumbwaiters, pneumatic tube systems and other like devices for the movement of supplies from the pharmacy to their desired hospital destination. The type or combination of equipment necessary will vary with each

CHARACTERISTICS OF RESILIENT FLOOR TILES

Type	Ease of Maintenance	Resistance			Advantages	Disadvantages
		To Moisture	To Alkali	To Oil & Solvents		
Asphalt	Fair*	Excellent	Excellent	Poor*	Lowest cost resilient tile Most resistant to cigaret burns Excellent choice for basement floors May be applied and used immediately	Least resilient and least comfortable tile Does not take as high polish as others Very poor indentation resistance Limited color range (dark)
Linoleum	Very Good	Poor	Fair to Poor	Excellent	More comfortable than asphalt Good warmth Low noise level	Can be used only on above-grade floors
Vinyl-Asbestos	Good	Excellent	Excellent	Good	Good wearing qualities at reasonable cost Inexpensive to maintain May be applied above, on or below grade Wider range of colors than asphalt	Only fair resilience and comfort
Cork	Fair	Fair	Fair	Fair	Excellent comfort, warmth, quietness	Can be used only on above-grade floors Soft, easily marred High cost
Rubber	Good	Good	Good	Poor	Almost as comfortable as cork Lustrous sheen Excellent indentation resistance Wide range of colors	High cost Usually unsuitable for below-grade locations Must be polished frequently to maintain high gloss
Vinyl	Very Good	Good	Excellent	Excellent	May be applied above, on or below grade Smooth and polished-looking Widest range of colors and styles	Most expensive of tiles

*New, grease-resistant variety shows good ease of maintenance and excellent solvent resistance.

hospital; therefore, it is recommended that advice be sought from the hospital's architect and/or the various manufacturers and distributors of such devices.

Plumbing

It is not expected that the pharmacist should be knowledgeable in the technicalities of the plumbing installation; however, he should be in a position to advise the architect and his plumbing consultant of the particular details and requirements of the pharmacy and the nature of the materials which will be disposed of through the various waste lines.

By so doing, the plans will properly specify acid resistant piping, adequate hot and cold water mixing valves, stainless steel or soapstone sinks, distilled water lines and faucets which will allow gallon jugs or carboys to be filled without the use of a connecting hose.

Finishes

a. Work Counters

Although many of the work counters will be constructed of stainless steel, others will not require such construction. For these units, Formica or a similar material is suggested as an efficient and durable surface.

b. Floors

The floors of the pharmacy proper should be resilient, smooth but not slippery, stain resistant and yet complimentary to the existing or proposed decor of the department. Many flooring materials are currently available which are highly satisfactory and economical. Some of the floor coverings currently in use are asphalt tile, vinyl tile, rubber tile and heavy duty linoleum. The Hospital Bureau, Inc.[7] has made available information on page 399.

In recent years, many architects and designers have introduced carpeting into the hospital pharmacy with aesthetic results. On the other hand, some of the installations have not been complementary to the operation of a hospital pharmacy. Carpeting has proven to be acceptable in the office, library, waiting room areas but has not been acceptable in the various work areas. Much of the complaint centers around the excessive generation of static electricity and the flammability of the carpet material.

Low relative humidity has always been the major problem in controlling static generation in carpets. The lower the relative humidity, the greater the problem. Thus, it is important to ascertain the kilovolts of static electricity that a carpet will generate at the normal building temperature and with a relative humidity of 10 to 20 per cent. Clearly, the lower the kilovolts generated, the more acceptable the carpet will be for pharmacy installation. The student is cautioned to the fact that a high humidity will also produce low kilovolt readings of static electricity. Obviously, a high humidity does not lend itself to the pharmacy area for a number of reasons associated with drug storage and personal comfort. Also, carpets that are advertised as being "static free" or "static proof" must be viewed with a jaundiced eye in view of the fact that such material does not exist. Static electricity is present, to some degree, in all materials.

With respect to flammability, the United States Public Health Service has promulgated carpet standards for hospitals and nursing homes using Hill-Burton funds. Carpets in these facilities must have a rating of not less than 75 using the Tunnel Test (ASTM Standard #E-84-61).

The floors of the manufacturing and parenteral solutions room should be supplied with a floor drain and covered with a durable paint or enamel. Recent literature describes the application of a vinyl epoxy latex coating to concrete floors which permits the routine use of soap and water for cleaning and yet does not crack and lift as do ordinary paints and enamels.

c. Walls

The walls of the pharmacy should be painted with a material which permits periodic washing without the danger of losing its original color. The selection of the appropriate color scheme is here left to the taste and discretion of the parties involved.

In the manufacturing and parenteral products rooms, painted wall surfaces do not usually withstand the constant washing necessary for the maintenance of the desired degree of asepsis. Accordingly, it is suggested that a ceramic tile, or other comparable material, be utilized in these areas.

SELECTED REFERENCES

BARKER, KENNETH N.: Planning a Hospital Pharmacy Facility, Am. J. Hosp. Pharm. *28*:6:423, 1971.

BROWN, THOMAS R., BARKER, KENNETH N., ROWLAND, F. HERRON, SMITH, MICKEY C., and MIKEAL, ROBERT L.: A National Survey of Planning for Hospital Pharmacy Facilities, Am. J. Hosp. Pharm. *28*:6:432, 1971.

SWENSSON, EARL S.: An Innovative Design in Hospital Pharmacy Facilities, Am. J. Hosp. Pharm. *28*:6:440, 1971.

OSTERBERGER, DAVID J.: Layout and Design for Mechanized Centralized Unit Dose Dispensing, Am. J. Hosp. Pharm. *28*:6:447, 1971.

BIBLIOGRAPHY

1. Minimum Standard for Pharmacies in Hospitals with Guide to Application, Am. J. Hosp. Pharm., *15*:11:992, 1958.

rapid dissemination of basic pharmacological research and as a source of research reference material.

This chapter will be concerned with the location, organization and contents of a pharmaceutical library.

Location

Ideally, the pharmaceutical library should be located within and as an integral division of the department of pharmacy. Although, if it becomes necessary for one reason or another to consolidate it with the regular hospital library then, rather than risk the chance of having no worthwhile facility, this alternative should be accepted.

The reasons for placing the pharmaceutical library in the pharmacy are many, but probably the most worthy is that an individual using the facility would have available to him on-the-spot consultation with individuals whose forte is information concerning drugs. Also, whenever a clinician's work requires data concerning drugs or drug therapy, he is, more likely than not, inclined to go to the pharmacy for the desired information. Clearly then, it is advantageous to both doctor and pharmacist to have the reference material at hand rather than consume more valuable time in going to the hospital library.

In addition, the pharmacy is the logical repose of all worthwhile drug related literature: the various journals, product reference and price catalogues, and special releases concerning withdrawal, toxicity or contraindications to the use of existing products.

Physical Facilities

Because the pharmaceutical library is usually restricted to the medical and nursing staffs, its dimensions will be determined by the size of the utilizing staff, the type of hospital, the number of textbooks, monographs and journals subscribed to as well as accessibility to the hospital library (if any) or to other medical libraries in the area.

Gartland[2] quoting the *Handbook of Medical Library Practice*[3] provides the following measurements as being useful in determining space requirements.

1. The reading area should allow 25 to 30 square feet per reader.
2. If rectangular tables are selected, they should measure 36 × 60 feet. These would then require 100 square feet of floor space for each. (Accommodates 4 readers.)
3. Circular tables measuring 48 inches in diameter and accommodating 4 readers also require 100 square feet of floor space.
4. Aisles:
   a. between tables—not less than 5 feet.
   b. between tables and walls—3 to 4 feet.

5. Shelf space:
   a. bound volumes—4 to 5 volumes per foot of shelf.
   b. reference tools—3 to 4 volumes per foot of shelf. An allowance of 7 inches per 3 foot shelf should be made for additions.

Selection of Contents

The pharmaceutical library should contain in it those volumes, monographs and journals dealing with pharmacy and its allied sciences. Volumes and other published materials dealing with the various clinical and preclinical subject areas should be reserved for the hospital medical library.

As a nucleus around which to add volumes, the library should contain the *United States Pharmacopeia* and the *National Formulary* and their supplements.

Pharmaceutical subjects which should be represented in the library include pharmacology, toxicology, pharmaceutical organic chemistry, pharmacognosy, physiology, anatomy and bacteriology. In addition, there should be included a dictionary, medical dictionary, abstract journals, and selected journals dealing with the above subjects. The various types of drug reference books should not be overlooked.

Since the library is to specialize in pharmaceutical subjects, certain pure pharmacy texts and journals should be included (see pages 387, 388, 407, 408, 409).

Most drug manufacturers provide in addition to their catalogues comprehensive literature concerning each of their products. It is strongly recommended that these be filed for ready reference. Those hospitals using the *American Hospital Formulary System* often file this type of literature according to the system of classification of drugs employed in the *Formulary*.

In January 1964, the American Society of Hospital Pharmacists commenced a new abstract publication entitled *International Pharmaceutical Abstracts*. In keeping with the recommendations of the Commission on Pharmaceutical Abstracts of the International Pharmaceutical Federation, the Society publishes the journal in English, issues it 24 times per year and provides a cumulative index twice annually.

International Pharmaceutical Abstracts includes abstracts of articles on product formulation and formulas; drug stability and storage; drug synthesis; pharmaceutical technology; pharmacognosy; pharmacology; biopharmaceutics; physical pharmacy; investigational drugs; drug evaluations; and history, ethics and sociology.

Some drug companies also produce films and projection slides covering a number of points of clinical interest. Certainly, a listing of these should be available in the pharmacy library and the pharmacist should be acquainted with the procedure for obtaining them for various clinical and nursing groups.

Of late, producers of pharmaceuticals have made available excellent plastic reproductions of various body organs which possess excellent teaching qualities. A collection of these should certainly be available from the pharmacy library to the school of nursing.

Federal publications, particularly those of the U.S. Department of Health, Education, and Welfare should always be obtained. One of the most recent issues for which every hospital pharmacist should have his hospital's name placed on the mailing list is *Investigational Drug Circular* issued by the Bureau of Medicine, Food and Drug Administration.

The Federal Food and Drug Administration publishes a journal containing its decisions and views. The name of the journal is *FDA Papers* and is available on a subscription basis from the Government Printing Office in Washington, D. C.

Many house organs contain excellent review articles of clinical interest to both nurse and physician. Accordingly, these should also be part of the pharmacy library.

The American Society of Hospital Pharmacists' *Drug Products Information File* (DPIF) is also a valuable addition to the library. The DPIF is a data bank composed of terms and code numbers for commercially available drug products. The drug data bank is organized to facilitate automatic processing of drug data. This multi-functional drug coding system is based on a 5-digit generic drug product number that identifies the generic drug product, a 6-digit brand drug product number which identifies a specific manufacturer's brand of drug, and a 5-digit brand drug product package number which extends the information to a specific package of a manufacturer's brand of drug product. In addition, each aspect of a drug product description such as route of administration, dosage form, strength, etc. is systematically coded.

Because of the versatility of the data bank, DPIF has been incorporated into applications such as inventory control; purchasing of drugs; formulary preparation; patient billing; drug therapy auditing; experimental drug information programs; adverse drug reaction programs; patient medication records, orders, summaries, charges and labeling.

With the trend towards the utilization of audio-cassettes for continuing education, the American Society of Hospital Pharmacists introduced VOICES 12/60. This is a monthly cassette tape communications program designed specifically for pharmacists, with particular emphasis on clinical and institutional pharmacy practice. Since this is a monthly continuing service, it constitutes the basis for a audio reference library.

The hospital pharmacist desirous of a single source to serve as a check list of possible publications is referred to the *Basic List of Books and Journals for Veterans Administration Medical Libraries,*[4] *The Guide To Information Sources for the Hospital Pharmacist*[5] and to the *World List of Pharmacy Periodicals.*[6]

The decision as to which textbook or journal is necessary for rendering good drug information service is a difficult one to make. Each hospital offering such a service may well have a different source library. The following is a listing used by one hospital and is offered as a guide to the practitioner seeking to create a drug information library:

American Drug Index

(Wilson, C. O. and Jones, T. E.) (Lippincott Co., Philadelphia, Pa.)

An alphabetical listing of drugs with cross-indexing by generic, brand and chemical names. Also included are the product composition, dosage forms and use.

American Hospital Formulary Service

(American Society of Hospital Pharmacists, Washington, D.C.)

Comprehensive presentation of drug monographs on selected commercially available drugs.

Dangerous Properties of Industrial Materials

(Reinhold Publishing Co. New York, New York)

The synonyms, descriptions, physical characteristics, hazards and countermeasures for approximately 12,000 common industrial and laboratory materials are listed.

deHaen Drugs In Use

(Paul deHaen, 11 West 42nd St., New York, New York)

Abstracts of clinical studies providing basic clinical data along with product information which is added by the abstract service.

Dispensatory of the United States of America

(Osol, A. and Farrar, G. E.) (Lippincott Co. Philadelphia, Pa.)

A collection of alphabetically arranged presentations on drugs and classes of drugs. Included in the descriptive matter is data on pharmacology, uses, contraindications, adverse effects and dosage.

Documenta Geigy Scientific Tables

(Konrad Diem, Editor)

(Geigy Pharmaceuticals, Ardsley, New York)

Contains tables of mathematical, physical and chemical data.

Extra Pharmacopoeia—Martindale Edition
(The Pharmaceutical Press, 17 Bloomsbury Sq., London, W.C. 1)
Drug monographs containing the usual information pertaining to physical and chemical properties, pharmacological activity and posology. A source of information for British and foreign drugs.

Facts and Comparisons
(P.O. Box 8 Baden Station St. Louis, Missouri)
Comparative listing of drugs to show composition, dosage forms and relative cost. Products are listed by therapeutic use.

FDA Clinical Experience Abstracts
(Dept. HEW, Food and Drug Administration Washington, D.C.)
Abstracts of clinical studies on drugs, devices, cosmetics, food additives, pesticides and nutrients with emphasis on adverse effects, hazards and efficacy.

FDA Suspected Adverse Reactions
(Dept. HEW, Food and Drug Administration Washington, D.C.)
Abstracts of unusual adverse reactions in single patients.

Handbook of *Non-Prescription Drugs*
(Griffenhagen, G. B., Editor)
(American Pharmaceutical Association, Washington, D.C.)
Compilation in tabular form of composition of over-the-counter products with accompanying descriptive monograph on each group of drugs.

Merck Index
(Merck & Co. Rahway, New Jersey)
Monographs of physical and chemical data about chemicals and drugs.

Organisch-Chemische Arzneimittel und ihre Synonyma
(Negwe, M., Editor)
(Akademia-Verlag, Berlin, Germany)
Tables of chemical structures, names and synonyms, and uses of organic chemicals. The book provides for a source of information on German drug products.

The Pharmacological Basis of Therapeutics 4th Ed.
(Goodman, L. S. and Gilman, A.)
(Macmillan Co., New York, New York)
Provides information relative to the activity, use and doses of drugs with particular emphasis upon the relationship of pharmacology to clinical practice.

PharmIndex
(Skyline Publishers P.O. Box 1029 Portland, Oregon)
A compilation of product information including composition, dosage forms, use and cost. Also included are review articles and investigational drug information.

Symptomatology and *Therapy* of *Toxicological Emergencies*

(Academic Press Inc., New York, New York)

Provides an alphabetical listing of toxic substances giving expected reactions and suggested treatment.

Unlisted Drugs

(Unlisted Drugs, Box 401, Chatham, New Jersey)

Contains a numeric and/or alphabetical listing of old and new drug items and for each is presented data pertaining to composition, action, dosage, manufacturer and pertinent reference source.

Drug Interactions

(Hansten, Philip D.)

(Lea & Febiger, Philadelphia, Pa.)

A clinically useful guide to drug-drug interactions and the effects of drugs on clinical laboratory results.

Clinical Toxicology 4th Ed.

(Thienes, C. H. and Haley, T. J.)

(Lea & Febiger, Philadelphia, Pa.)

A grouping of poisons according to their major toxic actions with accompanying method of treatment.

Hazards of *Medication*

(Martin, E. W., Editor)

(Lippincott Co., Philadelphia, Pa.)

A manual on drug interactions, incompatibilities, contraindications and adverse effects of drugs and drug products.

Drug Interactions—1

(American Society of Hospital Pharmacists, Washington, D.C.)

A compilation of abstracts pertaining to drug interactions.

Handbook of Drug Interactions

(Hartshorn, E. A.)

(Hamilton Press Inc., Hamilton, Illinois)

A compilation of articles on drug interactions which have been published in Drug Intelligence.

Drug Information Center

Of late, editors,[7] physicians,[8] pharmacists,[9-11] and administrators[12] have published much data concerning the use and need for adequate drug information in the treatment and care of patients. Many elaborate systems have been developed and put into use by pharmacists in the large teaching centers. In the small community hospital, it is not possible to install or staff such a drug information center. However, it is not impossible to provide the clinical staff with much vital information concerning the use and abuse of drugs, as well as information concerning the drug's chemical nature, mode of action, side effects, dosage forms, cost, and literature pertinent to its clinical use.

14

In addition, the hospital pharmacist is in a position to alert the physician of any untoward reactions encountered within the hospital from the use of the particular drug. All of this information can be provided the physician by the hospital pharmacist through the pharmacy library. This is possible because, in addition to the latest texts and journals, the hospital pharmacist is in daily touch with the medical service representatives of the major drug producers. Much vital literature and information can be gathered from this source if the hospital pharmacist will only avail himself of it. Once gathered, it should be properly catalogued and filed in such a manner as to make it readily available to all those desirous of making use of it.

Large university affiliated hospitals have developed and staffed a new division of the department of pharmacy which is commonly referred to as the **Drug Information Center.** This new concept in hospital pharmacy operations is usually located in a separate section of the pharmacy, contains a large number of reference texts, journals, reprints and brochures, may be equipped with electronic data processing equipment, and has a full-time director and adequate secretarial assistance.

In order to file the vast number of sources of information that are received by the unit, many hospital pharmacists have adopted the classification of drugs employed in the *American Hospital Formulary Service* and thus have a cross-reference between the files and the *Formulary*.

The Drug Information Center may also assume the responsibility of gathering information on all investigation use drugs in current use in the hospital; record all data on drug reactions in the institution; and may participate in the program of the local Poison Information Center. In some hospitals, the Drug Information Center publishes an Investigational Drug Bulletin and an Adverse Drug Reaction Report for the clinical staff.

The need for a reliable local source of drug information within a medical community is of inestimable importance in rendering effective clinical care to the patient. Thus, it behooves every hospital pharmacist to develop a local source of drug information irrespective of whether it be a modest pharmaceutical library or a comprehensive Drug Information Center. The main theme of either type unit should be—providing drug information when it is needed.

Recognizing the need for this type of service to be rendered by the hospital pharmacist, the American Society of Hospital Pharmacists, in 1968, issued a statement entitled *The Hospital Pharmacist and Drug Information Services.* In justification of the involvement of the hospital pharmacist in this endeavor, the statement cites the following:[13]

"1. Traditionally the service orientation of the pharmacist has been related to drugs—their efficacy, safety and control. Therefore, pharmacy encumbers by reason of tradition a special obligation to accept these challenges.
 2. Pharmacy is unique among the health professions in that it possesses an established, but unchallenged, capability to adapt its services for specific contributions to drug therapy. Full utilization of the hospital pharmacist's professional potential represents a more efficient and economical application of health manpower resources.
 3. There exists today a nucleus of hospital pharmacy practitioners who are engaged in the functional establishment of a service foundation for drug information activities and responsibilities. Increasing clinical involvement of the heretofore cloistered hospital pharmacist has precipitated a growing demand for this drug information support to those in immediate contact with drug care needs of the patient.
 4. Increasingly sophisticated concepts of pharmacodynamic and biochemical complexities of drug actions, a burgeoning drug literature, and the scientific and medicolegal difficulties attending clinical surveillance of drug experiences constitute adequate grounds for advocacy of interprofessional teamwork in the clinical use of drugs. Pharmacy's acceptance of its share of responsibility will lessen the formidable burden placed on other components of the health care community."

Clearly, if the profession of pharmacy is to accept the challenge and accompanying responsibility, its practitioners must be capable of performing in their new role. Within the ASHP's statement, the following performance guidelines are presented:[13]

"1. He demonstrates professional and technical competence in the evaluation, critical selection, and utilization of the drug literature. He presents to those whom he serves the maximum relevant information with a minimum volume of pertinent supporting documentation so as to permit independent, informed conclusions and decisions.
 2. His knowledge of institutional and extramural library facilities, literature utilization, and librarian services will permit his taking full advantage of all such resources available to him.
 3. He possesses written and verbal communication skills which enable him to contribute effectively to intra- and inter-institutional dialogue relative to pharmacotherapeutic information.
 4. He has the capacity for substantial contributions to the continuing education of all health professions.
 5. He is involved directly and indirectly in patient care with drugs as a contributor to its continuing quality and as a monitor of its characteristics.

6. He is familiar with electronic data processing methodology to the extent necessary for him to utilize its services for information storage, processing and retrieval.
7. He is qualified to provide professional services in support of the pharmacy and therapeutics committee.
8. He supports, complements and supplements the efforts of colleagues in pharmacy who are now attempting to marshal the knowledge, skills, scientific acumen and professional judgment necessary to bring appropriately effective pharmaceutical services of all types into the mainstream of patient care with drugs. Thus he contributes to and is an integral part of clinical pharmacy practice and the education of clinical pharmacy practitioners.
9. He contributes to the drug literature through appropriate participation in research activities which include, but are not restricted to, (a) clinical and pre-clinical drug studies, (b) surveillance of clinical drug experiences in his institution, and (c) experimentation in professional services."

A review of the literature reveals that drug information services within a hospital are beginning to be created on a more widespread basis. Some of these units are not as well developed as others, however they represent a trend. A good model of a comprehensive in-hospital drug information service is the unit operated within the University of Alabama Hospitals and Clinics.[14]

Regional drug information services or networks are, as yet, not very common. One that is in operation is the Michigan Regional Drug Information Network.[14] Some of the goals of the regional network include the development of a reproducible, standardized reporting system for auditing drug therapy, supplying of information to all hospitals, institutions and health professionals in the region and serving as a prototype for other medical centers and community hospitals wishing to develop similar services.

Specific objectives related to the latter goals were designed to provide:[14]

(1) An analysis of drug information and drug therapy relating to heart disease, cancer, stroke and related diseases and provision of this information to the physician;
(2) A drug information abstract service to physicians in the region regarding new developments in drug therapy and heart disease, cancer, stroke and related diseases;
(3) An analysis and evaluation of the regional utilization of drugs in the institutions served by the network and dissemination of this information to the respective medical staffs for audit; and
(4) A reduction in the lag time existing between the development of new information and the practical application of this information to patient care—.

Of interest to the student are the criteria set forth for participation by other units in the program.[14] They are as follows:

(1) That the director of the pharmacy department be interested in establishing a drug information center, be interested in the possibilities of affiliation with a larger center and be willing to continue the drug information center after the period of grant funding.

(2) That the hospital, in particular the pharmacy department, be willing to accept calls from physicians in the surrounding community and other health professionals and to answer these questions to the best of their ability.

(3) That the affiliated drug information center service an area of sizeable population and not impinge on other affiliate's area of coverage. It was also important that the surrounding community physicians related to this particular hospital for the health care of the community.

(4) That the administrative head of the hospital support a drug information center affiliated with the main center and be willing to continue support to the drug information center at the conclusion of the grant.

(5) That the members of the medical staff, preferably those affiliated with the Pharmacy and Therapeutics Committee, show an interest in support of the network.

(6) That the affiliate be willing to provide twenty-four hours a day, seven days a week coverage.

SELECTED REFERENCES

TERRY, LUTHER L.: The Crisis in Health Communications, Hospitals, J.A.H.A., *38*:12:2, 1964.

ADAMS, SCOTT: Hospital Libraries: Underdeveloped Base for Continuing Education. Hospitals, J.A.H.A., *38*:12:52, 1964.

GEISLER, RAYMOND H. and YAST, HELEN T.: A Survey of Current Hospital Library Resources, Hospitals, J.A.H.A., *38*:12:55, 1964.

KING, CHARLES M., JR. and FLACK, HERBERT L.: A Classification and Filing System for Hospital Pharmacy, Am. J. Hosp. Pharm., *18*:1:31, 1961.

HELLER, WILLIAM M.: Drug Information File Arranged According to AHFS Categories, Am. J. Hosp. Pharm., *18*:1:43, 1961.

SPERANDIO, GLEN J.: Hospital Pharmacy Notes No. 3. May–June 1960— How to Get the Most Out of Medical Literature, an insert in Tile and Till, 46, May–June, 1960.

HANAN, ZACHARY I. and JEFFREY, LOUIS P.: Drug Communications—A Pharmacist's Responsibility, Hosp. Pharm., *1*:1:10, 13, 1966.

CANADA, ANDREW JR.: Drug Information Service—Application to Immediate Patient Care, Hosp. Pharm., *1*:1:10, 13, 1966.

BIBLIOGRAPHY

1. DRYER, B. V.: Lifetime Learning for Physicians, J. Med. Ed., *37*: pt. 2, 1962.
2. GARTLAND, HENRY J.: Blue Print for a Professional Hospital Library, Hospitals, J.A.H.A., *38*:12:58, 1964.

3. DOE, J. and MARSHALL, M. L.: *Handbook of Medical Library Practice*, Chicago, American Library Association, 1956.
4. U.S. Veterans Administration, Basic List of Books and Journals for Veterans Administration Medical Libraries. Program Guide G-14 (Revised), Washington, D.C.: U.S. Government Printing Office.
5. Guide to Information Sources for the Hospital Pharmacist, 1960 Revision, Am. J. Hosp. Pharm., *18*:1:15, 1961.
6. ANDREWS, THEODORA: World List of Pharmacy Periodicals (From a Preliminary Listing by Sinifred Sewell), Am. J. Hosp. Pharm., *20*:2:43, 1963.
7. FRANCKE, LON E.: The Expanding Role of the Hospital Pharmacist in Drug Information Services, Am. J. Hosp. Pharm., *22*:1:32, 1965.
8. PELLEGRINO, E. D.: Drug Information Services and the Clinician, Am. J. Hosp. Pharm., *22*:1:38, 1965.
9. PARKER, PAUL F.: The University of Kentucky Drug Information Center, Am. J. Hosp. Pharm., *22*:1:42, 1965.
10. BURKHOLDER, DAVID F.: Operation of the Drug Information Center at the University of Kentucky, Am. J. Hosp. Pharm., *22*:1:48, 1965.
11. ANDERSON, R. DAVID and LATIOLAIS, CLIFTON J.: The Drug Information Center at the Ohio State University Hospitals, Am. J. Hosp. Pharm., *22*:1:52, 1965.
12. WITTRUP, RICHARD D.: The Responsibility of the Hospital for Drug Information Services, Am. J. Hosp. Pharm., *22*:1:58, 1965.
13. The Hospital Pharmacist and Drug Information Services, Am. J. Hosp. Pharm., *26*:7:381, 1968.
14. Drug Information Services: Two Operational Models, DHEW Publication No. (HSM) 72-3030 Stock No. 1721-0004 Superintendent of Documents, U.S. Printing Office, Washington, D.C. 20402.

Chapter

26

The Role of the Hospital Pharmacist in Educational and Training Programs

BECAUSE of the scope of their activity, their usually high professional standards, the academic accomplishments of the staff as well as their willingness to assume a teaching role has catapulted hospitals into a wide variety of teaching programs. These include undergraduate and graduate programs in medicine, teaching student nurses, licensed practical nurse programs, the training of technologists, physiotherapists, dietitians, administrative residents, social service workers and pharmacists.

Being an integral part of this academic setting, the hospital pharmacist is usually involved in one or more of these programs. It has been reported[1] that the major contribution made by the pharmacist to the hospital's teaching program is his role in the education of student nurses. The same publication further states that hospital pharmacists also take active roles in the training of graduate nurses, undergraduate pharmacy students as well as graduate students in hospital pharmacy programs.

As a matter of fact, the hospital pharmacist, because of his education, training and experience, does partake in both "internal" and "external" teaching ventures. This novel classification of the hospital pharmacist's teaching activity requires further elaboration.

Internal teaching programs are considered to be those which involve the training of student nurses; the conducting of seminars in therapeutics for graduate nurses, house staff members and senior medical staff; and assisting in the education of undergraduate pharmacy students, graduate pharmacy students and residents in hospital administration.

External teaching programs are considered to be those in which the hospital pharmacist is the guest lecturer or speaker, or possibly the sole instructor in charge of a specific course in a school or college.

Examples of external type programs are courses in colleges of pharmacy, refresher courses under the auspices of a college of pharmacy, seminars, institutes or conventions which are sponsored by professional associations.

Professional Education of the Hospital Pharmacist

In order that the hospital pharmacist effectively become engaged in the teaching and training of other personnel, he must himself be qualified by virtue of degrees as well as by experience.

Francke *et al.*[2] have shown that the majority of the chief pharmacists practicing today hold either a Graduate in Pharmacy (Ph.G.), Pharmaceutical Chemist (Ph.C.), or Bachelor of Science degree. A small number of practitioners also hold Master of Science, Doctor of Pharmacy, Doctor of Science, or Doctor of Philosophy degrees.

Because of the efforts of the colleges of pharmacy to graduate competent practitioners, it should not be too long before the trend will be towards the opposite end of the spectrum, namely, that the majority of the chief pharmacists will hold graduate degrees.

In the meantime, there does exist a shortage of hospital pharmacy practitioners and an attempt must be made to satisfy the need with what is available. In fact, the present graduate of the five-year curriculum, although holding only a Bachelor of Science degree, is reasonably well qualified to assume a certain amount of teaching responsibility particularly in those non-metropolitan, non-university affiliated community institutions. It is safe to say that, in these hospitals, relatively few members of the staff, with the exception of the medical and dental staff, hold graduate degrees.

The modern five-year program provides the pharmacist with a broad training in the biological, chemical, and pharmaceutical sciences. In addition an opportunity is provided for the acquisition of knowledge in the areas of statistics, management, marketing, and higher mathematics.

Those practitioners who presently hold the Master of Science degree (the present graduate degree in hospital pharmacy) have completed, in addition to the courses referred to in a sample five-year summary,[3] at least thirty-credit hours of graduate work in courses in hospital pharmacy, physical chemistry and advanced pharmacology. In addition, the curriculum requires a minimum of 2,000 clock hours of practice in hospitals to meet the *Accreditation Standard for Residency in Hospital Pharmacy,* approved by the Board of Directors of the American Society of Hospital Pharmacists in April of 1970 which provides the following definitions and qualifications:[12]

I. DEFINITION

A pharmacy residency in a hospital is a post-graduate program of organized training that meets the requirements set forth and approved by the American Society of Hospital Pharmacists in this Standard.

II. QUALIFICATIONS OF THE TRAINING HOSPITAL

A. The hospital shall be a general hospital accredited by the Joint Commission on Accreditation of Hospitals or the American Osteopathic Association.

B. Pharmacy residencies shall be conducted only in those hospitals in which the educational benefits to the resident are considered of paramount importance in relation to the service benefits which the hospital may obtain from the resident.

III. QUALIFICATIONS OF PHARMACY SERVICE

A. The pharmacy department shall be organized in accordance with the principles of good management under the direction of a legally qualified pharmacist and with sufficient appropriate personnel to carry out a broad scope of pharmacy services within the hospital and for the patient, and shall comply (where applicable) with all federal, state and local laws, codes, statutes and regulations.

B. There shall be at least one full time, legally qualified pharmacist for each resident.

C. The pharmacy department shall have adequate facilities to carry out a broad scope of service in the following areas of professional and administrative activity:

1. Departmental Administration
2. Outpatient Dispensing and Control
3. Inpatient Drug Distribution and Control
4. Formulation, Preparation and Control of Sterile Dose Forms
5. Formulation, Preparation and Control of Nonsterile Products
6. Drug Information Services
7. Clinical Services in Patient Care Areas

It is necessary that a regular and continuing experience be provided in these activities and it is not sufficient to create "artificial situations" for residents to obtain this experience.

If one of the designated activities or divisions of pharmaceutical practice is not available in the training hospital, arrangements shall be made with a hospital or facility acceptable to the AMERICAN SOCIETY OF HOSPITAL PHARMACISTS to provide the necessary experience.

D. The pharmacist-in-charge shall have the responsibility and the authority to carry out a broad scope of professional service.

E. The pharmacist-in-charge shall be a member of and actively participate in the pharmacy and therapeutics committee of the medical staff.

IV. QUALIFICATIONS OF THE PRECEPTOR

A. The pharmacist-in-charge of the hospital pharmacy shall be the preceptor of the residency training program and shall be subject to similar overall administrative control and guidance employed by the hospital for medical, dental, dietetic and other similar training programs.

B. The preceptor of the training program shall have completed a pharmacy residency in a hospital accredited by the AMERICAN SOCIETY OF HOSPITAL PHARMACISTS and have had two years of administrative experience in a hospital pharmacy, or have had at least five years experience in a pharmacy meeting the Minimum Standard for Pharmacies in Hospitals, a significant part of which experience should have been of an administrative nature.

C. The preceptor shall have demonstrated capabilities in the operation of a pharmacy service and made significant contributions to the development or improvement of hospital pharmacy practice.

D. The preceptor shall be an active member of the American Pharmaceutical Association and the AMERICAN SOCIETY OF HOSPITAL PHARMACISTS, and the local or state affiliated chapters of the SOCIETY. All other pharmacists on the staff should also hold active membership in these organizations.

V. QUALIFICATIONS AND SELECTION OF THE APPLICANT

A. The applicant shall be a graduate of a school of pharmacy accredited by the American Council on Pharmaceutical Education.
The applicant may begin residency training at the completion of the fifth academic year in those residency programs associated with a school of pharmacy in which the six-year pharmacy program is offered.

B. The applicant shall be recommended by his college faculty and/or previous employers.

C. The resident shall be a member of the American Society of Hospital Pharmacists.

D. Final approval of the qualifications of the applicant and his acceptance shall be the responsibility of the preceptor.

VI. RESIDENCY TRAINING SCHEDULE*

A. The resident shall participate in a predetermined and regular schedule under supervision in the following activities of pharmacy service for the minimum numbers of hours indicated:

1. Departmental Administration ....200 hr
2. Outpatient Dispensing and Control ....100 hr
3. Inpatient Drug Distribution and Control ....300 hr
4. Formulation, Preparation and Control of Sterile Dose Forms ....100 hr
5. Formulation, Preparation and Control of Nonsterile Products ....100 hr
6. Drug Information Service ....100 hr
7. Clinical Services in Patient Care Areas ......100 hr
8. Collateral and Interdepartmental Activities 100 hr
9. Lectures, Conferences and Seminars ......100 hr

B. The training schedule shall consist of a minimum of 2000 hours training time, extending over a period of 50 weeks or longer.

Each resident's activities shall be scheduled in advance.

Evidence sufficient to demonstrate implementation of the training schedule must be available for each resident in a manner and format which clearly delineates the scope and period of training.

VII. CERTIFICATION

A. An appropriate certificate indicative of successful completion of the prescribed residency shall be awarded to the resident by the hospital.

Having established a pharmacy residency program in the hospital, it is desirable to have the program accredited. The American Society of Hospital Pharmacists maintains an accreditation program under the direction of its *Council on Education and Training*. In April of 1970, the ASHP issued its *Statement on Accreditation of Pharmacy Residencies in Hospitals*. Because of its value to the practitioner in determining the quality of his educational program, it is hereinafter reproduced:[13]

Preamble

Hospital pharmacists have from the beginning of their formal association recognized the need for perpetuating and improving

---

* An elaboration upon this Standard, including specific activities in which the resident should receive instruction and experience, and specific criteria used in evaluation of hospital pharmacy residency training programs, is contained in the *Guide to Interpretation and Use for Accreditation Standard for Pharmacy Residency in a Hospital,* available from the Department of Education and Training, American Society of Hospital Pharmacists.

their specialty through organized training programs. Early in its history the AMERICAN SOCIETY OF HOSPITAL PHARMACISTS supported the development of training programs in hospital pharmacy and promulgated standards for residency in hospital pharmacy. To insure adherence to the principles and philosophy of these standards an accreditation program is established by the SOCIETY.

Objectives

The accreditation program shall have as its objectives (1) to improve the professional competency of hospital pharmacy practitioners through organized educational training programs; (2) to guide, assist and recognize those hospitals that wish to support the profession by operating such programs; (3) to provide criteria for the prospective resident in the selection of a program; and (4) to provide hospitals and related health agencies a basis for determining the level of competency of pharmacists in hospitals.

Definition

For the purpose of accreditation, the residency in hospital pharmacy is defined as an organized postgraduate training program, educational in nature, which meets the Accreditation Standard for Pharmacy Residency in a Hospital of the AMERICAN SOCIETY OF HOSPITAL PHARMACISTS. These programs shall be organized and conducted in such a manner as to develop special skills and competency in hospital pharmacy, far beyond the legal requirements for licensure.

Authority

The accreditation of hospital pharmacy residency programs is established by authority of the Board of Directors of the AMERICAN SOCIETY OF HOSPITAL PHARMACISTS under the direction of the Council on Education and Training.

All matters of policy relating to the accreditation program will be considered by the Council on Education and Training and will be submitted for approval to the Board of Directors of the SOCIETY

The Council on Education and Training shall review and evaluate applications and survey reports submitted. Recommendations of the Council will be referred to the Board of Directors for appropriate action.

Policies

The following policies shall apply to the accreditation program:
1. The accreditation program shall be conducted as a service of the AMERICAN SOCIETY OF HOSPITAL PHARMACISTS without charge to participating hospitals.
2. Hospitals desiring accreditation must voluntarily request evaluation of their program.

3. To be eligible for accreditation, a program must have been in operation for one year and have at least one graduate. (If accreditation is granted, it shall be retroactive to the date on which a valid and complete application, including all requested supporting documents, is received by the SOCIETY's Department of Education and Training.)
4. Accredited programs will be reexamined at least every three years.
5. Any major change in the organization of a program will be considered justification for reevaluation.
6. Programs shall be reviewed by an accreditation survey team consisting of at least two individuals, one of whom shall be the Director of the SOCIETY's Department of Education and Training. The other may be a member of the Council on Education and Training (preferably) or Board of Directors who is not from the same geographic area as the hospital being surveyed, or has no other conflict of interest which would prejudice him or cause him personal embarrassment.
7. A certificate of accreditation will be issued for a period not to exceed three years; however, the certificate remains the property of the AMERICAN SOCIETY OF HOSPITAL PHARMACISTS and shall be returned to the Society at any time accreditation is withdrawn or withheld.
8. Accredited programs without a resident in training for a period of three consecutive years will have accreditation withdrawn and must submit a new application and undergo reevaluation to regain accreditation.
9. Accreditation shall not be withdrawn without first notifying the hospital of the specific reasons why its program does not meet the SOCIETY's Accreditation Standard for Pharmacy Residency in a Hospital. In such instances, the hospital shall be granted an appropriate specified period of time to correct deficiencies.
10. The hospital shall have the right to appeal the decision of the Board of Directors.
11. Any reference by a hospital to accreditation by the SOCIETY in catalogues, bulletins, communications or other form of publicity shall state only the following: "(Name of Hospital) is accredited for residency in hospital pharmacy by the AMERICAN SOCIETY OF HOSPITAL PHARMACISTS."
12. A list of all accredited programs and residents in training shall be published periodically in the AMERICAN JOURNAL OF HOSPITAL PHARMACY.

Procedure

1. Application forms may be requested from:
    American Society of Hospital Pharmacists
    Department of Education and Training
    4630 Montgomery Avenue
    Washington, D.C. 20014
    These should be filled out in duplicate by the hospital seek-

ing accreditation. Return one copy of the application to the Society. Deadline dates for receipt of completed applications, including all requested supporting documents, are June 1 and December 1 of each year.

2. At a mutually convenient time the Society will send a survey team to review the hospital pharmacy and the residency program.

3. The application and the report of the surveyors will be reviewed and evaluated by the Council on Education and Training.

4. Recommendation will be made to the Board of Directors of the Society for appropriate action.

5. The hospital will be notified of any action taken by the Board of Directors not later than twelve months from the first deadline date following receipt of its completed application by the Department of Education and Training.

6. Hospitals wishing to appeal the decision of the Board of Directors must submit the appeal, in writing, to the Board of Directors within 60 days of receipt of notification.

Having established a sufficient background to permit the hospital pharmacist of today to assume a role in the teaching function of his hospital, it is necessary to dwell briefly upon the specific areas of internal and external teaching in which the hospital pharmacist may or should become involved.

Internal Teaching Programs

Training of Student Nurses

Much has been written concerning the role of the pharmacist in the teaching of student nurses. Some advocate that the hospital pharmacist should teach student nurses the entire course in pharmaceutical calculations and pharmacology; others propose that he undertake to teach certain aspects of these courses in conjunction with the nursing instructor.

How much or how little a hospital pharmacist teaches will depend upon the individual and the environment in which he operates. If the individual is capable and has so impressed the nurse educators by his daily actions and deeds, he will be invited, more likely than not, to assist in the teaching program. Once appointed to this responsibility, it behooves the hospital pharmacist to develop his phase of the program in strict compliance with the requirements set forth by the nursing accreditation authorities.

Furthermore, the prepared lectures should be updated each year —to include the latest developments in pharmacology and therapeutics; the nomenclature used and all references to weights and measures should be in accord with the hospital's drug formulary; and finally any reference to dosage, contraindications or cautions should also comply with the formulary unless the information to be presented supersedes the latest revision of the hospital formulary.

Many authors[4-6] have published special texts on the subject of pharmacology and therapeutics for nurses. These texts are in use in various schools of nursing and may serve as an excellent guide to the hospital pharmacist who undertakes the responsibility to teach these courses to student nurses.

In addition, hospital pharmacists should consult the various textbooks in pharmacology which are written for basic nursing students. Failure to do this may result in the preparation of a course, so sophisticated in content, that it will defeat the purpose of its presentation.

Seminars for Graduate Nurses, House Staff and Medical Staff

Although most pharmacists disseminate information to the members of the medical and nursing staffs via a pharmacy publication, there is still need for the direct or personal presentation which is afforded by conducting a seminar on the latest available therapeutic agents to the medical staff.

With regard to such a program, Sperandio[7] has stated that:

"The key to its success would be proper organization and presentation of the material. Ideally, the talk should be short (not over twenty minutes), complete, and concise. The subject should be covered in such a way that the audience can integrate all the facts and thereby obtain an appreciation of the many facets of drug therapy. Time should be allowed for discussion."

Frazier *et al.*[8] functioning as the 1954 Committee on Minimum Standards of the American Society of Hospital Pharmacists developed an outline of four lectures which may be presented by the hospital pharmacist to the resident staff.

Lecture One of this series concerns itself with an orientation to pharmacy services and covers such subject matter as:

> *a.* Location of the pharmacy
> *b.* A description of the physical plant
> *c.* Personnel
> *d.* Hours of operation
> *e.* Services provided by the department
> *f.* Hospital policies governing:
> > i. Formulary
> > ii. Use of generic names
> > iii. Use of the metric system
> > iv. Use of abbreviations
> > v. Use of research drugs
> > vi. Automatic stop orders
> > vii. Discharge medications
> > viii. Ordering narcotics and liquors

Lecture Two of the series is devoted to the philosophy and goals of the formulary system. In the course of the lecture, the hospital pharmacist should emphasize the composition of and the scope of the Pharmacy and Therapeutics Committee.

Lecture Three is suggested to take the form of a prescription clinic. Basically, this is an excellent suggestion and is highly recommended in view of the fact that very little attention is devoted to prescription writing in medical school classes. In the course of the lecture, the pharmacist should stress any Federal, state and hospital regulations governing the prescribing of drugs and the refilling of prescriptions. Past experience has also demonstrated that a short period of time devoted to a group criticism of prescriptions (projected onto a screen) which contain illegible writing, non-standard abbreviations, misplaced decimal points, misspelling of drug names and a mixture of English and Latin directions is extremely helpful in emphasizing the importance of accuracy in writing a prescription.

Lecture Four is reserved for a discussion of any topic of current interest to the staff. Suggested topics for this discussion include the following:

    i. Cost of medication
   ii. Incompatibilities of intravenous fluids
       and other injectable drugs
  iii. The new drug regulations
  iv. Drug interactions

Graduate nurses are encouraged to attend all in-service training programs offered within the hospital. These sessions are devoted to a wide spectrum of professional subjects. The hospital pharmacist should avail himself of the opportunity to present a few of the programs. His subject matter may consist of a discussion of new classes of therapeutic agents, incompatibilities of various drugs when added to intravenous solutions, drug storage and control, a review of the mathematics of pharmacy, or drug interactions.

Whatever the subject matter, it behooves the pharmacist to prepare the lecture adequately and where possible supplement the talk with slides, a short film, the distribution of an outline of the lecture, or the distribution of reprints or selected brochures describing the drugs lectured upon.

In addition, whenever new drugs are discussed, one should bring into the lecture room sample containers of the various forms which are commercially available. It is assumed that by actually handling, observing, smelling and where possible tasting the product, the nurse will be in a better position to detect an error should a mix-up in medication occur.

Training Undergraduate Students in Hospital Pharmacy

Blauch and Webster,[9] in The Pharmaceutical Curriculum, published in 1952 by the American Council on Education as a report for the Committee on Curriculum of the American Association of Colleges of Pharmacy, state:

> "It is a source of considerable surprise to note that only a few colleges of pharmacy have developed working arrangements with hospitals for teaching purposes. One finds colleges of pharmacy in universities which have also large teaching hospitals but in which the colleges have no connection whatever with the pharmaceutical service. No doubt this situation reflects the traditional educational emphasis on the retail pharmacy, which for a long time has been the principal means of pharmaceutical service. With the changes which are apparently impending in health service, the hospital pharmacy will almost certainly play an increasing role. Colleges of pharmacy may well note this fact and plan their instructions accordingly."

Since the publication of the above report, the American Association of Colleges of Pharmacy and the American Society of Hospital Pharmacists have approved a **Statement on the Abilities Required of Hospital Pharmacists.**[10] This statement lists six specialized areas of competence that should be considered in developing a curriculum for hospital pharmacy. These are as follows:

Specifically the well-qualified hospital pharmacist must have:

1. A thorough knowledge of drugs and their actions.
2. Ability to develop and conduct a pharmaceutical manufacturing program.
3. An intimate knowledge of control procedures.
4. Ability to conduct and participate in research.
5. Ability to conduct teaching and in-service training programs.
6. Ability to administer and manage a hospital pharmacy.

Therefore the Joint Committee of the American Association of Colleges of Pharmacy and the American Society of Hospital Pharmacists prepared, in January 1966, a **Syllabus for a Course in Hospital Pharmacy** and, in April 1966, these same organizations approved a **Suggested Guide to Curriculum Development for Hospital Pharmacy.**

With these tools in hand, the hospital pharmacist should take the initiative and meet with the college administration and faculty for the purpose of commencing a program in hospital pharmacy. At this meeting, the hospital pharmacist should point out the fact that his department offers the prospective student a wealth of experience in the professional practice of his profession.

Patient Teaching Program

This is one area of in-hospital teaching where the pharmacist can make a valuable contribution to the long term posthospital care of the patient. More frequently than not, patients leave the hospital with a variety of discharge medications with a meager knowledge of how they are to be used or, more importantly, how to recognize signs of toxicity or adverse reaction. This brief exposure to the medications is generally provided by the busy practitioner or a nurse.

Of late, those hospitals who have recruited clinical pharmacists to their staffs have developed extensive programs for the orientation of the patient to the subject of drug use both in the hospital and in the patient's home. These programs have consisted of patient counseling, development of instructional brochures, group conferences and closed circuit television presentations. Where the instruction needs to be individualized—as in the use of an individual's specific medication—the direct counseling technique is employed. However, where instruction of a general nature is to be given—such as how to detect adverse drug effects—the group discussion or television methodology is employed.

Training Clinical Pharmacists

With the development of this specialty within the profession of pharmacy, hospital pharmacists should work closely with the college of pharmacy and the college of medicine faculties as well as the various medical staff specialists in the conduct of such programs. Insofar as the clinical pharmacy programs are concerned, many schools have created specialization within the broad area of clinical pharmacy—pediatrics, clinical pharmacology, toxicology, drug information analysis and interpretation, infectious disease and geriatrics.

The hospital pharmacist, if he himself is unable to provide the training, should arrange to have the student acquainted with the contents of the medical record, drug history procedures, patient drug profile program, drug information center, poison control center, adverse drug reaction program and the opportunity to interface with interdisciplinary health care personnel such as physicians, dentists, nurses, dietitians and therapists. Of paramount importance, is the pharmacist's exposure to the patient—both ambulatory and hospitalized. Thus, the training of clinical pharmacists need not be limited to the hospital proper but may include the satellite health care centers, nursing homes, extended care facilities, home care programs and clinics.

Training Residents in Hospital Administration

Today, a relatively large number of universities maintain programs for the education of individuals desirous of a career in hospital administration. Candidates for the degree of *Master in Hospital Administration* must, in addition to the didactic requirements, serve a residency in an approved institution under the guidance of a preceptor.

While serving this residency, the neophyte administrator is exposed to the function and operation of every department in the hospital. Because it is at this time that the young administrator forms his opinion as to the organization and scope of the pharmacy department, as well as the responsibilities of the hospital pharmacist, the American Society of Hospital Pharmacists undertook, through its *Committee on Pharmacy in Hospital Administration Education,* to prepare a course outline to be used by the hospital pharmacist in presenting his image to the trainee in hospital administration.

In 1963, the then *Committee on Pharmacy in Hospital Administration Education* proposed an outline for the teaching of these students. The said outline is hereby presented in detail.[11]

I. Development of Hospital Pharmacy
   1. Influence of increased use of drugs
   2. Influence of the newer pharmaceuticals on the pharmacist's skills
   3. Influence of pharmaceutical associations
   4. Influence of all levels of pharmaceutical educational programs

II. Organization
   1. Establish a hospital department or purchase an outside service
   2. Personnel
      a. Education and qualifications
      b. Departmental organization
      c. Possibility of dual function in smaller hospitals: *e.g.* Pharmacist-Purchasing Agent; Pharmacist-Central Sterile Supply Coordinator
   3. Interdepartmental Relationships
      a. Administration
      b. Nursing
      c. Laboratories
      d. Miscellaneous
   4. Special relationship to the medical staff
      a. Pharmacy and Therapeutics Committee
      b. Control of research drugs
      c. Pharmacy bulletins

III. Physical Facilities and Design*
    1. General considerations
      a. Location
      b. Size
    2. Dispensing Areas
      a. In-patient
      b. Out-patient
      c. Ancillary supplies
    3. Compounding Areas
      a. Extemporaneous compounding
      b. Bulk compounding
      c. Sterile preparations
    4. Storage Areas
      a. General
      b. Narcotics
      c. Alcohol
      d. Special
    5. Administrative Areas
      a. Offices
      b. Library

IV. Responsibilities of the Pharmacist
    1. Administrative
    Budget, purchasing, inventory control, records, and reports
    2. Professional
    Dispensing, compounding, drug consultant role, teaching and research
    3. Legal
    Federal, state, local as they apply to alcohol, narcotics, dangerous drugs, poisons, pharmacy
    4. Ethical
      a. The patient
      b. The physician
      c. The hospital
      d. The community pharmacists

V. The Hospital Formulary System
    1. Guiding principles
    2. Philosophy of the Pharmacy and Therapeutics Committee
    3. The American Hospital Formulary Service
    4. The private formulary, its advantages and disadvantages

VI. Sources of Information†
    1. Pharmaceutical organizations

* Minimum Standard for Pharmacies in Hospitals, Am. J. Hosp. Pharm., *15*:4: 310, 1958.

†Special literature and reference material relative to the pharmacy department of a hospital are available to the administrative resident from the:

    American Society of Hospital Pharmacists
    4630 Montgomery Avenue
    Washington, D.C.

2. Pharmaceutical literature
   a. "Tentative Draft of An Outline for Teaching Students in Hospital Administration," Bull. Am. Soc. Hosp. Pharm., 8:357, 1951
   b. "Syllabus for a Course in Hospital Pharmacy," Bull. Am. Soc. Hosp. Pharm. 12:261, 1955.

External Teaching Programs

As has been previously stated, an external teaching program consists of any teaching activity performed by the pharmacist outside the hospital.

Most chief pharmacists in university-affiliated teaching hospitals hold appointments on the faculty of the associated college of pharmacy. In this capacity, the hospital pharmacist may and usually does teach courses other than hospital pharmacy. These include product development, preparation of parenteral products, sterilization technics and pharmacology.

Participation in seminars, institutes and refresher courses is another way in which the hospital pharmacist may carry on a teaching program. The sponsors of these programs do not necessarily have to be pharmaceutical organizations. As a matter of fact, participation in the activities of nursing, dietary, oxygen therapist and medical technologist associations does much to improve the professional stature of the hospital pharmacist.

Teaching, in its broadest interpretation, need not be restricted to personal lectures but may include the preparation of manuscripts for publication in the professional press. The subject matter may consist of the results of original scientific research in product development, sterilization technics; or comprehensive literature surveys in a particular area of hospital pharmacy; or the results of a study which improves the managerial and service rendering aspects of the department.

Some hospital pharmacists have been sufficiently progressive to obtain various grants-in-aid to support research in drug distribution technics or in studying the prescribing habits of physicians associated with large hospital clinics. Certainly this kind of basic study, when completed and published, serves as teaching material, for it is in this way that other pharmacists learn to improve the service they render to their institutions.

Drug Abuse Teaching Program

Hospital and clinical pharmacists can make a worthy contribution towards the education of the hospital's staff, employees, patients and students enrolled in the various teaching programs on the issues of drug abuse. In addition, the pharmacists should make themselves available to lecture on the subject to community agencies and other interested groups.

Generally, the drug information center of the department of pharmacy possesses the necessary drug abuse information as well as references to sources of additional teaching aids such as slides, films and film strips.

In addition to conducting lectures and conferences on the subject, displays can be prepared for showing in the hospital, local schools and in the library of the city or town. Also, training of out-of-hospital personnel who are interested in the drug abuse problem—school teachers, clergy men, law enforcement officials and members of the community at large—should be undertaken as part of the overall teaching program of the hospital pharmacy department.

SELECTED REFERENCES

PARKS, L. M.: Recruitment Tools, J. Am. Pharm. Assoc. Pract. Ed., *20*:5: 262, 1959.

FRANCKE, DON E.: The Philosophy and Objectives of Internship Training Am. J. Hosp. Pharm., *20*:4:172, 1963.

LACHNER, BERNARD J.: Role of the Hospital in Internship Training, Am. J. Hosp. Pharm., *20*:4:182, 1963.

FRAZIER, WALTER M.: The Responsibility of the Preceptor in Internship Training, Am. J. Hosp. Pharm., *20*:4:186, 1963.

PARKER, PAUL F.: The Extent of Facilities and Broad Scope of Service, Am. J. Hosp. Pharm., *20*:4:191, 1963.

LATIOLAIS, CLIFTON J.: The Use of Management Tools in Hospital Pharmacy Internship Training, Am. J. Hosp. Pharm., *20*:4:194, 1963.

FLACK, HERBERT L.: A Planned and Scheduled Experience Program as One Characteristic of Strong Training Programs, Am. J. Hosp. Pharm., *20*:4: 196, 1963.

GORRELL, JOHN and OLSZEWSKI, DELL: The Role of the Hospital Pharmacist in the Education of Medical Interns and Residents, Am. J. Hosp. Pharm., *23*:3:151, 1966.

BIBLIOGRAPHY

1. FRANCKE, D. E., LATIOLAIS, C. J., FRANCKE, G. N. and HO, N. F. H.: *Mirror To Hospital Pharmacy*, Easton, Penna., Mack Printing Co., p. 132, 1964.
2. Ibid., page 158.
3. Massachusetts College of Pharmacy Bulletin, Catalogue Number 1965-66 *54*:32, 1965.
4. FRAZIER, WALTER, *et al.*: 1954 Report of the A.S.H.P. Committee on Minimum Standards, The Bulletin, A.S.H.P., *12*:4:449, 1955.
4. FALCONER, MARY W. and PATTERSON, R. ROBERT: *Current Drug Handbook*, Philadelphia, W. B. Saunders Co., 1960.

5. WRIGHT, HAROLD N. and MONTAG, MILDRED: *A Textbook of Pharmacology and Therapeutics,* Philadelphia, W. B. Saunders Co., 1959.
6. MEHTA, H. R.:   *Pharmacy for Nurses,* St. Louis, C. V. Mosby Co., 1961.
7. SPERANDIO, GLEN J.:   Pharmacy Seminars Within the Hospital, *Hospital Pharmacy Notes* No. 5, September/October, 1960, Eli Lilly & Co., Indianapolis, Ind.
8. FRAZIER, WALTER *et al.*:   1954 Report of the A.S.H.P., Committee on Minimum Standards, The Bulletin, A.S.H.P., *12*:4:454, 1955.
9. BLAUCH, L. E. and WEBSTER, G. L.:   The Pharmaceutical Curriculum. A report prepared for the Committee on Curriculum of the American Association of Colleges of Pharmacy, American Council on Education, 1952.
10. Statement of Abilities Required of Hospital Pharmacists, Am. J. Hosp. Pharm., *19*:9:493, 1962.
11. Report of Committee on Pharmacy in Hospital Administration Education, Am. J. Hosp. Pharm., *20*:4:407, 1963.
12. Accreditation Standard for Pharmacy Residency in a Hospital, Am. J. Hosp. Pharm. *28*:3:189, 1971.
13. Statement on Accreditation of Pharmacy Residencies in Hospitals, Am. J. Hosp. Pharm., *28*:3:187, 1971.

Chapter

27

Preparation of the Annual Report

THE preparation of an annual report to the Administrator of the hospital on the activities of the department of pharmacy is one of the most important responsibilities of the hospital pharmacist. In addition, it is the pharmacist's duty to prepare the report in such a manner as to make it an informative yet analytical document covering the activities of the past fiscal year.

Present day managerial practices dictate that there must be adequate communication between all levels of management. It is said that without the free flow of proper information the particular enterprise cannot possibly progress to its maximal capacity. This basic principle of good management should obviously be applied in the hospital. Certainly, the hospital pharmacist can take the first step in the application of this basic principle by the preparation of a comprehensive annual report on the activities of his department.

Too many pharmacists, although they recognize this aspect of their work, refrain from the preparation of such a report because they feel that the administration is not interested in receiving one, or since no other department head submits a report, why should they be different.

The reader is hereby assured of the administration's desire for such a report and is also reminded that the pharmacist should be the leader in any movement, direct or indirect, which leads towards improvement of the hospital and the care which it renders to its patients.

The Format

There is no specific format which can be recommended for general use. The format should reflect the creativeness and the ingenuity of the author however, artwork and fancy design work should be avoided. Because the annual report properly belongs in the category of "business document," it should present such an appearance to the recipient.

In general, the report should be typewritten on white bond paper.

The typewriter ribbon should be black and the use of red letters or underlining should be avoided.

It is also recommended that the report document be properly identified as to content and author, therefore a front page showing this information as well as a table of contents are in order. Once the body of the report document is completed, all tables and pages should be numbered for the convenience of the reader.

Contents

Because each hospital and hospital pharmacy are different, so too are the contents of the reports submitted in each institution.

Accordingly, in the following discussion, a number of subjects will be covered which may be considered for incorporation into an annual report if they have application to the individual hospital or pharmacy department.

Some of the areas or subjects which may be incorporated into the pharmacist-in-chief's annual report are as follows:

I. *Introduction*

The introductory remarks should be brief and be confined to a statement of introduction and transmittal.

II. *The Pharmacy and Therapeutics Committee*

Because the pharmacist serves as the secretary of this committee he is in the best position to report on its activities. The report should include a statement on the present membership, the number of meetings held, programs undertaken by the Committee and plans for the new fiscal year.

III. *The Formulary*

A brief report on the hospital formulary is always in order. It should include a general review of the revisions made, that is, additions or deletions, and a statement concerning plans or the progress being made relative to a total revision and publication.

IV. *The Pharmacy Bulletin*

Comments on the pharmacy publication are desirable as a means of keeping the administration informed of this extracurricular activity. The pharmacist should briefly relate the number of times the paper was published during the past year and any truly worthy comments concerning the publication or its contents made by the professional staff.

V. *Teaching Activities*

If the pharmacist is engaged in the teaching programs of the hospital, the report should contain a resume of his activities in the teaching of student nurses, graduate nurses, interns and residents as well as the interns in the hospital pharmacy training program.

VI. *Professional Activities*
    Attendance at seminars, conferences or other professional meetings as well as a documentation of papers given or published are in order.

VII. *Personnel*
    Additions or departures from the staff may well be reported, particularly if those who have left have been appointed to positions of prestige and merit and to stress the accomplishments and the quality of the newcomers to the hospital staff.

VIII. *Business Statistics*
    This section of the report will probably comprise a large portion of the report if the pharmacist has had the foresight to accumulate the necessary data.
    Although some of the financial data which will be included in this section may also be provided to the Administration by the Comptroller, it should nevertheless be repeated here in order to present a total picture rather than force the busy administrator to seek the information in an ancillary document.
    The following will serve to acquaint the student and the hospital pharmacist with the type of statistical data which can be accumulated and presented in an annual report:

GENERAL STATISTICS

Opening Inventory Value ....
Closing Inventory Value ....
Rate of Inventory Turn-over ....
Income ....
Expenses ....
Ratio of Income to Expenses ....
Number of Pharmacists Employed ....
Average Income Generated/Pharmacist ....
Number of Hours of Service/Week ....
Gross Revenue/Hour of Service ....

IN-PATIENT PRESCRIPTION DATA

Number of Requisitions Dispensed ....
    a. Total Number of Items Ordered.....................
    b. Average Number Items/Requisition ....
    c. Total Dollar Value of Items Dispensed...........
    d. Cost to Hospital of (*c*) ....

OUT-PATIENT PRESCRIPTION DATA

Number of Ambulatory Patient
Prescriptions Dispensed ....
    a. New Prescriptions ....

    b. Refill Prescriptions ....

    c. Total Gross Income ....

        i. Cash ....

        ii. Charge ....

        iii. Free ....

    d. Average Price/Prescription ....

MANUFACTURING PROGRAM STATISTICS

Number of Products Manufactured ....

Number of Gallons of Liquids ....

Number of Pounds of Powders ....

Number of Pounds of Ointments ....

Number of Capsules (Hand filled) ....

Number of Capsules (Machine filled) ....

Number of Vials of Sterile Injectables ....

Number of Units of Large Volume Parenterals ....

Number of Units of Irrigating Fluids ....

The difference between the potential purchase price and the cost of manufacturing within the Hospital Pharmacy resulted in a savings to the Hospital of ....

UNIT DOSE AND IV ADDITIVE SERVICE

Number of Solid Dose Units Packaged ....

Number of Liquid Single Dose Units Packaged ....

Number of Syringes Pre-filled ....

Number of IV Additive Solutions Prepared ....

Number of Hyperalimentations Prepared ....

GENERAL HOSPITAL AND LABORATORY REQUISITION DATA

Number of Requisitions Filled ....

Number of Items Dispensed ....

Average Number of Items per Requisition ....

Dollar Value (based on cost to hospital) ....

IX. *Drug Information Center*

    A brief report concerning the addition of new subscriptions to journals or the purchase of new book or computer drug information services which may be of benefit to other segments of the hospital population should also be considered for inclusion.

X. *Drug Surveillance and Utilization Review*

    Because of the importance of these two aspects of drug control, the pharmacist's annual report should inform the administration of its effectiveness. This can best be accomplished by abstracting the minutes of the Drug Utilization Review Committee, if one is in existence, or that portion of the minutes of the Pharmacy and Therapeutics Committee dealing with the subject.[1,2]

XI. *Training Programs*

In order to obviate the impression that the Department of Pharmacy is solely a service unit, it is important to highlight the various teaching roles and functions of the department.

XII. *Proposed New Programs*

The report should be brought to a close with a brief discussion of proposed new programs or activities for the new fiscal year. These programs should not be discussed in detail in this report. The main purpose for including them here is to demonstrate that the pharmacist is always striving for better performance and higher goals and is not satisfied with a status quo policy no matter how satisfactory the past fiscal year may have been.

From the preceding discussion, it should be apparent to all concerned that the preparation of an annual report requires a great deal of preparation and planning. Properly prepared, it will enhance the professional stature of the pharmacist in the hospital.

SELECTED REFERENCES

RITA, SR. M.: Information Flow from Pharmacy to Administration, Hospitals, J.A.H.A., *38*:16:110. 1964.

LANTOS, R. L.: Responsibilities of the Chief Pharmacist to Hospital Administration, Hosp. Management, *85*:3:40, 1958.

STRICKER, SR. L.: Value of a Check List of Administrative Pharmacy Duties Am. J. Hosp. Pharm., *19*:1:18, 1962.

BIBLIOGRAPHY

1. LAVENTURIER, MARC: Utilization and Peer Review by Pharmacists, J. A.Ph.A., NS*12*:4:166, 1972.
   171, 1972.
2. BOISSEREE, VICTOR R. A Case Study in Peer Review, J. A.Ph.A. NS*12*:4:

Chapter

28

Safe Use of Medications in the Hospital

THE legal literature is replete with cases of injury or death caused by errors in the administration of medications. These unfortunate incidents are not restricted to occurrences within hospitals, but also in doctor's offices, clinics, retail pharmacies and in the home. Furthermore, these mistakes do not always show doctors, nurses or pharmacists as the primary cause of the error. For example, a central sterile supply room aide dispensed a bottle of boric acid solution instead of dextrose solution to the baby formula room—result, several infants died; a pharmacy helper dispensed sodium nitrite solution for sodium phosphate solution—result, two adults died. In both of the above cases, non-professional employees of the hospital were involved.

It would appear that, in the above instances, clearly defined hospital policies governing the handling, dispensing or distribution of drugs or related products may have prevented both tragedies. Furthermore, the lack of these policies could place the trustees, administrator, nurse and pharmacist in a vulnerable position with regard to law suits, both criminal and civil.

Because the hospital pharmacist is the best judge of whether or not safe practices are being followed in the handling, storage, administration or dispensing of drugs and related products, he must assume the mantle of responsibility for the development of the required policies for adoption by the administration and the hospital's board of trustees.

On September 27, 1957, the Coordinating Committee and Board of Trustees of the American Hospital Association voted as follows:

> "To urge through appropriate channels, that hospital pharmacists extend their responsibilities to include participation in programs dealing with the safe handling of drugs throughout the hospital."

Error-in-Medication—Defined

Seldom does a day pass in any large hospital but that some form of medication error is not reported. These errors, although not fatal or injurious to the patient, are nonetheless serious problems and must be coped with accordingly.

A review of the literature will reveal that there is a very wide range given as to the definition of a medication-error. Therefore, reports on the incidence of errors in one hospital or section of the country may not be comparable with those emanating from other hospitals in the same area or from another sector of the country.

In order to achieve some semblance of uniformity, it is suggested that hospital pharmacists consider the definition of medication-error as defined by R. David Anderson et al..[9]

> "The administration of the wrong medication or dose of medication, drug, diagnostic agent, chemical, or treatment requiring the use of such agents, to the wrong patient or at the wrong time, or the failure to administer such agents at the specified time or in the manner prescribed or normally considered as accepted practice."

Because of the comprehensive nature of the above definition, it may be difficult to determine a true error situation from that where the nurse's performance is acceptable but poor. Accordingly, Barker and McConnell[1] have developed the following definitions for types of errors:

    a. "Omissions—any dose not given by the time the next dose (if any) is due."

    b. "Wrong dosage—any dose either above or below the correct dosage by more than five per cent."

    c. "Extra dose given—any dose given in excess of the total number of times ordered by the physician."

    d. "Unordered drug given—the administration to a patient of any medication not ordered for that patient."

    e. "Wrong dosage form—any dosage form which is not included in the generally accepted interpretation of the physician's order."

    f. "Wrong time—any drug given 30 minutes or more before or after it was ordered, up to the time the next dose of the same medication was orderd. 'Prn' orders are not included."

    g. "Wrong administration— administration of a drug by a different route than was specified by the physician, such as giving by mouth a drug ordered intramuscularly."

Factors Contributing to Medication Errors

Many authors have published on this subject, and each has developed a check list by which the administrator or the pharmacist may evaluate the accident proness of his pharmaceutical service.[2,3] Amongst the most commonly cited factors which are stated to contribute towards the making of medication errors by both pharmacists and nurses are the following:

    a. Lack of a hospital pharmacist.

    b. Use of non-professional personnel in areas which may require professional judgment.

    c. Inadequate labeling of drug and chemical packages for the nursing station.

    d. Inadequate drug stations on the pavilions.

    e. Inadequate policies governing the reporting of incidents.

Corrective Measures

Lack of a hospital pharmacist

It is a well known fact that approximately 50 per cent of the hospitals in the United States do not employ a pharmacist on their staff.[4] This is a sad reflection upon the quality of care which most practitioners of medicine are forced to offer their patients. In addition, it is an open invitation for a serious medication error and subsequent litigation.

Recognition of the shortage of hospital pharmacists is hereby acknowledged, yet cannot be accepted as the excuse for not attempting to provide adequate pharmaceutical service.

Many solutions to this knotty problem have been described in the literature and include:

    1. The sharing of a pharmacist by two or more small hospitals.

    2. The combining of responsibilities which the pharmacist must carry such as pharmacist-purchasing agent, pharmacist-technician or pharmacist-administrator.

    3. The purchase of pharmaceutical service from a community pharmacy or possibly from a nearby large hospital.

Use of non-professional personnel in areas which may require professional judgment.

Lay personnel should, under no circumstances, be placed in positions or areas which may require the exercise of professional judgment. On the other hand, lay personnel should be used in the hospital in areas where they will not be required to act in the capacity of a professional person or in those departments where their acts are under the direct supervision of a professional person.

It is strongly recommended that the director of the pharmacy service develop a strong policy governing the role of lay persons performing in the pharmacy department. Once prepared, the policy should be recorded in the form of job descriptions and sections within the procedural manual.

Inadequate labeling of drug and chemical packages for the nursing station.

Unfortunately, too many individuals presume that the labeling of drugs and medications is a relatively simple matter and can, therefore, be assigned to lay employees. When this happens, medication containers become sloppy in appearance and lack the detail required by Federal and state laws, as well as the rules and regulations of the local boards of registration in pharmacy.

The basic concept of affixing a label to any container is to identify the contents and to relay to the user or consumer certain information which the manufacturer and the Government deem to be important. In fact, there should be little or no distinction between commercial medication containers and those dispensed by the hospital pharmacist to the nursing station. Both should bear information as to identity, strength, route of administration and cautions.

The medication label to be used in the hospital should be given considerable thought with respect to the information it is to convey, its size, color and adhesive quality. Many hospital pharmacists utilize only the generic name and metric system on the pharmacy label. Others use the generic name and immediately beneath place the trade name of the product. In addition, the apothecary weight equivalent to the metric system unit may also be displayed on the label. Some hospitals attempt to build into the label an additional safety factor through the use of a color coding system, namely labels printed with red ink on a white background indicate poisons; labels printed with blue ink on a white background indicate oral medications of a non-poisonous nature; green ink is reserved for topical products; black ink for nasal preparations; and purple ink for ophthalmic products.

The use of an auxiliary label is also encouraged in that it serves more readily to call attention to a specific point in relation to the medication. These auxiliary labels are readily available from a number of sources and may be affixed to the medication container in a variety of combinations.

Needless to point out, prescription container or other medication container labels must be neat, uniform, easy to read, unambiguous, comprehensive and factual. Labels should not be affixed one on top of the other for obvious reasons. Archambault[5] describes and pictures a "Label Position Indicator" which guarantees the uniform placement of labels upon containers. By the use of this simple device, medication containers will be labeled in exactly the same position thereby creating a uniform appearance on the medication station.

Inadequate drug stations on the pavilions.

Medication errors often occur when the nurse preparing the medication is distracted by the passing personnel, is unable to read adequately due to poor lighting, or is forced to go to several different cabinets to gather the materials necessary for the administration of the drug.

Many hospital architects and administrators have recognized this problem and in new construction provision is usually made for a medication room.

A medication room has been defined[6] as a room:

". . . used for the storage and preparation of medications."

Wagner[6] also provides that:

"This room should be enclosed for quiet, clear-glazed for observation both in and out, and sized to accommodate more than one person, because with team nursing, students, private-duty nurses, preoperative and postoperative care, several persons may often work here simultaneously."

The minimum requirements for a medication room are as follows:[6]

    i. Shallow or stepped shelves divided by some means for individual patient medication, with a system for readily changing patient identification.

    ii. A double-locked narcotics safe, with red warning light to indicate when the safe is unlocked, installed at eye level above the counter.

    iii. A counter having drawers underneath for storage of syringes and similar items, but open below without cabinets.

    iv. A bulletin board.

    v. A sink large enough for hand washing, equipped with gooseneck spout and blade handles, should be installed in the counter. This area should be equipped with paper towel dispenser, soap dispenser, and waste receptacle. A separate waste receptacle for broken glass and other non-burnable items should be provided.

    vi. A refrigerator mounted above the counter is more convenient, provides better visibility for drug storage, and allows greater ease in cleaning. An undercounter refrigerator with slide-out, removable tray shelves is acceptable.

In hospitals where a separate medication room is not possible, architects have seen fit to install commercial prefabricated drug stations off the main line of traffic or, where possible, to segregate the installation by a partition or sliding door arrangement.

15

These units are usually constructed of a non-magnetic stainless steel polished to a high finish. These are equipped with counter top space, sink, medicine shelves, medicine card rack, narcotic cabinet, biological refrigerator, medicine cup dispenser, illumination, syringe drawer and waste receptacles.

Although this type of unit is manufactured by a number of firms, probably the most widely known is the "Medi-Prep" unit (Fig. 94).

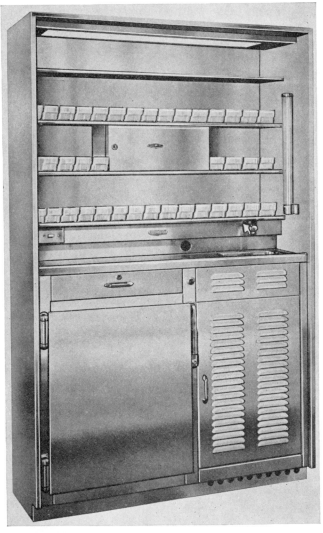

Fig. 94.   An example of a type of nursing station medication cabinet. This unit is manufactured by the Market Forge Co., Everett, Massachusetts and is known as the Medi-Prep Unit. There are different models of this unit commercially available. (Courtesy of Market Forge Co., Everett, Massachusetts.)

Inadequate policies governing the reporting of incidents.

Laxity in requiring a comprehensive report on each drug accident gives the employee the impression that nobody is interested, and therefore contributes toward the lowering of the standard of patient care. On the contrary, everybody from the nurse to the pharmacist, to the physician to the administrator is or should be interested in every single accident report in order to ascertain the extent of the injury to the patient as well as to initiate ways and means to prevent a recurrence.

This view is supported by the action taken by the Board of Trustees of the American Hospital Association on May 13, 1958[7] when it was voted—

> "To urge hospitals to establish an incident reporting system; further to urge adoption of the Incident Report, for use in conjunction with the incident reporting system . . ."

When used in conjunction with the above vote, the word "incident" was defined as follows:

> "An incident is any happening which is not consistent with the routine operation of the hospital or the routine care of the patient. It may be an accident or a situation which might result in an accident."

Where possible, the medication error report form should be a separate form from that of the typical incident report form. This is necessary because of the very nature of the information which is required. A medication error report form should be able to elicit the following information concerning each drug error: patient's name, hospital number, and location; name of the drug, its strength and route of administration; the time and date of the error; the name and title of the person making the error; the type of error—(1) omission, (2) wrong dose, (3) extra dose given, (4) unordered drug given, (5) wrong dosage form, (6) wrong time of administration, (7) wrong route of administration; the name of the doctor to whom the incident was reported; the name of the nursing supervisor to whom the incident was reported; a brief description of the treatment or the orders given by the doctor as a result of the error; and a statement by the nursing supervisor as to the measures taken by the Nursing Service to prevent such error from recurring.

Guidelines Relative to the Safe Use of Medications in Hospitals

The American Society of Hospital Pharmacists and its officers have always been concerned about safety practices and procedures in hospitals. Francke,[8] writing editorially, has summarized the history of the development of the Society's Committee on Safety Practices and Procedures and its subsequent publication of a series of guidelines for the safe use of drugs in the hospital.

This document represents one of the most important contributions made by the Society to improve and safeguard the care of hospitalized patients. Practitioners and students alike are urged to review its contents thoroughly and immediately proceed to implement its recommendations. Therefore, for the convenience of both, the *Guidelines Relative to the Safe Use of Medications in Hospitals,*[9] is hereby presented in full detail.

The following guidelines are presented for the use of professional personnel responsible for the safe handling of medications and diagnostic agents in hospitals. Recognizing that existing procedures may change, these guidelines are designed to provide a basis for formulating policies and procedures at the present time.

PREAMBLE

THE BOARD OF TRUSTEES OF THE AMERICAN HOSPITAL ASSOCIATION and the Executive Committee of the AMERICAN SOCIETY OF HOSPITAL PHARMACISTS in 1957 adopted the following significant position:

> To urge hospital pharmacists, through appropriate channels, to extend their responsibilities to include participation in programs dealing with the safe handling of drugs throughout the hospital.

Problems of medication safety are now the grave concern of the many persons involved with patient care. These include the hospital trustee, the physician, the administrator, the pharmacist, the nurse, and others. The multiplicity of drugs, the increased number and kinds of medications prescribed per patient, the increased number of both inpatients and outpatients who are being treated, and the ever-changing concepts of medical care make it mandatory that a system of safe medication practices be developed and maintained to insure that the patient receives the best possible care and protection.

In recent years, the rapid obsolesence of drugs, the availability of more specific drugs per disease entity, and the general increase in the prescribing of medications have placed a greater responsibility on pharmacy and nursing services in dispensing and administering medications.

The greatly increased use of medications has increased the hazard of possible error. The seriousness of the problem may be indicated by the fact that medication errors are among the leading causes of accidents in hospitals.

For the purpose of this statement, a medication error, though resulting from many possible causes, is defined as the administration of the wrong medicine or dose of medicine, diagnostic agent, or treatment requiring the use of such agent to a patient; or the administration of the medicine, agent, or treatment at the wrong time, or to the wrong patient; or the failure to administer such medication, agent, or treatment; or the failure to administer at the time specified or in the manner prescribed or normally considered as accepted practice.

SECTION I

LABELING and MEDICATION CONTAINERS— GENERAL

1.1 Drug labeling should be performed by a pharmacist or under the supervision of a pharmacist. Prescription labels and pharmacy stock labels should be used only by the hospital pharmacy. (See 1.16 and 4.14.)

1.2 The pharmacist should be consulted and should make recommendations concerning labeling, containers and storage of housekeeping items, insecticides, cleaners, and such.

1.3 Medication labels should be typed or machine-printed. Labeling with pen or pencil, use of adhesive tape or china marking pencils should be prohibited. A label should not be superimposed on a label.

1.4 The label should be legible, easily read, and free from erasures and strike-overs. It should be firmly affixed to the container. The label for stock containers should be protected from chemical action or abrasion.

1.5 Labels should bear the name, address, and telephone number of the hospital.

1.6 One order or prescription should be filled and labeled at a time.

1.7 The following or similar accessory labels and caution statements should appear where indicated:

    a. Poison
    b. Not to be taken internally
    c. Shake well before using
    d. For external use only
    e. For the eye
    f. For the nose
    g. For the ear
    h. Refrigerate at 2°–10°C (35°–50°F)
    i. Refrigerate after reconstitution
    j. Warning: Not for injection
    k. Do not use after ....
    l. Not to be swallowed
    m. Keep out of reach of children
    n. Keep from freezing
    o. Keep below freezing
    p. Caution: Potent Drug
    q. Research Drug

    *r. NONPROPRIETARY NAME
         Note for information of Staff:
         Prescription or order for (*Proprietary Name*) filled as per formulary policy; contents are same basic drug as prescribed, but may be of another brand.

    *s. NONPROPRIETARY NAME
         Note for information of staff:
         Contents may be used, per formulary policy, to fill prescriptions or orders for any of the following brands of the same basic drug:

         (Proprietary Name, Brand 1)
         (Proprietary Name, Brand 2)
         (Proprietary Name, Brand 3)

    t. Note change in color, size, or shape
    u. Other accessory labels providing special information such as dosage, side effects, or contraindications for investigational drugs may be used where necessary.

1.8   The metric system should be given prominence on all labels where both metric and apothecary systems are commonly used.

1.9   The name of the therapeutically-active ingredients should be indicated in compound mixtures.

1.10 Labels for medications should indicate the amount of drug or drugs in each dosage form unless otherwise indicated.

1.11 Drugs and chemicals in forms intended for dilution or reconstitution should carry directions for so doing. Whenever possible, dilutions and labeling should be done in the pharmacy.

1.12 Perishable drugs, such as antibiotics and biologicals, should clearly indicate the expiration date on the label.

1.13 The routes of administration should be indicated for parenteral medications whenever possible.

1.14 Numbers, letters, coined names, and unofficial synonyms and abbreviations should not be used to identify medications with the exception of approved letter or number codes for investigational drugs.

1.15 Only light-resistant, tight containers meeting U.S.P. standards should be used.

1.16 Medications if brought into the hospital by the patient or physician should be positively identified before use. Such medications should be checked by the hospital pharmacist with the originating pharmacy by prescription serial number. A supplemental label should be attached in the hospital pharmacy providing information required in Section II. Where no pharmacist is on duty, the physician should check with the issuing pharmacy and attach the supplemental label described above.

*Applicable to those hospitals operating under the formulary system as outlined in AHA-ASHP *Statement of Guiding Principles on the Operation of the Hospital Formulary System. See* AM. J. HOSP. PHARM., *17*:609 (Oct.), 1960.

1.17 Containers presenting difficulty in labeling, such as small tubes, should be labeled with no less than the prescription serial number, name of drug, strength, and name of the patient, and should then be placed in a larger carton or container bearing a label with the necessary information indicated in Sections II and III.

1.18 The label should conform with all applicable Federal, state, and local laws and regulations.

1.19 Floor stock medication labels should carry codes to identify source and lot number of medication.

SECTION II

LABELING and DISPENSING IN-PATIENT PRESCRIPTIONS

2.1 In addition to the recommendations outlined in Section I, the inpatient prescription labels should bear, as a minimum, the following information:

  a. Patient's full name
  b. Nonproprietary and/or proprietary name of the drug actually dispensed
  c. Strength
  d. Date of issue
  e. Name or initials of dispensing pharmacist

2.2 The prescription or in-patient order should have noted thereon, at the time dispensed, the source and batch identifying number of the medication and the initials of the dispenser.

2.3 For in-patient self-care medications, label as in Section III.

SECTION III

LABELING and DISPENSING OUT-PATIENT PRESCRIPTIONS

3.1 Medications to be dispensed to in-patients who are being discharged should be returned to the pharmacy for relabeling.

3.2 The out-patient prescription label should bear the following information:

  a. Patient's full name
  b. Prescription identification number
  c. Specific directions for use
  d. Date of issue
  e. Name or initials of dispenser
  f. Name of prescribing physician
  g. Where physician requests or hospital policy dictates, identity and strength should be on the label
  h. A "Keep out of reach of children" label
  i. Name, address, and telephone number of hospital

3.3   Prescriptions should have noted thereon, at the time dispensed, the source and batch identifying number of the medication and the initials of the dispenser.

3.4   An identifying check system to insure proper identification of out-patients should be established.

SECTION IV

CARE of DRUGS and DRUG CABINETS in NURSING UNITS

4.1   Medication centers should be functional and provide:

a. Adequate space so that drugs can be placed and arranged in accordance with 4.2
b. Adequate space to allow all container labels to be clearly visible
c. Adequate lighting so that labels can be clearly read
d. Adequate ventilation
e. Adequate work space protected from traffic and noise
f. Hot and cold running water
g. Sufficient equipment and supplies in readily usable form
h. Refrigeration
i. Inner-lockable narcotic cabinet
j. Adequate means for security

4.2   Medications should be placed in drug cabinets in accordance with an established plan for a particular hospital which provides standardized compartments for:

a. Internal medications
b. Narcotics, barbiturates, amphetamines
c. Poisons and external-use drugs
d. Emergency drugs
e. Ampuls
f. Investigational drugs

4.3   Drugs should be arranged alphabetically within the above mentioned groups insofar as possible.

4.4   Medication cabinets or rooms and narcotic compartments should be kept locked and the keys should be available only to the nurse in charge or her alternate.

4.5   Storage of drugs on mobile dressing carriages is discouraged unless properly secured.

4.6   Not more than one hypodermic tablet should be placed in a capsule for the purpose of protection against breakage or to facilitate counting or control.

4.7   Pharmacy should supply exact quantities for preparation of specific amounts of solution, or should preferably supply the finished preparation. Maintenance of bulk chemicals or stock drugs on the nursing units for preparation of solutions should be discouraged.

4.8   Separate storage facilities should be provided for:

    a. Test reagents
    b. General disinfectants and antiseptics
    c. Cleansing agents

4:9   Only drugs and the equipment for preparation and administration should be stored in medication cabinets.

4.10   Drug cabinets should be examined weekly or more often by the nurse in charge. Drugs which appear to have deteriorated, exceeded their expiration date, or are not being used should be returned to the pharmacy for proper disposition. Monthly, or more frequent, inspections should be made by the Directors of Pharmacy and Nursing Service or their delegates

4.11   Controlled drugs in the nursing unit shall be inventoried, recorded, and inspected in accord with an approved system.

4.12   Investigational drugs should be handled as directed in the Statement of Principles Involved in the Use of Investigational Drugs in Hospitals issued by the American Hospital Association and AMERICAN SOCIETY OF HOSPITAL PHARMACISTS

4.13   Reconstitution of antibiotics and other unstable drugs on the nursing unit should be kept to a minimum. They should be diluted in accordance with directions supplied by the pharmacy.

4.14   Antibiotics and other unstable drugs reconstituted on the nursing unit should carry a nurse-prepared label with essentially the following information:

    a. Expiration date
    b. Nurse's name or initials
    c. Dosage or strength per unit volume

4.15   Empty medication containers should be returned to the pharmacy.

4.16   Flammable or explosive liquids such as ether or acetone should be kept in as small supply as possible and in accordance with state and local fire regulations.

SECTION V

MEDICATION ORDERS

5.1   Medications should be given only on the written order of a physician. Exceptions to this policy should be covered by a written policy established by the Medical Board or Medical Staff of the hospital, as for example 5.2 and 5.3.

5.2   Emergency verbal orders may be accepted by a nurse. The physician should check the prepared emergency dose and container before the medication is administered. An order for the medication should be written by the physician at the earliest time possible.

5.3   *Stat* telephone orders may be accepted by a nurse. The order should be recorded on the doctor's order sheet, followed by the name of physician giving the order, the time, and the signature of the nurse receiving it. The nurse should repeat the order to the physician from her written record for confirmation. The physician should countersign this order on his next visit to the station. The nurse accepting a telephone order should be personally responsible for its execution.

5.4 Medication orders should be automatically cancelled under the following conditions:

    a. Patient goes to delivery room or operating room

    b. Transfer of patient to another service

    c. In accordance with written policy of the Medical Board adopted in connection with the Automatic Stop Order statement of the Joint Commission on Accreditation of Hospitals

    d. In accordance with written policy of the Medical Board adopted in connection with Suggested Regulations for Handling Narcotics in Hospitals by the AMERICAN SOCIETY OF HOSPITAL PHARMACISTS and approved by the American Hospital Association

5.5 The physician will specify the time a stat or single order was written. After the nurse administers the medication, she should write, "Given," the time administered, and her signature.

5.6 Medication orders should be legibly written and should include:

    a. Name of medication

    b. Dosage expressed in the metric system, except in instances where dosage is commonly expressed otherwise

    c. Signature of the physician

    d. Frequency of administration, if other than oral

    f. Date and hour

5.7 The use of abbreviations and chemical symbols in the writing of medication orders is discouraged and, if used, should be limited to those agreed upon and jointly adopted by the nursing, pharmacy, and medical staffs of a particular hospital.

5.8 Any question arising from a medication order, including the interpretation of illegible order, should be referred to the physician writing the order. The nurse should not be expected to attempt to carry out the order until the question is resolved.

SECTION VI

MEDICATION CARDS

6.1 A medication card should be made and used for the preparation and administration of all medications and should carry essentially the following information:

    a. Patient's first and last names
    b. Location of patient and hospital number
    c. Name of drug
    d. Dosage
    e. Route of administration if other than oral
    f. Frequency of administration
    g. Time(s) of administration
    h. Any special precautions or observations
    i. Initials of nurse preparing or verifying the medication order
    j. Expiration date of order
    k. Date card made out

6.2   The medication card should be clearly written in ink or printed and verified by the nurse against the physician's order.

6.3   Cards for "Delayed" or "Omitted" medications should be removed from the regular medication card file and placed in a designated place.

6.4   On assuming charge of a patient unit, the nurse should check the medication cards against the doctor's order to insure the following:

    a. All cards are in their proper place
    b. Cards for "Delayed" or "Omitted" medications have been removed
    c. Cards for medications to be resumed following "Omit" or "Delay" are returned to their proper place in the file
    d. Cards for discontinued orders are removed and destroyed

SECTION VII

PREPARATION of MEDICATIONS for ADMINISTRATION

7.1   Ascertain that prescribed dose has not previously been administered.

7.2   Select medication card(s) or drug(s) to be administered.

7.3   Check medication card(s) for expiration time and date and omission.

7.4   Arrange medication cards with medicine cups in the order in which medications are to be administered. Use a separate cup for each medication unless otherwise ordered.

7.5   Expose each medication card singly while preparing the medication.

7.6   Give full attention while preparing medication.

7.7   Select drug and compare it to medication card.

7.8   Ascertain that the container is completely and properly labeled, including strength when indicated. Never use unlabeled medications.

7.9   Read the label three (3) times

     a. Before removing from shelf
     b. Before measuring or preparing the dose
     c. Before replacing on shelf

7.10 Medications prepared for administration, but not used, should be discarded.

7.11 The pharmacist should be contacted when there is a question regarding the mixing of medications in the same syringe or container.

7.12 A copy of the hospital formulary, an up-to-date incompatibility chart for possible parenteral medication mixtures, and an antidote chart should be maintained at each nursing station.

7.13 Pharmaceutical calculations required in the administration of medications should be checked by another nurse or, if possible, with the pharmacist.

7.14 The metric system, to the extent possible, should be used in prescribing, administering, and recording medications. Approximate metric and apothecary equivalents and information for computing dosage should be readily available on the nursing unit.

SECTION VIII

ADMINISTRATION of MEDICATIONS

8.1 Medications should be administered only if information regarding the drug is available in the form approved by the Pharmacy and Therapeutics Committee. The nurse should know and consider:

     a. General use of the drug
     b. Therapeutic action
     c. Usual dosage
     d. Factors modifying the dosage
     e. Factors modifying the effects
     f. Untoward actions, side effects, precautions, and contraindications
     g. Antidote, if known
     h. Medium, route and frequency of administration
     i. Signs of deterioration of drug

8.2 Medications should be prepared and given as near the specified time as possible.

8.3 The patient for whom the medication is intended should be positively identified by checking the identification band or hospital number, or by other means as specified by hospital policy.

8.4 The person administering the medication should stay with the patient until the medication has been taken. Exceptions to this rule are selected medications which may be left at the patient's bedside on the physician's written order.

8.5   All medications should be administered by the person who has prepared the dose. For exceptions to this rule, see (5.2) (8.8).

8.6   Parenteral medications which are not to be mixed in a syringe should be given in different sites.

8.7   The administration of blood and blood derivatives should be the responsibility of the physician. The physician should be responsible for starting intravenous and subcutaneous infusions, for administering all intravenous medications, and for adding medications to flowing intravenous fluids. Exceptions should be covered by written policy established and endorsed by the Medical Board of the hospital, which policies should be in compliance with existing state nursing, pharmacy, and medical practice acts and regulations, or rulings of the office of the state attorney general.

8.8   In instances when the administration of medications is delegated to another person, the nurse should assume the responsibility for supervision of the procedure.

SECTION IX

RECORDING of MEDICATIONS

9.1   All administered medications or omitted medications should be recorded on the patient's medical record according to an established procedure.

9.2   Hospital policy should determine the responsibility for recording medications administered by the physician.

SECTION X

MEDICATION ERRORS

10.1   Each hospital should set up a clear statement of policy for all medication errors. Such policy should include:

a. Reporting
b. Recording
c. Review
d. Channel for analysis and necessary action
e. Written report

10.2   If an error occurs in the administration of medication, the physician and the proper administrative representative should be informed immediately.

10.3   A written report, in accordance with hospital policy, should be prepared and sent to the proper hospital officials within 24 hours.

Drug Interaction Surveillance

The safe use of medications in hospitals, extended care facilities and nursing homes goes beyond the assurances that the appropriate drug has been dispensed and that the label information is correct. Generally, the introduction of a unit dose system into the operation tends to eliminate many of the errors in medication administration and, at the same time, provides the ultimate in drug control, packaging and dispensing.

To assure the patient and physician of total drug safety, it is essential that the pharmacist maintain a drug interaction surveillance program. Such a program should include a method to check on drug-drug and drug-laboratory test reactions. Because more than one mechanism may be involved, and because each mechanism may be quite complex, the classification of drug interaction mechanisms is very difficult and the practice thereof constitutes a form of specialization in pharmacy. However, the average practitioner of hospital pharmacy can maintain adequate surveillance by instituting a program of working from a direct copy of the physician's original order sheet; preparing a patient drug profile (PDP); and a drug interaction reporting form (DIRF).[10] These combined with the judicious selection and use of the latest textbooks on the subject will assure all concerned that proper drug safety techniques are being practiced.[11,12]

SELECTED REFERENCES

BARKER, KENNETH N.: The Demonstration and Evaluation of an Experimental Medication System for the U. A. M. C. Hospital, Vols. 1 and 2, Drug Systems Research University of Arkansas Medical Center, Little Rock, Arkansas, July 1967.

BARKER, K. N., KIMBROUGH, W. W. and HELLER, W. M.: A study of Medication Errors in a Hospital, University of Mississippi, Oxford, Mississippi, 2nd Printing, 1968.

STEVENS, ROBERT M. and WOLFERT, REUBEN R.: A Random Filing System for In-patient Medication Records, Am. J. Hosp. Pharm. 26:5:290, 1969.

BENNETT, BERKLEY V.: Patient Safety is Everyone's Responsibility, Hosp. Form. Mgt. 7:1:24, 1972.

BIBLIOGRAPHY

1. BARKER, KENNETH N. and McCONNELL, WARREN E.: The Problems of Detecting Medication Errors in Hospitals, Am. J. Hosp. Pharm., 19:8:361, 1962.
2. ARCHAMBAULT, GEORGE F.: Pharmacy Accidents Can Be Prevented, Hospitals, J.A.H.A., 31:7:68, 1957.
3. SCHLOSSBERG, ELI: Sixteen Safeguards Against Medication Errors, Hospitals, J.A.H.A., 32:19:62, 1958.
4. ANON.: Hospitals, J.A.H.A., Guide Issue (Agust 1, Part II), 38:513, 1964.
5. ARCHAMBAULT, GEORGE F.: Labels for Nursing Station Medication Containers, Hospitals, J.A.H.A., 32:18:50, 1958.
6. WAGNER, CHARLES: Planning the Patient Care Unit in the General Hospital, Public Health Service Publication No. 930-D-1, U.S. Government Printing Office, Washington, D.C.

 7. ANON.: Incident Reporting System, Hospitals, J.A.H.A., *32*:15:46, 1958.
 8. FRANCKE, DON E.: Safety Practicies and Procedures (An Editorial), Am. J. Hosp. Pharm., *19*:11:553, 1962.
 9. ANDERSON, R. DAVID *et al.*: Guidelines Relative to the Safe Use of Medications in Hospitals, Am. J. Hosp. Pharm., *19*:11:577, 1962.
10. ARNOLD, THOMAS R.: Drug Interaction Reporting in a Small Hospital, Hospital Pharmacy, *7*:3:79, 1972.
11. HANSTEN, PHILIP D.: *Drug Interactions,* Lea & Febiger, Philadelphia, 1971.
12. HARTSHORN, EDWARD A.: *Handbook of Drug Interactions,* Drug Intelligence Publications, Hamilton Press Inc., Hamilton, Illinois.

Chapter

29

The Small Hospital, Nursing Homes and Part-Time Pharmacists

NEARLY 2500 hospitals in the United States do not employ either a full-time or a part-time pharmacist to provide pharmaceutical services to their patients and physicians. In these institutions, non-pharmacist personnel handle the drugs which do not require compounding. All others are purchased from local community pharmacies.[1]

It is sometimes overlooked that these very same drugs which are daily handled by untrained hospital personnel are required, by law, to be dispensed in the retail pharmacy or the large hospital by duly qualified, licensed pharmacists. By permitting this double standard to exist, trustees, administrators, pharmacists, and pharmacy law enforcement officers are, in effect, denying the small hospital's patient high quality pharmacy service. In addition, the institution's officers and administration are openly inviting both criminal and civil actions should a serious drug accident occur within the hospital.

The American Hospital Association, the American Society of Hospital Pharmacists and the American College of Apothecaries have held that the size of the hospital should not in any way limit or deprive the patient of the pharmacy service to which he is entitled.[2]

Although the ideal goal to ensure adequate pharmaceutical services in all hospitals, irrespective of size, is to place a pharmacist on each staff, we fully realize that this would be a utopian state. Accordingly, a more practical approach must be sought.

Fortunately, a number of far-sighted, economically and safety minded small hospital administrators have explored and developed a number of plans for the provision of adequate pharmaceutical services with their institutions.

In this chapter, we shall concern ourselves with the study of the

MODEL NURSING HOME-PHARMACIST RETAINER AGREEMENT

Whereas, the _____ (hereinafter referred to as "Nursing Home") desires to provide
(name of Nursing Home)
quality pharmaceutical services to its inpatients; and

Whereas, _____ (hereinafter referred to as "Pharmacist") is a pharmacist in good
(name of Pharmacist)
standing licensed to practice his profession under the laws of this state;

Now, therefore, on this _____ day of _____, 196___, in consideration of the mutual agreements and prom-
(date)   (month)
ises hereinafter set forth, the parties hereto agree:

1. The _____ Nursing Home agrees to retain Pharmacist and Pharmacist agrees to provide Nurs-
ing Home with pharmaceutical services. Nursing Home agrees that during the period of this retainer that Pharmacist shall
have the exclusive right to furnish medication and all related medical and health supplies and devices which Pharmacist is
legally and professionally qualified to provide.

2. The retainer of Pharmacist shall commence on the date of this Agreement and shall continue for _____
(months, years) from the date hereof. Subject to this Agreement continuing in full force and effect for said period, Pharmacist shall have the option to continue his retainer hereunder for an additional like period by giving Nursing Home written
notice of his intention so to do not less than _____ days nor more than _____ days prior to the expiration of the initial
term. Upon the exercise of this option by Pharmacist, all of the terms and conditions of this Agreement shall continue in
full force and effect for such additional period, except the option to continue the retainer.

3. During the period of the retainer hereunder, Pharmacist shall serve Nursing Home and shall perform any and all
services in pharmaceutical matters required or requested in connection with the operation of the Nursing Home premises
located at _____, including compliance with all regulatory requirements to meet the conditions or
(street address)
standards of participation in any governmental medical or health assistance programs. Pharmacist will perform such other
services of an advisory or educational nature which are related to pharmaceutical services or for which his education,
training, and experience as a pharmacist are especially suited, without further compensation other than that provided for in
this Agreement.

4A. Pharmacist shall devote such time, energy, and skill as his duties hereunder shall require and shall, at least quarterly, or at any time upon request, submit a report of principal activities performed and to be performed by him for Nursing Home, and shall render such assistance as may be requested by Nursing Home in reviewing the provisions and activities relating to pharmaceutical services in connection with governmental inspections or voluntary accreditation programs.

4B. Pharmacist shall devote not less than _____ hours but not more than _____ hours per _____ (week, month, year)
to the performance of his duties under this retainer which shall include all time expended in preparing reports of activities
performed or to be performed by him for Nursing Home and time expended in reviewing the provisions and activities relating to pharmaceutical services in connection with governmental inspections or voluntary accreditation programs.

5A. Nursing Home shall pay to Pharmacist as fees for his professional services under this retainer an aggregate of
$ _____ . (_____ dollars) per _____ (month, year), in addition to the actual cost of medication sup-
(number)   (spell out)
plied. Nursing Home shall reimburse pharmacist monthly for the actual cost of medication dispensed to patients upon written
statements of account.

5B. Nursing Home shall pay to Pharmacist his usual and customary fee for each prescription order dispensed to Nursing Home patients which shall not be greater than that Pharmacist charges other noninstitutionalized patients. In addition,
Nursing Home shall pay Pharmacist for his professional consultation and other services performed on Nursing Home premises a retainer in the aggregate sum of $ _____ , (_____ dollars) per _____ (month, year).
(number)

5C. Nursing Home shall pay to Pharmacist his actual cost of ingredients plus a professional fee of $_____
(number)
(_____ dollars) for each prescription order dispensed to Nursing Home's patients. In addition, Nursing Home shall
pay Pharmacist for his professional consultation and other services performed on Nursing Home premises a retainer in the
aggregate sum of $_____ (_____ dollars) per _____ (month, year).
(number)

6. Nursing Home agrees to provide Pharmacist with office and pharmacy space needed in performing the services of
his retainer and with such secretarial service as may be required. Nursing Home agrees to reimburse Pharmacist for expenditures made on behalf of Nursing Home for reference works, physical equipment, and supplies other than drugs needed
in performing his professional duties upon written statements of account rendered monthly: Provided, however, that any
expenditure in excess of $_____ for any one item shall first require the approval of the Nursing Home.

7. Pharmacist is retained and employed by Nursing Home only for purposes and to the extent set forth in this Agreement, and his relation to Nursing Home shall, during the period that this retainer is in effect, be that of an independent
practitioner, and Pharmacist shall be free to dispose of such portion of his time, energy, and skill not required in the performance of his duties hereunder in such manner as he may choose and to such persons, firms, or corporations as he deems
advisable. Pharmacist shall not be considered under the provisions of this Agreement or otherwise as having an employee
status or as being entitled to participate in any plans, arrangements, or other benefits pertaining to pension, or other em-
ployee-benefit plans.

8. Pharmacist agrees to obtain and maintain a suitable professional liability policy to provide adequate coverage
against mistake or neglect in the performance of his professional services under this retainer.

9. Nursing Home shall make such arrangements as may be necessary to assure Pharmacist of effective and actual control of drugs and related supplies, and the records pertaining thereto, under policies and procedures developed in accordance
with sound pharmaceutical practices.

10. Pharmacist shall arrange to provide the services of another pharmacist to perform the obligations of this retainer
during any absence, vacation or other limited periods when Pharmacist is not personally available.

11. This agreement may be terminated by either party at any time for good and sufficient cause provided the alleged
grounds for termination have been presented in writing at least 30 days prior to the effective date of the termination.

In witness whereof, Nursing Home has caused this agreement to be executed through its duly authorized representative
and Pharmacist has accepted its terms and promises on this _____ day of _____, 196_____.

Name of Nursing Home _____

By: (Signature) _____

Title: _____

Signature of Pharmacist _____

FIG. 95. Model Nursing Home-Pharmacist Retainer Agreement of the type
recommended by the American Pharmaceutical Association and the American
Society of Consultant Pharmacists.

457

four principal methods of handling drugs in the hospital without a full-time pharmacist. These same methods may be utilized in the nursing home or extended care facility with minor modification.

Methods of Handling Drugs in Hospitals Without a Full-Time Pharmacist

The four principal methods of handling drugs in hospitals without a full-time pharmacist are as follows:

1. A community pharmacist contracts to provide a full pharmaceutical service to the hospital and he, or his duly licensed agent, goes to the institution and actively participates in performing the service contracted for (Fig. 95).
2. A community pharmacist contracts to provide drug merchandise only. He does not go to the hospital. In this situation, other hospital personnel, principally nurses, function in the institution as drug dispensers or distributors.
3. Pharmacy service in the small hospital is provided by the department of pharmacy of a nearby large hospital.
4. No pharmacist is involved in the hospital's drug service, which is carried on by nurses, technicians or aides.

Small Hospital-Community Pharmacist, The Full Responsibility Relationship

It has been reported[2] that to insure that a part-time pharmaceutical program in the small hospital will succeed, the following are essential:

1. "a compact, adequate (but not necessarily large) separate drug room."
2. "a pharmacist on active duty in the hospital on an average of three hours per day."
3. "a direct telephone service between the small hospital's drug room to the independent pharmacy for consultation services."
4. "stand-by delivery service from the independent pharmacy to the hospital."
5. "the availability of an emergency telephone number and service for the use of the hospital at all hours."

Since this initial attempt was made to develop ground rules for the quasi professional-commercial relationship between the small hospital and the community pharmacist, the American Hospital Association and the American Society of Hospital Pharmacists have cooperated in the development of the following *Suggested Principles of Relationship Between Smaller Hospitals and Part-Time Pharmacists* [3]

SUGGESTED PRINCIPLES OF RELATIONSHIP BETWEEN SMALLER HOSPITALS AND PART-TIME PHARMACISTS WHO PROVIDE PHARMACEUTICAL SERVICES

Approved by the Board of Trustees of the American Hospital Association and the Executive Committee of the American Society of Hospital Pharmacists
February, 1959

Preamble

ALL HOSPITALS should be cognizant of the contribution made by a sound and organized pharmaceutical service for improved patient care and treatment. The introduction annually of numerous potent drugs requires that all hospitals have the full or part-time service of a registered pharmacist. In small hospitals which cannot obtain or afford a full-time hospital pharmacist, the services of a pharmacist on a part-time or consultative basis may be obtained.

If the services of a hospital pharmacist of another hospital are not obtainable, the services of a local registered pharmacist should be utilized whenever possible. When pharmaceutical service from a local pharmacy is considered, the part-time pharmacist and the hospital might consider certain guiding principles of affiliation. The Principles of Relationship Between Smaller Hospitals and Part-time Pharmacists are suggested to achieve the objective of better patient care.

Basic Principle

1. *The pharmaceutical service of the hospital shall be organized and maintained primarily for the benefit of hospital patients.*

In any hospital, the individual elements which are maintained and coordinated are all subordinate to the main objective of providing care to the sick and injured. Any function either newly added or strengthened, as in this instance drug or pharmaceutical services (from any source whatever or by any arrangement), must be in agreement with this basic principle.

Organization

1. *The hospital pharmaceutical service should be under the direction of a professionally competent legally qualified pharmacist.*

The hospital must exercise due care in its selection of personnel. The hospital safeguards the patient and its public trust by fixing the responsibility for its varied functions by appointing adequately qualified individuals.

2. *A part-time pharmacist, as a professional member of the hospital staff and as the head of a hospital function or department, must assume the responsibilities involved.*

Recognition as a member of the hospital organization will be in direct proportion to the responsibility which the individual is capable of accepting on a part-time basis.

3. The part-time pharmacist shall be responsible to the proper administrative authority of the hospital for developing, supervising and coordinating the activities of the pharmaceutical services to hospital patients and departments.

With hospital affiliation, an attendant responsibility is placed on the part-time pharmacist to preserve the unity and coordination of the hospital's component activities as directed by the administrator in policies laid down in behalf of the public which the hospital governing board represents. Thus the part-time pharmacist subscribing to a hospital connection in terms of relationships, is primarily responsible to the hospital administrator for those services provided to hospital patients and departments.

Rules, regulations and procedures regarding drug services to hospital patients and departments should not be counter to or in opposition to the hospital's policies for patients as interpreted and approved by the hospital administrator in behalf of the medical staff, and of the hospital governing board and the public it represents.

4. The organization of hospital pharmaceutical services, the relationship to the hospital and its elements, and the specific services to be provided should be outlined and reviewed periodically by the hospital administrator and the part-time pharmacist who provides pharmaceutical services to hospital patients and departments.

To keep abreast of changing developments or staff demands for high standards of service and to obviate misunderstandings, relationships should be outlined initially and reviewed periodically. This appears to be particularly necessary in those situations where certain elements of services are provided on the hospital premises, and others in varying degrees emanate from sources away from the hospital environment arranged by delegation to others who may be unfamiliar with hospital safeguards and policies.

5. The organization of pharmaceutical services should include the utilization of an organized Pharmacy and Therapeutics Committee responsible for the development of rules and regulations pertaining to professional policies related to pharmaceutical services for hospital patients.

Following the usual practice in hospitals, the medical and pharmacy staffs acting in an advisory capacity are the most qualified to recommend to the hospital such policies as relate to selection, evaluation and distribution of drugs used in the hospital. The composition and specific objectives of the Pharmacy and Therapeutics Committee as well as its appointment may be developed to best meet the needs of the hospital and its standards.

Functions

1. The primary functions of the service provided by a part-time pharmacist should be to furnish drugs with sufficient dispatch so that patient care will not be hindered, to provide adequate safeguards for the patient and hospital personnel, and to provide therapeutic agents of respected quality.

Responsibilities do not begin or end with filling prescriptions or furnishing drugs remotely from the hospital. The well-rounded and minimum responsibility might include such personal services by the part-time pharmacist as staff education related to safeguards in use of drugs on the premises, contribution to educational or research programs where extant, provision of maximum consultation services to nursing and medical staffs, inspection of drug storage and distribution throughout the hospital, attendance at committee and department meetings, preparation of fiscal and professional reports where necessary, maintenance of an approved stock of emergency drugs, provision for 24-hour drug services, elimination of waste, etc.

2. *Records concerned with hospital patient services should be maintained separately, preserved for the period prescribed by legal or hospital requirements, and be readily available.*

Such records as narcotic, barbiturate, alcohol, prescription, and requisition requests differ between hospitals and retail pharmacy practice. Identification with a hospital transaction or treatment may be of prime importance.

3. *The relationship between the hospital and the part-time pharmacist in the function of drug procurement or purchasing for both patient and general hospital use should be based on fixed responsibilities and meet the following principles on Business Relationships.*

The smaller hospital generally purchases supplies through a modified central channel in the organization. The need for expert evaluation of specifications in the drug field is recognized. Hospitals contributing services to indigent patients enjoy special price privileges, and drugs in this category ethically should not be diverted to other outlets. The complexity in the area of procurement and possibility of abuses by either the hospital or the part-time pharmacist require careful evaluation of the procedure.

a. That basis of financial arrangement between a hospital and part-time local pharmacist should be followed which would best meet the local situation. It is recognized that no one basis would seem applicable or suitable in all instances.

The hospital and the part-time pharmacist must have a thorough appreciation of each other's business systems and controls. This may involve detailed exploration.

b. Arrangements involving services to patients through voluntary insurance, indigent patients, or employees should be established in accordance with accepted hospital relationships and philosophies involving such programs.

Some insurance plans vary between localities, and in some instances the so-called "no-pay or part-pay" patients comprise a sizable number of persons. Special financial arrangements in accord with hospital policy for other services provided may be required.

c. Arrangements for a regular schedule for the personal services of the part-time pharmacist on the hospital premises should be made on a flexible basis related to time spent and services provided.

The hospital schedule and its 24-hour service to patients demands a varying amount or period spent during regular visits or to meet emergency requirements. In general, an average amount of time may be considered initially. Such an arrangement should be included in a plan, even though many services are provided remotely from the hospital premises.

d. Solicitation of patients or rendering services to the medical staff for their private practice through hospital channels by any person connected with the hospital is unethical.

The privilege of hospital affiliation should not be used to gain unfair advantage over other members of the profession. Patients and physicians are attracted to a particular pharmacy because of its known merit and established reputation for satisfactory service. Implied or open solicitation through hospital connections should not be indulged in by part-time pharmacists.

e. Relationships between a part-time pharmacist and the hospital are considered on the merit of reputable, prompt service to patients at reasonable cost, ability to serve the hospital in all phases of pharmacy service demanded by hospital requirements, and should subscribe to the suggested principles.

In communities where several pharmacies are available, a hospital may hesitate to engage the services of any one pharmacist because of pressures and ill-feeling against the hospital by other pharmacists. Intra-professional rivalry should not place the hospital in a position of not raising its own pharmacy service standards. The hospital as a community institution should be allowed the privilege of judging its future relationships for expanded services on the basis of a part-time pharmacist's ability to provide those services in the spirit in which patient care is provided in that hospital.

Conclusion

These Principles of Relationship Between Smaller Hospitals and Part-time Pharmacists for Hospitals are suggested. These recommended guides for further development and discussion are a beginning for those hospitals and pharmacists who wish to explore possibilities for developing higher standards of pharmaceutical service in institutions without full-time pharmacists.

A combination of such principles and the Minimum Standard for Pharmacies in Hospitals can provide both smaller hospitals and part-time pharmacists a working basis for a higher level of pharmaceutical service.

Small Hospital-Community Pharmacist, The Partial Responsibility Relationship

Under this plan, the community pharmacist contracts to provide the small hospital with prescription orders and other drug merchandise. He does not agree to partake in any of the routine activities normally engaged in by the hospital pharmacist.

An agreement of this type usually provides that the nurse or the physician telephone to the community pharmacist the patient's drug needs. The compounded prescription is then to be delivered to the hospital with a properly identified charge slip. The hospital then bills and collects for the prescription medication along with the routine hospital charges. At the end of a specified billing period, the community pharmacy renders to the hospital a detailed bill of all prescriptions and other drug stocks less a previously agreed upon discount from the total charges. This discount, therefore, provides the community hospital with a small income from its drug service to compensate for its expenses in the billing and collection of the drug charges.

Responsibilities of Community or Consulting Pharmacists To Extended Care Facilities and Small Hospitals

Since most extended care facilities and small hospitals do not employ full time pharmacists, many of them contract for such service. Pharmacists who agree to provide such a service are required by the Medicare law to assume certain responsibilities and perform specific functions. These go far beyond the dispensing of prescriptions for patients but include an interdisciplinary approach towards the provision of consulting pharmaceutical service.

Dispensing Prescriptions for Extended Care Facilities and Small Hospital Patients

Extended care facilities, nursing homes and small hospitals do not maintain a full service pharmacy on the premises. Thus, the medical staff relies upon community pharmacists to dispense medications from the local pharmacy and have them delivered to the facility. The labels on these prescriptions, in addition to the customary information, should also indicate:

> a. Name of Medication
> b. Strength
> c. Name of Manufacturer
> d. Lot and/or control number

The above information is desirable in the event of a drug recall.

Consulting Pharmaceutical Service

Generally, the community or consulting pharmacist is expected to work with the organized medical staff, the Director of Nursing and the Administrator for the purpose of establishing written policies and procedures for the control and utilization of medications in the facility.

These policies are normally referred to as the *Policy and Procedural Manual for Pharmacy Services* and should include, among others, the following subject headings:

1. Automatic "Stop Order" policy.
2. Control system for alcohol and spiritous liquors.
3. Control system for all drugs covered by the Controlled Substances Act of 1971. This Act controls the use of narcotics, barbiturates, amphetamines and certain stimulant and depressant medications.
4. Controls for the use of research drugs.
5. Control of physician's drug samples.
6. Policy governing self administration of medications.
7. Emergency drug kits

   a. Contents
   b. Inspection procedure.

8. Reporting of medication errors.
9. Reporting of adverse drug reactions.
10. Periodic inspection of nursing station medication cabinets to insure—

    a. That external medications are kept apart from internal use drugs.
    b. That biological refrigerator has a thermometer, that temperature range of refrigerator is 35.5° to 50° F. (Ice cube section used for small pox, yellow fever, measles and polio vaccines, if stocked, and of types requiring below freezing storage.) Biologicals may also be kept in general use refrigerator providing they are stored in a separate box.
    c. That there are no outdated medications (antibiotics, biologicals, etc.)
    d. That medication cabinets are kept locked.
    e. That Metric-English weight and measure conversion charts are at each nursing station medication center.
    f. That working text references on drug uses, side effects and contraindications, such as the American Hospital Formulary Service of the American Society of Hospital Pharmacists are at nursing station medication centers.

11. Policy on medication labeling.
12. Policy and procedure on removal of medications from pharmacy or drug room in absence of pharmacist.
13. Policy and procedure on medications to be taken home by the patient.
14. Pharmacy or store room inventory control system including the dating of stocks on receipt.
15. Macroscopical (light-testing) examination of parenterals.
16. Policy concerning additives to parenterals.

17. The creation and activities of the Pharmacy and Therapeutics Committee including the keeping of written minutes of meetings.
18. The establishment and maintenance of a formulary or drug list.
19. Fire control provisions.
20. Qualification of pharmacists and experience requirements.
21. Policy on record keeping.
22. Policy on Poison Control Center Communications and references.
23. Audit of narcotics and other "controlled' drugs at nursing stations.
24. An "official" (medical staff approved) list of medical abbreviations applicable to drug administration and dispensing.
25. Application of FDA medication lot number recall "alarm" to the facility.
26. Policy and procedures relative to the writing and signing of medication orders.

Small Hospital-Large Hospital Pharmacy Relationship

Many large hospitals often provide assistance to the smaller hospitals by providing pathology and radiology services. In addition, the small hospital often sends to the larger hospital various specimens of human fluids for comprehensive or special laboratory procedures. Since the avenue of cooperation is opened by the above, is there any reason why the large hospital cannot also provide pharmaceutical coverage?

The pharmacy service between the two hospitals can be handled in the same manner that a retail pharmacist would assume full responsibility for the pharmacy service. In this case it is much simpler for telephone service between the two institutions is open around-the-clock, the pharmacist who is on-call at the larger hospital may also cover the small hospital; and finally the inventory of the large hospital is usually more than adequate to provide for emergency items for the small hospital.

This type of arrangement is mutually advantageous to both hospitals in that it provides the smaller hospital with the services of experienced hospital pharmacists and permits the larger hospital with another opportunity to contribute to the over-all improvement of medical care in the community.

Suggested Program for Small Hospitals with no Pharmacy or Pharmacist Relationship

Hospitals in this category of having no pharmacy or pharmacist relationship usually rely upon other personnel to handle their daily services. Although nurses are primarily engaged in this practice, it is a known fact that aides and technicians are also utilized.[1]

Drugs used by these institutions are usually stored in a small room, often referred to as the "drug room." Invariably, it is overcrowded, with no semblance of inventory control.

Even under these conditions, the hospital administrator can undertake a simple program to improve his pharmacy service even though he is unable to secure the minimal services of a part-time pharmacist. The proposed program consists of the following steps:

1. The administrator should call a meeting of representatives of his medical and nursing staffs for the purpose of reviewing the present drug inventory and selecting the medications which the hospital should keep and at the same time ascertain those items not in the inventory but which should be procured.
2. Merchandise in the drug room, not on this list, should be discarded or, where possible, exchanged for medications which have been requested to be added to the inventory.
3. A subscription to the American Hospital Formulary Service should be entered because this will make available to the administrator, doctor and nurse a single, concise and authoritative source of information on the drugs carried in the drug room.
4. All of the drugs and related diagnostic agents should then be purchased in the smallest units possible in order that they may be dispensed to the nursing station without repackaging or labeling (both of which are pharmacy acts). Strip packaging is ideally suited for this type of dispensing.
5. If at all possible, place the responsibility for the drug room in the hands of the hospital's most competent nurse or nursing supervisor.
6. Make some arrangement with the local pharmacy for the purchase of prescriptions calling for mixtures of medications for individual patients.
7. The administrator should meet with his medical and nursing staff at least twice a year in order to keep the inventory current and maintain the interest of all concerned in this aspect of patient care.

Because this program requires the purchase of medications in small individual use packages, the cost per dose of the medication will necessarily be higher to both the hospital and to the patient. This, however, should not deter the administrator from undertaking such a program for in exchange for this slightly higher cost per dose of medication he is providing as safe a pharmaceutical service as is possible under the circumstances.

Pharmacy's Role in Nursing Homes—Extended Care Facilities

The United States Public Health Service in its Nursing Home Standards Guide defines the term nursing home as—

> "a facility or unit which is designated, staffed and equipped for the accommodation of individuals who are not in need of hospital care but who are in need of nursing care and related medical services which are prescribed by or performed under the direction of persons licensed to provide such care or services in accordance with the laws of the state in which the facility is located."

With the advent of Medicare, a great deal of attention has been focused on the nursing home and the role which it must play in the care of our elderly citizens.

The Nursing Homes and Related Facilities Branch, Division of Medical Care Administration, Public Health Service published a report on licensed nursing homes[4] and related facilities which showed that as of June 1965, there were 18,958 facilities with 760,441 beds in the country who were providing either nursing home services, personal care with nursing services, or plain custodial care.

Other statistics that are of interest are that in 1975 there may be as many as 25 million people in this country who will be sixty-five years of age or older; that an additional 70,000 nursing home beds are under construction and that the average nursing home will have approximately 66 beds with a range of 40- to 100-bed capacity.

Clearly then, these patients will require medical, nursing and pharmaceutical services in a volume which is far greater in scope and concentration than we are able to provide due to the personnel shortages within these three professions.

Thus many community pharmacists and hospital pharmacists will have to do double duty in order for the profession of pharmacy to meet its obligation to these patients.

The relationship between the community pharmacist and/or the local hospital pharmacist would be similar to that of servicing a small community hospital. Since these have been presented earlier in the chapter they will not be repeated here.

Public Law 89–97 provides for certain conditions for a pharmaceutical service in the extended care facility. For the convenience of the reader these are hereinafter reproduced and will serve as guidelines for those pharmacists who do respond to the call for pharmaceutical service in the nursing home.

Condition of Participation For
Extended Care Facilities

PHARMACEUTICAL SERVICES

WHETHER DRUGS ARE GENERALLY PROCURED FROM A COMMUNITY PHARMACY OR STOCKED BY THE FACILITIES, THE EXTENDED CARE FACILITY HAS METHODS AND PROCEDURES FOR ITS PHARMACEUTICAL SERVICES THAT ARE IN ACCORD WITH ACCEPTED PROFESSIONAL PRACTICES.

Standard A
Procedures for Administration of Pharmaceutical Services

The extended care facility provides appropriate methods and procedures for the obtaining, dispensing and administering of drugs and biologicals, developed with the advice of a staff pharmacist, a consultant pharmacist, or a *pharmaceutical advisory committee* which includes one or more licensed pharmacists.

FACTOR 1. If the extended care facility has a pharmacy department, a licensed pharmacist is employed to administer the pharmacy department

FACTOR 2. If the facility does not have a pharmacy department, it has provision for promptly and conveniently obtaining required drugs and biologicals from community pharmacies.

FACTOR 3. If the facility has only a drug room where bulk drugs are stored:

(i) The consultant pharmacist is responsible for the control of all bulk drugs and maintains records of their receipt and disposition.

(ii) The consultant pharmacist dispenses drugs from the drug room, properly labels them and makes them available to appropriate licensed nursing personnel. Wherever possible, the pharmacist in dispensing drugs works from the prescriber's original order or a direct copy.

(iii) Provision is made for emergency withdrawal of medications from the drug room.

FACTOR 4. An emergency medication kit approved by the facility's group of professional personnel is kept readily available.

Standard B
Conformance With Physician's Orders

All medications administered to patients are ordered in writing by the patient's physician. Oral orders are given only to a licensed nurse, immediately reduced to writing, signed by the nurse and countersigned by the physician within 48 hours. Medications not specifically limited as to time or number of doses, when ordered, are automatically stopped in accordance with written policy approved by the physician or physicians responsible for advising the facility on its medical administrative policies.

FACTOR 1. The charge nurse and the prescribing physician together review monthly each patient's medications.

FACTOR 2. The patient's attending physician is notified of stop order policies and contacted promptly for renewal of such orders so that continuity of the patient's therapeutic regimen is not interrupted.

FACTOR 3. Medications are released to patients on discharge only on the written authorization of the physician.

Standard C

Administration of Medications

All medications are administered by licensed medical or nursing personnel in accordance with the Medical and Nurse Practice Acts of each State.

Each dose administered is properly recorded in the clinical record.

FACTOR 1. The nursing station has readily available items necessary for the proper administration of medication.

FACTOR 2. In administering medications, medication cards or other State approved systems are used and checked again the physician's orders.

FACTOR 3. Medications prescribed for one patient are not administered to any other patient.

FACTOR 4. Self-administration of medications by patients is not permitted except for emergency drugs on special order of the patient's physician or in a predischarge program under the supervision of a licensed nurse.

FACTOR 5. Medication errors and drug reactions are immediately reported to the patient's physician and an entry thereof made in the patient's clinical record as well as on an incident report.

FACTOR 6. Up-to-date medication reference texts and sources of information are provided, such as *ASHP Hospital Formulary* and *Physicians Desk Reference.*

Standard D

Labeling and Storing Medications

Patients' medications are properly labeled and stored in a locked cabinet at the nurses' station.

FACTOR 1. The label of each patient's individual medication container clearly indicates the patient's full name, physician's name, prescription number, name and strength of drug, date of issue, expiration date of all time-dated drugs, and name, address and telephone number of pharmacy issuing the drug. It is advisable that the manufacturer's name and the lot or control number of the medication also appear on the label.

FACTOR 2. Medication containers having soiled, damaged, incomplete, illegible, or makeshift labels are returned to the issuing pharmacist or pharmacy for re-labeling or disposal. Containers having no labels are destroyed in accordance with State and Federal laws.

FACTOR 3. The medications of each patient are kept and stored in their originally received containers and transferring between containers is forbidden.

FACTOR 4. Separately locked, securely fastened boxes (or drawers) within the medicine cabinet are provided for storage of narcotics, barbiturates, amphetamines and other dangerous drugs.

FACTOR 5. Cabinets are well lighted and of sufficient size to permit storage without crowding.

FACTOR 6. Medications requiring refrigeration are kept in a separate, locked box within a refrigerator at or near the nursing station.

FACTOR 7. Poisons and medications "for external use only" are kept in a locked cabinet and separate from other medications.

FACTOR 8. Medications no longer in use are disposed of or destroyed in accordance with Federal and State laws and regulations.

FACTOR 9. Medications having an expiration date are removed from usage and properly disposed of after such date.

Standard E

Compliance With Laws Controlling Narcotics, Etc.

The extended care facility complies with all Federal and State laws relating to the procurement, storage, dispensing, administration and disposal of narcotics, hypnotics, amphetamines, certain psychosomatic medications, and other legend drugs.

FACTOR 1. A narcotic record is maintained which lists on separate sheets for each type and strength of narcotic the following information: date, time administered, name of patient, dose, physician's name, signature of person administering dose, and balance.

Drug Safety in the Nursing Home and Extended Care Facility

The consultant pharmacist serving the nursing home and the extended care facility has the obligation of ensuring safe medication practices in the facility. This goes far beyond the accepted procedures of proper dispensing and labeling of medications and their containers. The horizon for the initiation of control measures is limitless and depends upon the ingenuity of the consultant. However, two tried and true methods are readily available.

First, the consultant pharmacist should maintain a patient drug profile on each and every patient in the unit. Again, these profiles vary

PBBH

I. GENERAL INFORMATION	Frequency		

TPR————————— —————————   Diet: Regular —————————   Activities of Daily Living:

BP ————————— —————————   Special: specify—————————   Bathing: —————————————

Intake ————————— —————————   —————————————   Eating: —————————————

Output ——————— — —————————   Fluids: —————————   Mobility: —————————————

Date	II. Medications		III. Diagnostic Tests				
			Date Ord.	X-ray	Date Done	Lab.	Date Done
				EKG			
				Special			

IV.

No.—————————————   Adm. Date ————————————————   Religion ———————————— SIL —————————

Name —————————————————   Adm. Diagnosis ——————————————————————————————

FORM 241

Fig. 96.   Patient profile form in use in one institution.

with the facility and the pharmacist however. Reference to Figure 96 provides the pharmacist with one type of profile. Some of the items on this profile may appear to be superfluous to some yet they have proven useful on occasion. These are the data on "religion" and SIL (Seriously ill list). The religion information has been useful whenever the patient was likely to have blood or blood products prescribed and the use of such products was against his religious beliefs. The data indicating whether or not the patient was considered so ill as to warrant placement on the seriously ill list may be of use to the pharmacist in his discussions with the physician and nursing staff. In addition, it helps to emphasize the urgency with which changes in the therapeutic regimen must be made.

Second, the routine inspection of the nursing station is of great importance in that it helps to remove out-dated and deteriorated medications from the medication closet and helps to check to see that products are properly labeled and stored. A sample check list is presented in Figure 97.

PETER BENT BRIGHAM HOSPITAL
Nursing Unit Inspection Guide

Unit_____   Department of Pharmacy   Routine_____
Date_____   Follow-up_____

A. INDIVIDUAL PATIENT DRUGS:
    1. Present arrangement and space allotment for inpatient med-
        dications is satisfactory . . . . Yes___ No___
    2. All drugs have been returned to pharmacy for credit fol-
        lowing discontinuation or patient discharge . . . . . . Yes___ No___
    3. All labels on medication containers are accurate, are
        not defaced, and necessary accessory labels are present . Yes___ No___
    4. Injectable medications are properly labeled as to date
        of reconstitution, concentration, expiration date (in
        addition to patient room-number, name and date). . . . .. Yes___ No___
    5. Drugs requiring refrigeration are properly stored . . . . Yes___ No___

B. CHARGE FLOOR STOCK DRUGS:
    1. Stock level for each item is adequate . . . . Yes___ No___
    2. All items have charge voucher attached . . . . Yes___ No___
    3. All items are appropriately labeled and stored . . . . .. Yes___ No___

C. FREE FLOOR STOCK-DRUGS:
    1. Present arrangement and space allotment for floor stock
        is satisfactory . . . . Yes___ No___
    2. All items are properly labeled . . . . Yes___ No___
    3. All labels are in satisfactory condition . . . . Yes___ No___
    4. Internal drugs are separated from external drugs . . . . Yes___ No___
    5. All items are in adequate supply . . . . Yes___ No___

D. EMERGENCY STOCK DRUGS:
    1. Emergency box is in proper place . . . . Yes___ No___
    2. Emergency cart is ready for use . . . . Yes___ No___
    3. All drugs are in date . . . . Yes___ No___

E. REFRIGERATED DRUGS:
    1. All drugs are in the appropriate compartment . . . . Yes___ No___
    2. All drugs are properly and completely labeled
        (expiration date, concentration, reconstitution date
        etc.) . . . . Yes___ No___

F. NARCOTICS, BARBITURATES AND CONTROLLED SUBSTANCES:
    1. The narcotic drawer is locked . . . . Yes___ No___
    2. The key is with the Head Nurse (or nurse in charge) . . . Yes___ No___
    3. All drugs are currently being used . . . . Yes___ No___

Notes and comments as a result of discussion of inspection form with
Nurse:_____
_____
_____
_____

All Drugs Removed from the Unit have been reviewed with the Nurse.

Signed:
_____ Pharmacist_____Nurse

Copy-1 - Pharmacy   Copy-2 - Nursing Unit   Copy-3 - Nursing Unit

FIG. 97.   Sample Nursing Unit Inspection Guide.

SELECTED REFERENCES

Nursing Homes and Related Facilities, Fact Book, U. S. Public Health Service, Washington, D. C., Government Printing Office, 1963.

KABAT, HUGH: Drugs, Medicare and the Nursing Home, Nursing Homes, *15*: 10, 1966.

Conditions of Participation for Home Health Agencies, U. S. Dept. of Health, Education and Welfare, Washington, D. C., Government Printing Office (HIM 2 1966).

CASHMAN, JOHN W.: Nursing Homes in the Medicare Program, J. A. Ph. A., *6*:236, May, 1966.

McDONALD, ROY J.: Nursing Homes Today, J. A. Ph. A., *6*:239, May, 1966.

ECKEL, FRED M.: Pharmacist's Key to Nursing Home Inservice Training, J. A. Ph. A., *6*:258, May, 1966.

Pharmaceutical Services in the Nursing Home, 6th Ed., American Pharmaceutical Association, Washington, D.C., 1972.

BIBLIOGRAPHY

1. FRANCKE, D. E., LATIOLAIS, C. J., FRANCKE, G. N. and HO, N. F. H.: *Mirror To Hospital Pharmacy*, p. 169, American Society of Hospital Pharmacists, Washington, D.C.
2. Extending Pharmacy Services in Smaller Hospitals, Am. Prof. Pharm., *22*: 6:540, 1956.
3. Suggested Principles of Relationship Between Smaller Hospitals and Part-Time Pharmacists, Am. J. Hosp. Pharm., *16*:3:124, 1959.
4. Conditions of Participation for Extended Care Facilities, U. S. Dept. Health, Education and Welfare, Washington, D. C., Government Printing Office (HIM 3 1966).

Chapter

30

Professional Practices and Relations

THE hospital pharmacists of this country can, and in many instances do, carry on a professional and public relations program. The literature is replete with evidence of the need of promoting pharmacy to its kindred professions and to the public.

Hospital pharmacists are in an excellent position to do the profession a great service because of their daily contact with the members of the allied professions and a sizeable segment of the public.

Opportunities for a Public Relations Program

The hospital pharmacy in an average size hospital is the focal point for about 15 to 20 physicians each day in addition to a number of nurses, technicians, and other allied specialists. Therefore, hospital pharmacists can promote pharmacy by instituting and following through with a good professional relations program. Obviously, the execution of such a program will cost very little from a monetary standpoint but will call for an investment of time and effort on the part of those participating. Moreover, despite the tremendous amount of money spent by the drug industry in promoting their products to physicians, there are some doctors who just will not be detailed, will not read their direct mail or journal advertising or who cannot be contacted; but there are relatively few doctors who do not have hospital affiliations and, therefore, they can be contacted by the hospital pharmacist.

Walsh and Hassan[1] have stated that a reasonable program of professional promotion for hospital pharmacy involves the application of the following:

1. Publishing and distributing a pharmacy bulletin (Chapter 6).
2. Cooperating in hospital teaching program (Chapter 26).
3. Taking an active role in administrative committee work.
4. Taking an active role in pharmaceutical organizations.
5. Cooperating with the medical research staff.

6. Maintaining an adequate reference library (Chapter 25).
7. Cooperating with community pharmacists (Chapter 29).
8. Accepting speaking engagements.
9. Preparing hospital pharmacy displays.
10. Developing and maintaining the hospital formulary (Chapter 5).
11. Maintaining an efficient, professional pharmacy.
12. Being a safety expert (Chapter 28).
13. Maintaining a well-controlled manufacturing section (Chapter 21).
14. Making special promotional efforts.

Participate in Administrative Committee Work

There seems to be no limit to the number and kind of committees on which the hospital pharmacist may serve. This type of work offers him the opportunity of demonstrating his ability and college training in the medical sciences as well as business administration. Many hospital pharmacists are currently serving on such committees as the Current Practice Committee, Safety Committee, Infection Control Committee, Antibiotics Committee and the Administrative Policy Committee.

Those pharmacists who feel that they are too busy to undertake these extra-curricular activities soon find that they are excluded from the professional group within the hospital. This is brought about by the fact that the failure to participate in the problems of the hospital and related professions implies that the pharmacist is either not knowledgeable or is uninterested in the welfare of the institution and indirectly the patient.

Membership in Professional Associations

There are a number of associations which represent the various segments of American pharmacy. Of these, the *American Pharmaceutical Association* purports to represent the profession as a whole; the *American Society of Hospital Pharmacists* represents the hospital pharmacist; the *American College of Apothecaries* speaks for the professional pharmacist; the *National Association of Retail Druggists* represents the retail store owner plus a number of other associations representing manufacturers, wholesalers, colleges of pharmacy and the various scientific disciplines of pharmacy.

Certainly, the minimal membership which the hospital pharmacist should hold should be in the *American Pharmaceutical Association* and the *American Society of Hospital Pharmacists*. It is also desirable for him to belong to his regional and local pharmaceutical associations.

Many hospital administrators advocate personal membership in state and national hospital associations. If the pharmacist finds it possible to become a member of these groups, it not only enhances his professional stature, but also gives him an opportunity to learn about and understand the problems of his professional associates, thereby better qualifying him for his own position.

It has been stated[1] that approximately 63 per cent of the practicing physicians of the United States belong to the *American Medical Association,* whereas about 20 per cent of the practicing pharmacists belong to the *American Pharmaceutical Association.*

Clearly then the pharmacists of America, and more particularly the hospital pharmacists, must make every effort to strengthen our professional organizations in order that they may provide all branches of pharmacy with the leadership and services essential to a growing profession.

In addition, the mere joining of our professional associations is not sufficient. It is mandatory that in order to ensure developmental growth of both the individual and the association, each member must take an active role in the sponsored programs and committee assignments.

Cooperate with Medical Research Staff

Clinical research, as it is conducted today, requires the cooperation of all of the allied health services. Pharmacy is no exception. The hospital pharmacist can become an integral part of this research in a number of ways.

1. He can be of invaluable assistance to the busy physician by controlling the inventory and distribution of the investigative material.

2. He can maintain an accurate record on the chemistry, pharmacology, posology, and toxicology of the compounds being studied. This information is oftentimes vital to another physician who is called in an emergency to treat a patient who is taking the research drug when the original investigator cannot be located.

3. By suggesting and preparing better vehicles or physical forms of the new compounds undergoing trial.

4. The astute pharmacist will offer to develop and operate a double or triple blind study for the clinical evaluation of the research drug.

5. Because the pharmacist is usually a member of local social or fraternal groups, he is in an excellent position to assist the physician in the recruiting of normal human subjects for controlled *in vivo* studies of investigational use drugs.

Cooperate with Local Pharmacists

This phase of the program requires delicate handling on the part of those concerned. Many times the cry is heard from the community practitioner of pharmacy that the hospital pharmacist is not cooperative and is driving him into bankruptcy because of the low prices quoted in hospitals for many medications. This fighting between the ranks is uncalled for and can be eliminated if both parties will learn to cooperate with and not compete against each other.

Some means of cooperation between retailer and hospital pharmacist are as follows: loaning each other products, making available from the hospital pharmacy special formula medications, supplying copies of prescriptions when legal restrictions do not apply, and finally, supporting organizations and legislation sponsored by the community pharmacists.

A step in the right direction was taken when the *American Pharmaceutical Association* and the *American Society of Hospital Pharmacists* joined together to create a *Commission to Study Outpatient Hospital Pharmacy Service.*

Among the elements to be studied by the commission will be (1) the hospital pharmacy in essential patient service, (2) the need for the public to have medications dispensed by pharmacists, (3) professional opportunities in community and hospital pharmacy, (4) the effect of the number of community and hospital pharmacies on professional opportunities, (5) effects of location on status, and (6) legal implications.

Maintain an Efficient Professional Pharmacy

A clean, well-organized pharmacy with alert personnel can do much towards the furtherance of professional and public good will. It makes no difference where the pharmacy is located, how old it is, or how little equipment it has; it can still reflect cleanliness, organization, and alertness of personnel. The effect of a good library and reference files, and committee participation have already been discussed.

Accept Speaking Engagements

The hospital pharmacist is usually the unseen but essential member of the hospital health team. Patients expect and get his services; however, they seldom if ever get to know anything about the role played by the hospital pharmacist.

Therefore, the public relations aspect of the recommended program can be greatly benefited if the hospital pharmacist will give a part of his free time to the addressing of civic, fraternal, and church organizations.

Another means of creating good professional relations is to be of service to the pharmaceutical manufacturers by accepting invitations to appear on their sales training programs.

It goes almost without saying that hospital pharmacists should welcome a chance to appear on refresher course programs offered by the colleges of pharmacy, or on the programs of local, regional or national hospital and pharmaceutical associations.

Hospital Pharmacy Displays

The old Chinese proverb of "one picture is worth a thousand words" can be readily applied to this part of the program.

A display in the hospital lobby during *National Pharmacy Week* can do a great deal for both public and professional relations. Displays depicting the role of hospital pharmacy in the hospital picture can be of inestimable value when arranged in conjunction with local nursing and medical meetings or conventions.

Be a Safety Expert

According to Miss Nina Craft, Director of Nursing Services and Education, Los Angeles County General Hospital, Los Angeles, California (see Am. Prof. Pharm. p. 730, Sept., 1953), "Fifty per cent of the accidents to patients due to drug administration could have been eliminated for the nurses by the pharmacists." For a detailed discussion on drug safety see Chapter 28.

Special Promotional Efforts

This category is intended to allow for the ideas born as a result of deep thought and, in some instances, imagination. One such promotional effort was the distribution of Christmas cards imprinted with names of the pharmacy staff and sent out to the various departments and staff members.

Another promotional effort was the distribution of hand lotion and hand cream manufactured in the hospital pharmacy to each new female employee of the hospital.

Participation in Comprehensive Health Care Programs

The preparation and formulation of a health services delivery system designed to meet the legislative and administrative guidelines developed by the Federal Government has been delegated to the local community. In this setting providers of all facets of health care are expected to interface and work cooperatively with the consumer to develop new systems for the delivery of comprehensive medical care at reasonable cost. As a result thereof, programs such as the Regional Medical Programs (RMP), Model Cities Demonstration Act, Health Maintenance Organizations (HMO's), Home Care Services and neighborhood health centers have developed. In July of 1973, the Federal Government introduced Professional Service Review Organizations (PSRO's) and Certificate of Need (CofN) requirements for the review of medical care and utilization and for the determination of need for new facilities, equipment and services. In addition, a number of new prepaid health insurance plans have come upon the scene. Pharmacists, pharmacy as a profession and colleges of pharmacy must be prepared to participate in the planning, organization and operation of these units if pharmacy is to be included in the reimbursement rate for the so-called "comprehensive health care services."[2]

Of primary importance to the institutional pharmacist, is the position taken by the American Hospital Association as is evidenced by the following excerpts from its *Statement* on *Health Care for the Disadvantaged*:

> "The fullest possible involvement of hospitals in the delivery of community health services is in the best interests both of the citizens of the community and the hospital. It guarantees an improvement in the total fabric of health care."[3]

From the point of view of having an experienced force participate in the planning of community health needs, the *Statement* provides:

> "The hospital is the key community center of high quality health services. The hospital, together with its medical staff, is the health resource that has demonstrated great success in assembling sophisticated equipment and expert personnel. It has also encouraged the introduction of the improvement of elements of community control, and internal quality checks, and administrative and organizational knowledge. These factors qualify it to assume leadership in improving health care for all, rich and poor, urban and rural."[3]

Although it is not possible to provide the student with a detailed discussion of all of the concepts for providing comprehensive health care to all Americans, it is important to touch upon some of the better known and utilized plans. In this connection, the American people have decided that the right to optimal health care is necessary for all people to enjoy their constitutional right to life, liberty, and the pursuit of happiness. To achieve this, a great deal of thought and study went into various methodologies and there merged a general consensus that the ideal health system should achieve the following goals:[4]

> a. Accessibility.
> b. Availability.
> c. Acceptability to the consumer and provider.
> d. Phased implementation, assuring that the system is able to accept the increased demand before money is poured into health care.
> e. Minimal government regulation.
> f. Consumer participation in the cost and in the organization of services.
> g. Quality assurance.
> h. Cost predictability.

Health Maintenance Organizations

On February 18, 1971, President Richard M. Nixon delivered a special message to the Congress titled "Building a National Health Strategy." In it he stated:[5]

> "In recent years, a new method for delivering health services has achieved growing respect. This new approach has two essential attributes. It brings together a comprehensive range of medical services in a single organization so that a patient is assured of convenient access to all of them. And it provides needed services for a fixed contract fee which is paid in advance by all subscribers."

> "Such an organization can have a variety of forms and names and sponsors. One of the strengths of this new concept, in fact, is its great flexibility. The general term which has been applied to all of these units is 'HMO'—Health Maintenance Organizations."

Thus, it is clear that a Health Maintenance organization (HMO) is based upon four principles:[5]

> a. "It is an *organized system* of health care which assures the delivery of
> b. "an agreed upon set of *comprehensive health maintenance* and *treatment services* for
> c. "a voluntarily *enrolled group* of persons in a geographic area and
> d. "is reimbursed through a pre-negotiated and fixed periodic payment made by or on behalf of each person or family unit enrolled in the plan."

Continuing Care Service—Home Care Service

In addition to being responsible for inpatient care, the hospital must also help to provide a matrix in which seemingly disparate parts of the health care rendered can be linked into an organic whole—a health care network. Thus, hospitals, particularly those in the medical center setting, have developed continuing care and home care services.

The Continuing Care Service is the link between the hospital, nursing home, extended care facility or rehabilitation facility. At times, it can include the patient's home. The service generally plans for the full range of continuing care needs of patients after discharge from the hospital.

The Home Care Service provides continuing medical care of the patient when he has been discharged to his home. Such a service coordinates the activities of the patient's physician, the visiting nurse and brings into the home environment the services of the dietitian and social service workers.

Prepaid Health Care Programs

Comprehensive prepaid medical care insurance programs are generally available to all economic groups and provide inpatient and outpatient care in accord with the scope of the program. The nation's two largest such programs are the Kaiser-Permanente on the west coast and the Health Insurance Plan of Greater New York.

Two novel programs have been developed on the east coast; the *Harvard Community Health Plan* (HCHP) and *Health Inc.*

The HCHP differs from the west coast and New York plan in that it is sponsored by a medical school and its arrangements for the provision of hospital and medical services is through four of the medical schools affiliated teaching hospitals. In addition, HCHP has developed contractual relationships with Blue Cross and private insurance carriers for the marketing of the "Plan" thereby precluding the need for HCHP to become an insurance carrier.

Health Inc., on the other hand, is a private, non-profit corporation dedicated towards the development of a mechanism for providing health care for all low-income groups in a specified geographic area in cooperation with municipal, state and federal government.

Drug Rehabilitation Programs

Because of the widespread abuse of drugs, this area of endeavor is quite popular on the community front. Accordingly, participation in these programs by the individual who knows most about drugs—the pharmacist—is mandatory in order to preserve good public and professional relations. In addition to drug abuse educational programs, the pharmacist should encourage these members of the program to study and participate in the following areas:

  a. Drug abuse problems treated in the hospital.
  b. Legal and ethical issues involved in treating drug abuse.
  c. Medical and psychiatric approaches to the treatment of drug abuse.
  d. Problems associated with detoxification, especially with concurrent medical or surgical disease.
  e. The use of various drugs in detoxification programs.
  f. Drug abuse treatment programs in the urban and suburban areas served by the hospital.

Drug Consultation Programs

One study on the significance of drug consultation programs conducted by pharmacists to the discharged hospital patient concluded that discharged patients who had such consultation, showed less deviation from prescribed drug regimens and had fewer medication problems at home than did patients who had not been accorded this service.[6]

Obviously, drug consultation programs are important from the point of view of patient safety, however, a great deal of good public relations benefit can accrue to the hospital from this professional practice.

In discussing drug therapy with the patient, the following points are recommended for discussion by Cole and Emanuel:[6]

  1. "Determination of medication already being taken which may duplicate or interfere with newly prescribed medications.
  2. The optimum dosage administration schedule to be followed.
  3. Measures to be taken in the management of side effects of the prescribed medications.
  4. The importance of administering all doses of the medications as prescribed."

Summary

The points and the program that have been discussed are basic signs that can be followed on the road to better professional relations between all branches of the medical profession and the laymen.

Better understanding, however achieved, always leads to better and mutual respect.

A better program of professional relations will help us as pharmacists to better serve the needs of humanity. Perhaps the great Dr. Albert Schweitzer summed up what should be our real objective when he said:

> "I do not know what your destiny will be, but one thing I do know: The only people who will be really happy are those who will have sought and found how to serve."

SELECTED REFERENCES

ARCHAMBAULT, G. F.:   Pharmacy Human Relations, Hosp. Progress, *40*:83, 1959.

YOUNG, K. C.:   A Code of Professional Conduct for Pharmacy, Hosp. Forum, *3*:37, 1960.

ARCHIN, M.:   A Public and Professional Relations Program for Hospital Pharmacists, Part I., Hosp. Forum, *3*:31, 1960.

Ibid: *3*:31, 1960.

An Institute on HMO's—Health Maintenance Organizations. M.H.A. Newsletter Supplement, Vol. XXIII No. 2—February 1972, Massachusetts Hospital Association, Burlington, Massachusetts 01803.

Pharmacy Foundations and HMO's, The VOICE of the Pharmacist, Vol. XV No. 19—March 3, 1972, American College of Apothecaries, 874 Union Ave., Memphis, Tenn. 38103.

BIBLIOGRAPHY

1. WALSH, R. A. and HASSAN, W. E.:   A 14 Point Program for Promoting Professional and Public Relations by the Hospital Pharmacist, The Bulletin Am. Soc. Hosp. Pharm., *13*:4:315, 1956.

2. EMANUEL, SR. D.C. and BARR, MARTIN: The Role of Wayne State University College of Pharmacy in the Development of an Innovative and Comprehensive Health Care Program, J.D.Ph.A., NS*11*:10:551, 1971.

3. ———: Statement of Health Care for the Disadvantaged 5-60, American Hospital Association, Chicago, Illinois 60611 (1970).

4. AINSWORTH, THOMAS H., JR.: The Significance of the HMO Concept to Hospitals and to the Hospital System, M.H.A. Newsletter Supplement, Vol. XXIII No. 2, February 1972, Massachusetts Hospital Association, Burlington, Massachusetts 01803.

5. ———: Health Maintenance Organizations, The Concept and Structure, U.S. Dept. of Health, Education and Welfare, Health Services and Mental Health Administration, 5600 Fishers Lane, Rockville, Md. 20852.

6. COLE, PHILIP and EMANUEL, SR.: Drug Consultation: Its significance to the Discharged Hospital Patient and Its Relevance as a Role for the Pharmacist, Am. J. Hosp. Pharm. *28*:12:954, 1971.

Index

Page numbers in *italics* indicate illustrations. Page numbers followed by "t" indicate tables.